FERTILITY AND CONTRACEPTION IN THE HUMAN FEMALE

The Authors

JOHN A. LORAINE

D.Sc., M.B., Ph.D., (Edin.), F.R.C.P.E.

Director, Medical Research Council Clinical Endocrinology Research Unit;
Honorary Consultant Endocrinologist, Royal Infirmary, Edinburgh;
Associate in Endocrinology, Western General Hospital, Edinburgh;
Honorary Senior Lecturer, Department of Pharmacology, University of Edinburgh.

E. TREVOR BELL

B.Sc. (Dunelm), Ph.D. (Edin.)

Formerly Member of Scientific Staff Medical Research Council, Clinical Endocrinology Research
Unit, Edinburgh. Currently Seinor Lecturer, Department of Physiology, University of Manchester

FOREWORD BY

SIR DUGALD BAIRD,

B.Sc., M.D., F.R.C.O.G.

Formerly Regius Professor of Midwifery, University of Aberdeen

Fertility and Contraception in the Human Female

John A. Loraine
E. Trevor Bell

FOREWORD BY
Sir Dugald Baird

E. & S. LIVINGSTONE LTD
EDINBURGH AND LONDON
1968

©

E. & S. LIVINGSTONE LTD., 1968

SBN 443 00567 2

PRINTED IN GREAT BRITAIN

FOREWORD

A FEATURE of contemporary Britain is the changing attitude to sex and reproduction and evidence of a strong desire to understand its physiological, behavioural and social aspects. A more liberal policy towards abortion, contraception and family planning is enshrined in recent legislation. The introduction of a hormonal method of contraception completely controlled by the woman herself marks another milestone in her emancipation and puts her on an equal footing with men in her sex life. No doubt this is only the forerunner of many more changes bringing new problems in their wake and one would wish to be able to recognise possible pathological tendencies in society as early as possible.

Much or our knowledge of reproductive physiology is derived from the study of animals, because observations on the human subject pose difficult problems, as, owing to the length of human gestation, they require long term, continuous research. One of the advantages in Britain of the Medical Research Council Units is that they provide whole time careers in clinical research. Dr. Loraine and his colleagues in the Clinical Endocrinology Research Unit in Edinburgh are very favourably situated to make contributions in the field of human reproductive physiology. The work is bound to be painstaking and time-consuming and until recently the methods of studying hormonal function have been somewhat crude and inexact, but new and improved techniques are constantly being developed. This book brings together information on these and their clinical application. It is based on the original work of Dr. Loraine's Unit, from which illustrative cases are cited, and contains an extensive and critical review of the literature. It is reassuring that practical application of laboratory work is receiving so much attention. Clinical problems such as dysmenorrhoea, amenorrhoea, infertility, the menopause and contraception are all discussed, as also are the wider problems of world population increase.

The assumption of an ever-increasing responsibility for our own destiny in the reproductive field as in many others makes it imperative that we take decisions for action only after the most careful study of the facts. The long term consequences usually take time to reveal themselves, although there has been little interval between the sudden fall in infant mortality resulting from modern chemo-therapy in underdeveloped countries and the population explosion which this initiated.

Dr. Loraine and his colleagues have made in this book a valuable contribution to understanding some of the most urgent problems of our time.

Aberdeen, 1968   DUGALD BAIRD

PREFACE

THERE are few areas of medical research in which progress in the past decade has been so rapid as that involving reproduction in the human female. Important advances in the field during this time have included a more rational approach to the treatment of problems of infertility, a better understanding of the endocrinology of the menstrual cycle and of abnormal gynaecological conditions and, above all, the development of new and efficient methods of birth control, notably by the oral contraceptive pill and by the intra-uterine device.

The purpose of this book is to present a reasonably comprehensive account of the subjects of fertility and contraception as they appear to the authors in the year 1967. Particular attention is given to data accumulated during the 1960's, but, where relevant, some of the earlier work is also reviewed. As implied in the title the subject matter of the book deals almost exclusively with studies in the human, results of animal experiments being discussed only in sections in which comparable information in women is not available.

The first two chapters are concerned with the physiology of the ovary and with the mechanisms controlling ovulation. The third describes recent advances in methods for the quantitative determination of hormones and their metabolites in blood and urine, special attention being given to the oestrogens, androgens and human pituitary gonadotrophins. The fourth and fifth chapters are devoted to the normal menstrual cycle, the former dealing with hormone assays in normally menstruating women and the latter with other factors which are believed to be under hormonal control. Advances in the endocrinology of gynaecological disorders are discussed in Chapter VI, special attention being given to recent findings in patients with amenorrhoea, dysmenorrhoea and oligomenorrhoea. Chapters VII and VIII deal respectively with the gonadotrophic hormones and Clomiphene, compounds capable of stimulating ovarian function and of producing ovulution in a proportion of women suffering from infertility. The ninth and tenth chapters are devoted to methods of birth control, the former reviewing the field of oral and the latter of intra-uterine contraception. The final chapter describes certain aspects of the world population crisis and emphasizes the desperate need for remedial action in this, the major problem of the twentieth century.

The authors are especially grateful to the Medical Research Council without the generous support of which the studies conducted in the Clinical Endocrinology Research Unit, and described in many of the chapters, would not have been possible. Our sincere thanks are also due to Mr. S. F. Lunn for checking the references quoted in the bibliography. The secretarial help of Mrs. Sheila Callan, Mrs. Nancy McCalman, Miss Ena McKay, Miss Dorothy Murphy and Miss Olive J. Spode is gratefully acknowledged. We are much indebted to our publishers, Messrs. E. & S. Livingstone, for their constant co-operation and for ensuring the rapid publication of this book.

JOHN A. LORAINE

Edinburgh 1968   E. TREVOR BELL

CONTENTS

CHAPTER I

The Ovary: Some Anatomical, Biological and Biochemical Considerations

INTRODUCTION

ANY book dealing with fertility and contraception in women must include a description of the gross anatomy of the human ovary, and this constitutes the first topic for consideration in this chapter. There follows a discussion of the development of the ovarian follicle and corpus luteum, such sections being incorporated because knowledge of these processes is essential for the proper understanding of the physiology of the menstrual cycle and the pathology of abnormal gynaecological conditions. The final portion of the chapter is concerned with some of the biological and biochemical effects on the ovary of the pituitary gonadotrophins, follicle-stimulating and luteinising hormones. The lactogenic hormone, prolactin (luteotrophin), is not discussed because the role of this substance in the formation and maintenance of the corpus luteum both in the human and in various animal species is at present controversial.

Detailed information on some of the subjects considered herein is available from a number of sources. Thus, classical descriptions of the anatomy and histology of the human ovary, together with the changes occurring during the normal menstrual cycle, have been provided in various textbooks including those by Maximow and Bloom (1957), Novak and Woodruff (1962) and Ham (1965). During the 1960's several review articles dealing with the physiology and biochemistry of the ovary have been published, among the more comprehensive of which are papers by Eik-Nes (1964), Savard *et al.* (1965), Richardson (1966 *a b c d*), Short (1967) and Blandau (1967).

GROSS ANATOMY OF THE OVARY

The normal human ovary is a flattened structure shaped like a bean. It measures 2·5 to 5·0 cm. in length, 1·5 to 3·0 cm. in width and 0·6 to 1·5 cm. in thickness. In women during reproductive life the organ consists essentially of three components—the *follicle*, the *corpus luteum* and the *stroma* or *interstitial tissue*.

The ovary is organised into two main areas known respectively as the *cortex* and the *medulla*. The former contains the follicles and associated structures together with the stromal tissue, while the latter is composed primarily of a connective tissue matrix which surrounds the main ovarian blood vessels and lymphatics. The ovary is covered by the germinal epithelium which is thought to be derived from the coelomic epithelium, and consists of a single layer of cuboidal cells. During the early stages of development some of the cells, instead of remaining cuboidal in shape, become larger and more rounded, and some authorities consider these to be the actual germ cells. Although the suggestion has been made that in the human female the germ cells ultimately give rise to the ova, this point has not yet been definitely established (see Arey, 1965).

The younger the subject the more numerous are the primary ovarian follicles. Thus it is claimed (Baker, 1963) that during intra-uterine life the human ovary may contain up to 6,500,000 germ cells. By the time of birth the number has been reduced by the process of atresia to some 2,000,000 of which approximately half are atretic. At puberty the count probably does not exceed 10,000 (Mears 1965). Reduction in numbers takes place throughout the whole of reproductive life, and by the age of 50 few if any ova remain. The ovary of a woman who has recently passed the menopause is characterised by the relative absence of primary follicles, of follicles in various stages of normal development and of recent corpora lutea. In the postmenopausal era the ovaries gradually shrink and eventually consist almost entirely of fibrous tissue. It has been estimated that during reproductive life only some 350 to 400 ova mature and are extruded, the remainder disappearing through atresia. No reliable information is at present available regarding the process whereby a given ovum is selected for maturation and subsequent extrusion, and this remains a most important subject for future investigation (see Sturgis, 1961).

DEVELOPMENT OF THE FOLLICLE

The *primordial follicle* is a spherical structure with a diameter of approximately 45 μ. It consists essentially of a relatively large ovum surrounded by a single layer of flattened epithelial cells, constituting the *membrana granulosa*. The nucleus of the ovum is large and centrally placed ; its cytoplasm is pale and contains " yolk " granules which are evenly dispersed throughout. The epithelial cells of the membrana granulosa are the first to show that a primary follicle is about to develop. Such cells become definitely cuboidal in shape, subsequently being stratified into several layers (see Figure 1). Immediately afterwards a central cavity or *antrum* forms. The ovum becomes situated at one pole of the follicle and is surrounded by an accumulation of granulosa cells, termed the *cumulus oöphorus* or *discus proligerus*. The granulosa cells do not contain blood vessels, being dependent for their nutrition on a highly vascular layer of connective tissue cells, the *theca interna*, by which they are surrounded. Outside the theca interna is a layer of rather condensed ovarian stroma known as the *theca externa*. It must be emphasised that, although the cells of the theca interna are of connective tissue origin, they are highly sensitive to hormonal

3

influences ; some of them may take on an epithelial appearance, being known then as *theca lutein cells.*

The *mature Graafian follicle* is an easily recognizable structure rarely exceeding 8 mm. in diameter. It is surrounded by the theca externa which, as in the developing follicle, is merely a layer of condensed ovarian tissue. Next is the theca interna,

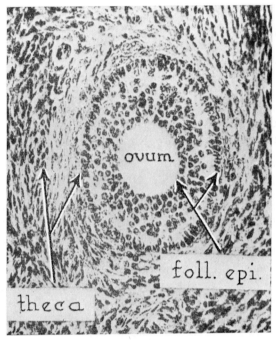

FIG. I

Photomicrograph of primary ovarian follicle prior to the stage of antrum formation.

(From Ham, 1965.)

a highly vascular layer derived from connective tissue, the cells of which are rich in lipoid and even before ovulation resemble the lutein cells of the corpus luteum (see p. 8). The membrana granulosa of the mature follicle consists of a number of layers of round or polyhedral cells ; these have darkly staining nuclei which are centrally placed. With the growth of the granulosa there frequently form small areas of cystic degeneration with clear central cavities ; the latter are surrounded by granulosa cells and are generally known as the bodies of Coll and Exner.

In the maturing follicle the antrum is ovoid in shape and is filled with a clear fluid termed the *liquor folliculi*. At one pole of the follicle is the well developed cumulus oöphorus in which the ovum is embedded (see Figure 2). The innermost layer of granulosa cells immediately surrounding the ovum is arranged in a radial form and constitutes the *corona radiata*. Within the

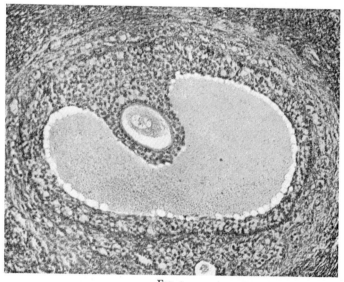

FIG. 2

Photomicrograph of maturing Graafian follicle illustrating well developed cumulus oöphorus, ovum and antrum.

(From Novak and Woodruff, 1962.)

corona radiata is a refractile membrane, the *zona pellucida*, and between the latter and the ovum is the tiny *perivitelline space*. The ovum contains a nucleus or *germinal vesicle* and a nucleolus.

In Figure 3 is shown a schematic representation of a mature follicle. Follicular development culminates in ovulation, which is considered separately in Chapter II. This event is followed by the formation of the corpus luteum.

DEVELOPMENT OF THE CORPUS LUTEUM

After ovulation has occurred the follicle generally collapses. The small opening from which the ovum has been shed (the stigma) becomes plugged with fibrous tissue and the stage is now set for the formation of the corpus luteum. The majority of the granulosa is not shed at the time of ovulation, the ovum carrying with it only the zona pellucida and a small proportion of the cells of the cumulus oöphorus.

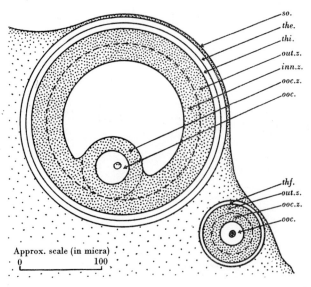

Approx. scale (in micra)
0   100

Fig. 3

Schematic diagram of primary and maturing follicle.

so. = surface of ovary; the. = theca externa; thi. = theca interna; out. z. = outer zone of membrana granulosa ; inn. z. = inner zone of membrana granulosa ; ooc. z. = oocyte zone or discus proligerus ; ooc. = oocyte ; thf. = theca folliculi.

(From Bullough, 1942.)

It is now agreed that the characteristic lutein cells of the corpus luteum originate from the granulosa cells of the original follicle. Immediately after ovulation these cells are relatively large, oval or polyhedral in shape and laden with lipoid material. Vascularisation of the corpus luteum now takes place, the chief feature of this process being the penetration of the granulosa cells by thin-walled blood vessels arising from the theca interna. These pass vertically through the length of the granulosa and open into the lumen, which they fill partially with blood.

Pari passu with the vascularisation of the corpus luteum the structure of the granulosa cells alters. They begin to show the characteristics of genuine lutein cells, becoming large and

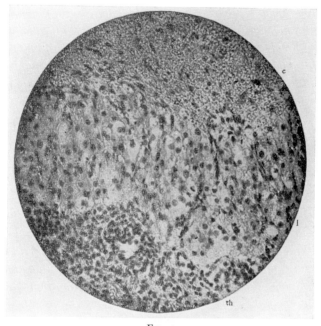

FIG. 4

Photomicrograph of early corpus luteum showing vascularisation.

(From Novak and Woodruff, 1962.)

polyhedral in shape with small nuclei and vacuolated cytoplasm. At the same time the cells of the theca interna undergo regression, becoming much smaller and losing their lipoid content; eventually they are indistinguishable from ordinary connective tissue cells. The theca interna with its associated blood vessels grows in the form of trabeculae which divide the lutein zone into large cellular compartments.

7

The corpus luteum usually attains maturity some ten days before the next menstruation. By this time its diameter is from 1·0 to 1·5 cm. and it contains a cavity. Sometimes the latter is relatively large and is filled with a light yellow fluid ; more frequently it is small and partly organized. In the mature corpus luteum the lutein zone has become very broad and is traversed by trabeculae originating from the theca interna and

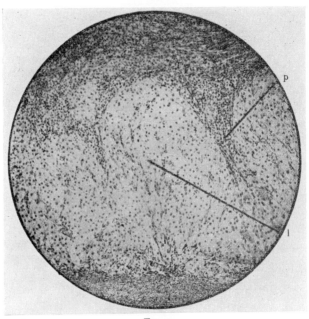

FIG. 5

Photomicrograph of mature corpus luteum showing lutein (1) and theca lutein or paralutein (p) cells.

(From Novak and Woodruff, 1962.)

containing many blood vessels. Changes now occur in some of the cells of the theca interna in the trabeculae which become definitely epithelial in appearance and are sometimes referred to as theca lutein or paralutein cells.

From three to seven days prior to the onset of the next menstruation regression of the corpus luteum begins to take place. The essential features of this process are an increase in the lipoid content of the cells and increasing fibrosis of the lutein zone, this being followed in some weeks by hyalinisation. Eventually these changes result in the formation of the *corpus albicans* which consists of an amorphous convoluted hyalinised area surrounding a central plug of cicatricial tissue.

In Figure 4 is shown a section of the corpus luteum at the early stage of vascularisation ; Figure 5 illustrates the mature structure. A schematic representation of the sequence of events occurring in the ovary during follicular development and corpus luteum formation is provided in Figure 6.

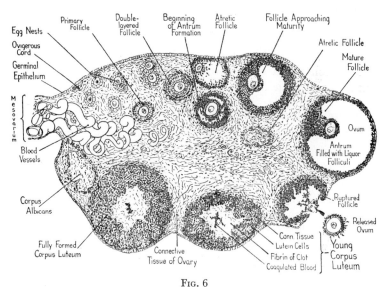

FIG. 6

Schematic diagram illustrating changes in the ovary during follicular development and corpus luteum formation.

(From Patten, 1953.)

BIOLOGICAL AND BIOCHEMICAL EFFECTS OF GONADOTROPHIC HORMONES ON THE OVARY

It is now generally accepted that in man the majority of the effects of the anterior pituitary on the ovary are mediated by its two gonadotrophins, the follicle-stimulating hormone (FSH) and the luteinising hormone (LH). Both of these substances are proteins and have been obtained in a highly

9

purified form from the pituitary glands of various species including the human. A considerable amount of information is now available on the chemical nature of FSH and LH, and for details of the present position in this field the reader is referred to publications by Loraine and Bell (1966), Apostolakis and Loraine (1967), Butt (1967 *a b*) and Hartree (1967).

Much work has been reported in the literature on the biological and biochemical effects of purified preparations of FSH and LH on the ovaries of various animal species. However, at the time of writing, comparable information in human subjects is so meagre as to be virtually nonexistent, and this is obviously an area which will require intensive investigation in the future. In the ensuing section the biological actions of the gonadotrophins will be illustrated by studies in rats and mice, while biochemical effects will be described in bovine, rabbit and human ovaries.

1. Some Biological Effects of FSH and LH

This subject has interested investigators since the 1940's, and classical early papers in the field include those of Fevold (1941) and Greep *et al.* (1942). More recent publications include articles by Woods and Simpson (1960), Carter *et al.* (1961), Papkoff (1965), Lostroh and Johnson (1966), Eshkol (1967) and Eshkol and Lunenfeld (1967). Important review articles have been contributed by Richardson (1966 *a b c d*) and Greep (1967).

Recently, Lostroh and Johnson (1966) have made a reappraisal of the effects of purified ovine FSH and LH on the ovary and uterus of the hypophysectomised rat ; a summary of their conclusions is given in Table 1. It will be noted that high dosages of FSH caused the formation of small antra in the follicles while comparable dosages of LH produced repair of the ovarian interstitial tissue. Neither hormone given alone was capable of stimulating steroid production as judged by uterine weight increase, but combinations of FSH and LH caused uterine enlargement presumably resulting from the secretion of oestrogens by the ovary. FSH given alone failed to produce luteinisation of the follicles, but this occurred when the two hormones were administered in combination. The data of Lostroh and Johnson (1966) are in general agreement with those reported many years previously by Fevold (1941) and Greep et al. (1942).

Eshkol (1967) and Eshkol and Lunenfeld (1967) have studied the effect on the histology of the mouse ovary and uterus of a gonadotrophin derived from postmenopausal urine and containing both FSH and LH (Pergonal:Serono) and of a highly purified urinary FSH containing little or no LH. The

TABLE 1

EFFECTS OF OVINE FSH AND LH ON THE OVARY AND UTERUS OF THE HYPOPHYSECTOMISED RAT

(After Lostroh and Johnson, 1966)

Material administered	Dosage µg./day	Ovarian weight mg.±S.E.	Uterine weight mg.±S.E.	Ovarian histology	
				Follicles	Interstitial tissue
Saline		9·0±0·7	23·5±1·3	no antra	atrophic
FSH	1	9·7±0·8	23·9±1·7	no antra	atrophic
FSH	3	20·5±1·5	22·5±0·7	small, small to medium antra	atrophic
LH	1	6·3±0·6	20·8±0·9	no antra	complete repair
LH	20	10·4±0·8	19·7±1·2	no antra	complete repair
FSH + LH	1 / 20	12·0±0·8	25·2±2·3	no antra	complete repair
FSH + LH	3 / 1	29·0±3·6	83·5±9·1	medium to large antra	complete repair
FSH + LH	3 / 20	35·3±3·9	82·0±5·3	medium to large antra	complete repair

results they obtained are similar to those of Lostroh and Johnson (1966) and are illustrated in Figure 7. Their experiments indicated that, following the administration of Pergonal, follicular growth in the ovaries was considerably stimulated and uterine weight was increased some threefold over control values ; the uterus also showed marked histological evidence of stimulation. When the animals were injected with the highly purified preparation of FSH, follicular growth was again apparent ; however, the uterus remained small and infantile in character, its histological appearance being similar to that of uninjected controls.

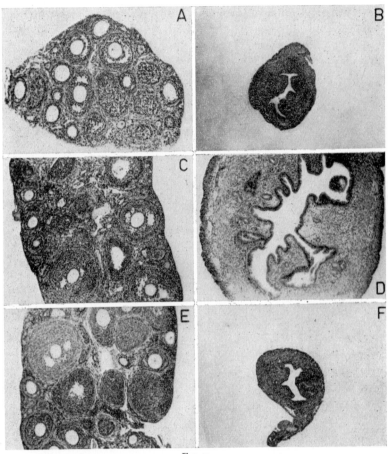

Fig. 7

Photomicrographs of ovaries and uteri of untreated mice (A and B), of animals receiving Pergonal (C and D), and of mice treated with a purified FSH preparation (E and F).

(From Eshkol, 1967.)

2. Some Biochemical Effects of FSH and LH

(*a*) EFFECTS ON STEROIDOGENESIS. These have so far been studied mainly in the case of LH. It is now generally agreed that in the human ovary steroidogenesis can occur in the follicles, interstitial tissue and corpora lutea. Virtually no information is currently available on steroidogenesis in the first two of these tissues, and accordingly the ensuing discussion will be restricted to experiments performed with corpora lutea. Much of the pioneer work in this field has been conducted by Savard and his co-workers in Miami, U.S.A. on whose findings the present section is based (see Hammerstein *et al.*, 1964 ; Rice *et al.*, 1964 ; Marsh and Savard, 1966 ; Savard, 1967).

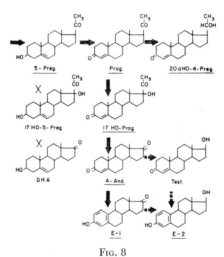

FIG. 8

Pathway of steroid biosynthesis in human corpus luteum.
(From Savard, 1967.)

Differences in the pattern of steroid biosynthesis between the human and bovine corpus luteum have been emphasised by Savard (1967). Whereas the latter species synthesises from acetate pregnenolone, progesterone and 20β-hydroxypregn-4-en-3-one as its main steroids, the former produces a much more complex mixture of compounds including pregnenolone, progesterone, 20α-hydroxypregn-4-en-3-one, 17-hydroxyprogesterone, Δ⁵-androstenedione, oestrone and oestradiol (see Figure 8). When LH is added to either human or bovine corpora lutea an increase in steroid production occurs, and

Savard (1967) believes that the hormone acts at a point or points in the steroid biosynthetic pathway which are common to the two types of gland.

The exact site of action of LH on the steroid biosynthetic chain has not yet been established with certainty (see Savard *et al.*, 1965 for review). Some investigators believe that one such site is on the enzymes responsible for the cleavage of the side chain of the cholesterol molecule. Steps in the transformation of cholesterol to Δ^5-pregnenolone and progesterone are shown in Figure 9. The data of Hall and Koritz (1964), working with the bovine corpus luteum, indicate that three

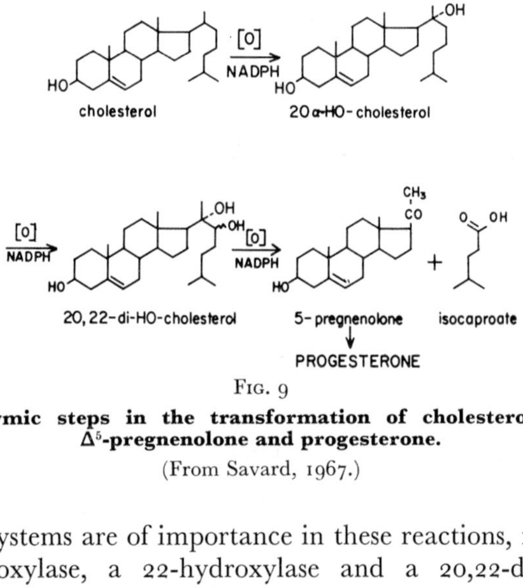

FIG. 9

Enzymic steps in the transformation of cholesterol to
Δ^5-pregnenolone and progesterone.

(From Savard, 1967.)

enzyme systems are of importance in these reactions, namely a 20α-hydroxylase, a 22-hydroxylase and a 20,22-dihydroxy desmolase ; only the first of these is thought to be rate limiting. Comparable work on the side chain cleavage of cholesterol in the human ovary has not yet been reported and will be awaited with interest. Savard *et al.* (1965) and Armstrong (1967), using bovine corpus luteum and rabbit ovarian interstitial tissue respectively, have suggested sites of action of LH other than that involving the side chain cleavage of cholesterol, and have postulated that the hormone may act at an early stage in the biosynthetic pathway, probably between acetate and cholesterol. Further work is necessary to prove or disprove

14

this interesting suggestion. A diagrammatic representation of possible sites of action of LH on the bovine corpus luteum is given in Figure 10.

The mechanism whereby LH produces its effect on steroid biosynthesis is at present far from clear (see Marsh and Savard, 1966). One possibility is that the hormone could activate the enzyme, adenyl cyclase, causing increased formation of adenosine-3'-5'-monophosphate (cyclic AMP) from adenosine 5-triphosphate (ATP). Alternatively LH could inhibit the phosphodiesterase which normally destroys cyclic AMP. The structural formulae of cyclic AMP and of ATP are shown in

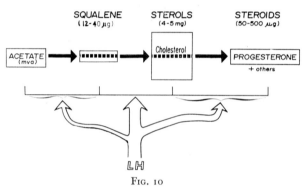

FIG. 10

Possible site of action of LH in the bovine corpus luteum slice.

mva. = mevalonic acid. (From Savard, 1967.)

Figure 11. Marsh *et al.* (1966) have demonstrated that under the influence of LH the rise in cyclic AMP levels in the bovine corpus luteum precedes by some fifteen to twenty minutes the increase in progesterone synthesis. This finding, along with other evidence summarised by Savard (1967), suggests that cyclic AMP may be an important factor in the mechanism of action of LH. However, much further work in this area is required before any definite conclusions can be drawn. It must be emphasised that the hypothesis implicating cyclic AMP in the mechanism of action of protein hormones is not new, having originally been proposed by Haynes *et al.* (1960) for ACTH in relation to adrenal steroidogenesis.

(*b*) OTHER EFFECTS. At the time of writing virtually no information exists on the effects of FSH on any biochemical parameter in the human ovary and data in animal species are also sparse. In particular, the effects of this hormone on the biochemistry of follicular growth are quite obscure and obviously merit close attention in the future.

In addition to its actions on steroidogenesis LH is probably responsible for the occurrence of ovulation (see p. 20). As will be emphasised in Chapter II, the precise mechanism whereby this event is brought about is still unknown. LH may also produce changes in tissue permeability, blood flow and intermediary metabolism in the ovaries (see Richardson, 1966 *a b c d*). However, research in these areas is still at a very preliminary stage indeed, and a critical review of the subject is not warranted at the present time.

FIG. 11

Structural formulae of ATP and cyclic AMP.

SUMMARY AND CONCLUSIONS

A description is given of the gross anatomy of the human ovary, and it is emphasised that the number of primary follicles diminishes with increasing age.

Stages in the development of the follicle and of the corpus luteum are reviewed, attention being given to the morphological differences between the primary and mature follicle and between the maturing and regressing corpus luteum.

Biological effects of FSH and LH on the ovaries are discussed. It is concluded that purified FSH produces follicular growth, that purified LH causes repair of interstitial tissue, and that, for uterine stimulation, a combination of the two hormones is required.

Sites of action of purified LH on ovarian steroid biosynthesis are considered, and the possible role of cyclic AMP as a mediator of LH action is described.

It is emphasised that little or no information is currently available regarding the manner by which FSH produces its effects on the ovaries.

REFERENCES

APOSTOLAKIS, M. & LORAINE, J. A. (1967). In *Hormones in Blood.* Second ed. Eds. Gray, C. H. and Bacharach, A. L. New York : Academic Press. Vol. I p. 273.

AREY, L. B. (1965). *Developmental Anatomy.* Philadelphia : Saunders.

ARMSTRONG, D. T. (1967). In *Recent Research on Gonadotrophic Hormones,* p. 188. Eds. Bell, E. T. and Loraine, J. A. Edinburgh : Livingstone.

BAKER, T. G. (1963). *Proc. Roy. Soc. B.* **158,** 417.

BLANDAU, R. J. (1967). *Clin. Obstet. Gynecol.* **10,** 347.

BULLOUGH, W. S. (1942). *J. Endocrinol.* **3,** 150.

BUTT, W. R. (1967 *a*). In *Recent Research on Gonadotrophic Hormones,* p. 129. Eds. Bell, E. T. and Loraine, J. A. Edinburgh : Livingstone.

BUTT. W. R. (1967 *b*). *Hormone Chemistry,* p. 103. London : Van Nostrand.

CARTER, F., WOODS, M. C. & SIMPSON, M. E. (1961). In *Control of Ovulation,* p. 1. Ed. Villee, C. A. New York : Pergamon.

EIK-NES, K. B. (1964). *Physiol Rev.* **44,** 609.

ESHKOL, A. (1967). In *Recent Research on Gonadotrophic Hormones,* p. 202. Eds. Bell, E. T. and Loraine, J. A. Edinburgh : Livingstone.

ESHKOL, A. & LUNENFELD, B. (1967). *Acta Endocrinol.* **54,** 91.

FEVOLD, H. L. (1941). *Endocrinology,* **28,** 33.

GREEP, R. O. (1967). *J. Endocrinol.* **39,** ii.

GREEP, R. O., VAN DYKE, H. B. & CHOW, B. F. (1942). *Endocrinology,* **30,** 635.

HALL, P. F. & KORITZ, S. P. (1964). *Biochemistry,* **3,** 129.

HAM, A. W. (1965). *Histology.* Fifth ed. London : Pitman.

HAMMERSTEIN, J., RICE, B. F. & SAVARD, K. (1964). *J. Clin. Endocrinol. Metab.* **24,** 597.

HARTREE, A. S. (1967). In *Recent Research on Gonadotrophic Hormones,* p. 130. Eds. Bell, E. T. and Loraine, J. A. Edinburgh : Livingstone.

HAYNES, R. C., Jr., SUTHERLAND, E. W. & RALL, T. W. (1960). *Recent Prog. Hormone Res.* **16,** 121.

LORAINE, J. A. & BELL, E. T. (1966). *Hormone Assays and their Clinical Application.* Second ed. Edinburgh : Livingstone.

LOSTROH, A. J. & JOHNSON, R. E. (1966). *Endocrinology,* **79,** 991.

MARSH, J. M. & SAVARD, K. (1966). *J. Reprod. Fertil. Suppl.* **1,** 113.

MARSH, J. M., BUTCHER, R. W., SAVARD, K. & SUTHERLAND, E. W. (1966). *J. Biol Chem.* **241,** 5436.

MAXIMOW, A. A. & BLOOM, W. (1957). *A Textbook of Histology.* Seventh ed. Philadelphia : Saunders.

MEARS, E. (1965). *Handbook on Oral Contraception.* London : Churchill.

NOVAK, E. R. & WOODRUFF, J. D. (1962). *Gynecologic and Obstetric Pathology.* Fifth ed. Philadelphia : Saunders.

PAPKOFF, H. (1965). *Acta Endocrinol.* **48,** 439.

PATTEN, B. M. (1953). *Human Embryology.* New York : McGraw-Hill.

RICE, B. F., HAMMERSTEIN, J. & SAVARD, K. (1964). *J. Clin. Endocrinol. Metab.* **24,** 606.

RICHARDSON, G. S. (1966 a). *N. Engl. J. Med.* **274,** 1008.
RICHARDSON, G. S. (1966 b). *N. Engl. J. Med.* **274,** 1064.
RICHARDSON, G. S. (1966 c). *N. Engl. J. Med.* **274,** 1121.
RICHARDSON, G. S. (1966 d). *N. Engl. J. Med.* **274,** 1183.
SAVARD, K. (1967). In *Recent Research on Gonadotrophic Hormones*, p. 184. Eds.
Bell, E. T. and Loraine, J. A. Edinburgh : Livingstone.
SAVARD, K., MARSH, J. M. & RICE, B. F. (1965). *Recent Prog. Hormone Res.* **21,** 285.
SHORT, R. V. (1967). *Ann. Rev. Physiol.* **29,** 373.
STURGIS, S. H. (1961). In *Control of Ovulation*, p. 213. Ed. Villee, C. A. New
York : Pergamon.
WOODS, M. C. & SIMPSON, M. E. (1960). *Endocrinology*, **66,** 575.

CHAPTER II

Morphological and Biochemical Changes Associated with Ovulation

INTRODUCTION

THE literature contains many publications dealing with the subject of ovulation. Morphological changes occurring in the ovary prior to this event are now well established but, in contrast, the precise physiological and biochemical mechanisms responsible for ovulation remain to be elucidated. Furthermore, it must be emphasised that, until now, knowledge of the factors controlling ovulation has been obtained solely by experiments in various animal species, information in the human female being so fragmentary as to be virtually non-existent.

The aims of the present chapter are two-fold. Firstly, a brief description of the macroscopic and microscopic changes associated with ovulation will be given ; subsequently the various hypotheses which have been put forward to explain this process will be discussed. Much of the present account is based on data reported in five major review articles which have been published over the past eight years (see Zachariae, 1959 ; Young, 1961 ; Asdell, 1962 ; Blandau, 1966 ; 1967).

ANATOMICAL CHANGES ASSOCIATED WITH PRE-OVULATORY SWELLING AND OVULATION

It is generally agreed that in the pre-ovulatory phase of the oestrous cycle and probably also in the human menstrual cycle the Graafian follicle grows steadily up to the time of pre-ovulatory swelling. In some animal species, notably the rabbit, sheep, guinea-pig and rat, there is rapid follicular growth for some 10 to 12 hours prior to ovulation, during which time considerable amounts of follicular fluid accumulate (Hammond, 1927 ; Hunt, 1934 ; Myers et al., 1936 ; Boling et al., 1941 ; Rowlands and Williams, 1943 ; Rowlands, 1944 ; Bell and Lunn, 1967). However, in other species, e.g. the cat and the ferret, this process may take as long as 25 to 30 hours (Robinson, 1918 ; Dawson and Friedgood, 1939, 1940). The fluid accumulating during the pre-ovulatory phase is generally referred to as *secondary follicular fluid* ; this term is used to distinguish it from the fluid present before this phase. The main characteristic of the secondary follicular fluid is its relatively low viscosity.

Another important feature of pre-ovulatory growth is the separation of the ovum and corona radiata from the underlying membrana granulosa (stratum granulosum). As the time of ovulation approaches the membrana granulosa at the base of the follicle becomes thicker than at the apex. In a proportion of follicles destined to ovulate, folding of the membrana granulosa occurs, and sometimes spaces filled with fluid appear between the theca interna and the basement membrane of the membrana granulosa. Häggquist (1921), in experiments conducted in the human female, and Asdell (1962) in the cow have reported that, immediately prior to ovulation, the membrana granulosa is invaded by capillary loops. According to Asdell (1962) such an invasion does not take place in the monkey, rabbit and rat.

In Figure 12 which is taken from an article by Blandau (1966) changes in the oestrous cycle in the rat are illustrated. The major stages shown are (i) the development of the antrum (1 to 4), (ii) the separation of the cumulus oöphorus from the underlying stratum granulosum (5), (iii) the formation

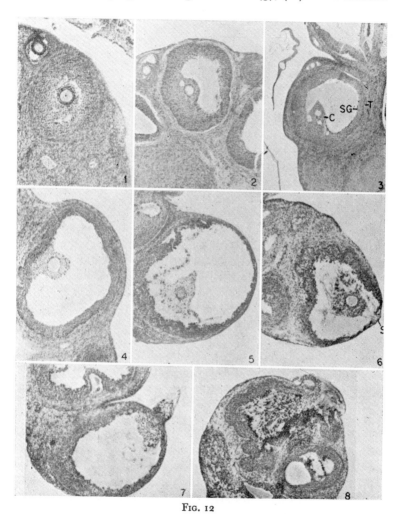

FIG. 12

Stages in the oestrous cycle in the rat.

C = cumulus oöphorus ; SG = stratum granulosum ; T = theca ;
S = stigma. (From Blandau, 1966.)

of the stigma (6), (iv) the rupture of the follicle with expulsion of the ovum (7) and (v) the collapse of the follicle after the occurrence of ovulation (8).

There is general agreement that the first macroscopic indication that ovulation is about to occur in the formation of the macula pellucida or *stigma*. One of the first descriptions of the stigma was given by Walton and Hammond (1928) in the rabbit. In this species a thin translucent secondary cone forms at the centre of the stigma and rupture of the follicle occurs within the cone. The ewe has a relatively large stigma and shows the presence of several secondary cones (McKenzie and Terrill, 1935, 1937). Careful studies of ovulatory stigmata in a variety of animal species have indicated that these structures are circumscribed in area and are avascular. Elongated stigmata are encountered in birds and amphibia (Bartelmez, 1912 ; Phillips and Warren, 1937 ; Rugh, 1935) while in rats and rabbits the structures may be oval or spherical (Walton and Hammond, 1928 ; Hill *et al.*, 1935).

The elegant experiments of Blandau (1955) have demonstrated that it is possible to predict the site of stigma formation if the surface of the ovulatory follicle in the living rat is examined. There is first a decrease in blood flow in a circumscribed area ; this is followed by a reorganisation of the capillary network to form a definite ring of vessels around the edge of the stigma (see Figure 12). Capillary blood flow within the area of the stigma itself then ceases, resulting in the formation of a circumscribed pale area. If relatively high magnification is employed it will be seen that the superficial germinal epithelium in the area covering the stigma sloughs off ; subsequently the thin stroma beneath separates exposing a clear pellucid membrane. The latter rapidly forms a secondary cone which begins to protrude above the surface of the follicle. The membrane lining the secondary cone becomes stretched and thinned out ; soon it ruptures and so allows the follicular contents to flow out. On the basis of his studies in rats Blandau (1955) has concluded that the time of extrusion varies in individual animals from 11 seconds to 12 minutes ; in the majority of cases extrusion occurs within one to three minutes. When the ovum is released along with the follicular fluid the walls of the antrum gradually collapse.

The process of ovulation has been observed in a limited number of species other than the rat. Studies in the rabbit have been reported by Walton and Hammond (1928), Kelly (1931), Hill *et al.* (1935), Markee and Hinsey (1936) and Smith (1937), in the cow by Umbaugh (1949), and in the human by Decker (1951) and Doyle (1951).

On the basis of the observations described above it is now conceded that ovulation generally does not occur in an explosive manner. According to Walton and Hammond (1928) the flow of follicular fluid from the antrum in the rabbit is " steady and continuous ". The experiments of Markee and Hinsey (1936) in the same species demonstrated that as the tip of the follicular stigma opened the contents flowed out slowly. Blandau (1955), whose careful studies in rats constitute a classical investigation in this field, found that in the majority of the animals the contents of the follicle flowed out slowly and gradually, while in a small proportion the ovulation was of a more explosive type. Two ovulations in the human female have been described by Doyle (1951) ; on both occasions the contents of the follicle were extruded slowly.

SUGGESTED HYPOTHESES TO ACCOUNT FOR THE OCCURRENCE OF OVULATION

These fall into two main groups :

(1) Hypotheses based on alterations in intrafollicular pressure.

(2) Hypotheses involving the effects of enzymes.

1. Hypotheses Based on Alterations in Intrafollicular Pressure

Rouget in 1858 was among the first to postulate that rupture of the follicle was a direct result of an increase in follicular pressure. He concluded that such an increase was caused by contraction of the smooth muscle present in the ovarian stroma. Waldeyer (1870) considered that increased intrafollicular pressure resulted from hypertrophy of the theca interna, while Heape (1905) took the view that the main factors were vasodilation and haemorrhage from capillaries. Thomson (1919) concluded that the immediate cause was an increased secretion of follicular fluid.

The importance of smooth muscle in the induction of ovulation in a variety of animal species has been stressed by numerous investigations including Pflüger (1859), Aeby (1861), Heape (1905), Von Winiwarter and Sainmont (1909), Guttmacher and Guttmacher (1921) and Corner (1921). However, the hypothesis that smooth muscle contraction is the major factor producing ovulation has been challenged by other workers notably Hammond and Marshall (1925), Schröder (1930), Ammann (1936) and Claesson (1947). Of especial significance are the experiments of the last mentioned investigator who, using histological, histochemical and biophysical techniques, demonstrated that the Graafian follicle was not surrounded by smooth muscle in various animal species including the cow, pig, rabbit and guinea-pig.

Blandau and Rumery (1963), Espey and Lipner (1963) and Rondell (1964) have reported experiments in which intrafollicular pressure in rats and rabbits has been measured ; a summary of the results obtained has been given by Blandau (1966). Micropipettes were introduced into the follicles of exteriorised ovaries of anaesthetised animals, and the observation was made that ovulation was usually not associated with a marked increase in follicular hydrostatic pressure. The range for follicular pressure quoted by Blandau and Rumery (1963) in follicles of varying sizes was from 19·0 to 23·1 cm. of water ; these results are similar to the figures reported by Landis (1934) who estimated hydrostatic pressure in the mesentery of the rat. An important contribution to this field is the publication of Espey and Lipner (1963) in which intrafollicular pressure in the rabbit ovary was measured. These workers observed a close correlation between intrafollicular pressure and arterial blood pressure and noted that, prior to ovulation, no marked alterations occurred in either parameter. Following ovulation, intrafollicular pressure fell from a mean figure of approximately 17 mm. to 5 mm. Hg.

The chemical composition of follicular fluid and its relationship to the occurrence of ovulation have been studied by numerous investigators amongst whom are Lutwak-Mann (1954), Perloff et al. (1955), Caravaglios and Cilotti (1957), Zachariae and Jensen (1958), Jensen and Zachariae (1958) and Zachariae (1959). The main interest of Zachariae and his

24

co-workers (see Christiansen *et al.*, 1958 ; Jensen and Zachariae, 1958 ; Zachariae and Jensen, 1958 ; Zachariae, 1959) was in the mucopolysaccharide content of the ovary which they estimated during the period of follicular growth and at the time of ovulation. They found that immediately prior to ovulation formation of sulphomucopolysaccharides ceased, this coinciding with depolymerisation of acid mucopolysaccharides. The latter were studied in considerable detail and were found to consist mainly of hyaluronic and chondroitin sulphuric acids. On the basis of their evidence Zachariae and his colleagues considered that the enzyme producing depolymerisation in the pre-ovulatory phase was hyaluronidase. The occurrence of depolymerisation was found to be associated with a marked rise in colloid osmotic pressure. This in turn caused water imbibition, a factor which might be responsible both for follicular growth and for subsequent rupture of the follicle. The hypothesis proposed by Zachariae and his associates to explain ovulation is that the process is essentially one of endosmosis in which the accumulation of increased follicular fluid causes rupture of the walls of the antrum. This concept is not supported by the data of Lutwak-Mann (1954) who, on the basis of observations in the cow, noted that the chemical composition of the follicular fluid was similar to that of the plasma.

2. Hypotheses Involving the Effects of Enzymes

Various research workers including Schochet (1915, 1920), Petry (1943), Moricard and Gothie (1946), Kraus (1947), Jung and Held (1959) and Espey and Lipner (1965) have postulated that ovulation occurs as a result of enzymic degradation of the follicular wall. According to Moricard and Gothie (1946), pituitary gonadotrophic hormones cause a diastase to be secreted into the antrum ; this digests the follicular wall and leads to rupture of the follicle. In 1959 Jung and Held reported the presence of proteolytic enzymes and of acid and alkaline phosphatases in follicles of various sizes in the pig. The three enzymes were found in higher concentration in the small follicles, and it was suggested that they might be associated with the occurrence of ovulation. On the other hand, Kraus (1947) whose investigations were performed in rabbits, concluded that proteolytic enzymes were of little significance in the causation of ovulation.

Espey and Lipner (1965), using the exteriorised rabbit ovary, studied the effect of the intrafollicular injection of a number of enzymes on the rupture of the Graafian follicle. The substances investigated included collagenase, nargase, pronase, trypsin, chymotrypsin, peptidase, ficin, papain, lysozyme and hyaluronidase. Changes in the follicle similar to those observed during a normal ovulation were produced by preparations of bacterial collagenase and by the proteases, pronase and collagenase. On the basis of their evidence showing similarities between enzymatically induced rupture of the follicle and coitally induced ovulation, Epsey and Lipner (1965) postulated that the structural changes preceding follicular rupture might be the result of proteolysis. Furthermore, they suggested that if proteolysis were indeed responsible, stigma formation would follow as a result of generalised changes in the follicular wall.

3. Comment

It is obvious from the foregoing discussion that no single hypothesis can adequately explain the processes involved in follicular rupture and ovulation. Another point to emerge is that, in spite of the fact that research in this area has been in progress for more than a century, the evidence produced to date is far from conclusive. Studies on the mechanisms involved in ovulation both in human subjects and in experimental animals would appear to be especially relevant in the 1960's in view of the availability for clinical use of compounds which are capable both of stimulating and of inhibiting ovarian function (see Chapters VII, VIII and IX). It can only be hoped that research in this field will be considerably expanded in the future and that solutions will be found to a number of important problems which have remained controversial for a considerable period of time.

SUMMARY AND CONCLUSIONS

A description is given of the anatomical changes occurring in the ovary immediately prior to ovulation. There is now agreement that the first indication that ovulation is likely to take place is the formation of the stigma.

Direct visualisation of the ovaries in various animal species and in the human female has demonstrated that the process of ovulation is generally not explosive in nature. The two main hypotheses which have been adduced to account for ovulation depend on changes in intrafollicular pressure and on enzyme action. Neither hypothesis provides a completely satisfactory explanation for this event.

REFERENCES

AEBY, C. (1861). *Arch. Anat. Physiol.* 635.
AMMANN, K. (1936). *Histologie des Schwein-Eierstockes unter besonderer Berücksichtigung des Ovarialzyklus.* Frauenfeld.
ASDELL, S. A. (1962). In *The Ovary*, Vol. 1, p. 435, Eds. Zuckerman, S., Mandl, A. M. & Eckstein, P. New York : Academic Press.
BARTELMEZ, G. W. (1912). *J. Morphol.* **23**, 269.
BELL, E. T. & LUNN, S. F. (1967). *J. Endocrinol.* In press.
BLANDAU, R. J. (1955). *Fertility Sterility*, **6**, 391.
BLANDAU, R. J. (1966). In *Ovulation*, p. 1, Ed. Greenblatt, R. B., Philadelphia : Lippincott.
BLANDAU, R. J. (1967). *Clin. Obstet. Gynecol.* **10**, 347.
BLANDAU, R. J. & RUMERY, R. E. (1964). *Fertility Sterility*, **14**, 330.
BOLING, J. L., BLANDAU, R. J., SODERWALL, A. L. & YOUNG, W. C. (1941). *Anat. Record*, **79**, 313.
CARAVAGLIOS, R. & CILOTTI, R. (1957). *J. Endocrinol.* **15**, 273.
CHRISTIANSEN, J. A., JENSEN, C. E. & ZACHARIAE, F. (1958). *Acta. Endocrinol.* **29**, 115.
CLAESSON, L. (1947). *Acta. Anat.* **3**, 295.
CORNER, G. W. (1921). *Contributions to Embryol.* **13**, 119.
DAWSON, A. B. & FRIEDGOOD, H. B. (1939). *Anat. Record*, **75**, Suppl. 1, 74.
DAWSON, A. B. & FRIEDGOOD, H. B. (1940). *Anat. Record*, **76**, 411.
DECKER, A. (1951). *Fertility Sterility*, **2**, 253.
DOYLE, J. B. (1951). *Fertility Sterility*, **2**, 474.
ESPEY, L. L. & LIPNER, H. (1963). *Am. J. Physiol.* **205**, 1067.
ESPEY, L. L. & LIPNER, H. (1965). *Am. J. Physiol.* **208**, 208.
GUTTMACHER, M. S. & GUTTMACHER, A. F. (1921). *Bull. Johns Hopkins Hosp.* **32**, 394.
HÄGGQUIST, G. (1921). *Anat. Anz.* **54**, 264.
HAMMOND, J. (1927). *The Physiology of Reproduction in the Cow*, p. 226, Cambridge : Cambridge University Press.
HAMMOND, J. & MARSHALL, F. H. A. (1925). *Reproduction in the Rabbit.* Edinburgh : Oliver and Boyd.
HEAPE, W. (1905). *Proc. Roy. Soc. B.* **76**, 260.
HILL, R. T., ALLEN, E. & KRAMER, T. C. (1935). *Anat. Record*, **63**, 239.
HUNT, R. (1934). *Trans. Roy. Soc. Edinburgh*, **58**, 1.
JENSEN, C. E. & ZACHARIAE, F. (1958). *Acta. Endocrinol.* **27**, 356.
JUNG, G. & HELD, H. (1959). *Arch. Gynaekol.* **192**, 146.
KELLY, G. L. (1931). *J. Fla. Med. Ass.* **17**, 422.
KRAUS, S. D. (1947). *Western J. Surg.* **55**, 424.
LANDIS, E. M. (1934). *Physiol. Rev.* **14**, 404.
LUTWAK-MANN, C. (1954). *J. Agric. Sci.* **44**, 477.
McKENZIE, F. F. & TERRILL, C. E. (1935). *Anat. Record*, **61**, Suppl. p. 58.

McKenzie, F. F. & Terrill, C. E. (1937). *Res. Bull. Mo. Agric. Exp. Sta.*, No. **264.**
Markee, J. E. & Hinsey, J. C. (1936). *Anat. Record,* **64,** 309.
Moricard, R. & Gothie, S. (1946). *Compt. Rend. Soc. Biol.* **140,** 249.
Myers, H. I., Young, W. C. & Dempsey, E. W. (1936). *Anat. Record,* **65,** 381.
Perloff, W. H., Schultz, J., Farris, E. J. & Balin, H. (1955). *Fertility Sterility,* **6,** 11.
Petry, G. (1943). *Fermentforsh.* **17,** 184.
Phillips, R. E. & Warren, D. C. (1937). *J. Exp. Zool.* **76,** 117.
Pflüger, E. (1859). *Arch. Anat. Physiol.* 30.
Robinson, A. (1918). *Trans. Roy. Soc. Edinburgh,* **52,** 303.
Rondell, P. (1964). *Am. J. Physiol.* **207,** 590.
Rouget, C. (1858). *J. Physiol. Paris,* **1,** 320.
Rowlands, I. W. (1944). *J. Endocrinol.* **3,** 384.
Rowlands, I. W. & Williams, P. C. (1943). *J. Endocrinol.* **3,** 310.
Rugh, R. (1935). *J. Exp. Zool.* **71,** 163.
Schochet, S. S. (1915). *Anat. Record,* **10,** 447.
Schochet, S. S. (1920). *Surg. Gynecol. Obstet.* **31,** 148.
Schröder, R. (1930). *Handb. Mikr. Anat. Menschen.* **VII:** 1, 329.
Smith, J. T. (1937). *Am. J. Obstet. Gynecol.* **27,** 728.
Thomson, A. (1919). *J. Anat.* **54,** 1.
Umbaugh, R. E. (1949). *Am. J. Vet. Res.* **10,** 295.
Von Winiwarter, H. & Sainmont, G. (1909). *Arch. Biol.* **24,** 627.
Waldeyer, W. (1870). *Eierstock und Ei.* Leipzig : Engelmann.
Walton, A. & Hammond, J. (1928). *Brit. J. Exp. Biol.* **6,** 190.
Young, W. C. (1961). In *Sex and Internal Secretions*, Vol. **1,** p. 449, Ed. Young, W. C., Baltimore : Williams and Wilkins.
Zachariae, F. (1959). *Acta Endocrinol.*, Suppl. **47.**
Zachariae, F. & Jensen, C. E. (1958). *Acta. Endocrinol.* **27,** 343.

CHAPTER III

Hormonal Methods for the Assessment of Ovarian and Pituitary Gonadotrophic Function

INTRODUCTION

THIS chapter deals with techniques for the quantitative determination of oestrogens, progesterone, pregnanediol, pregnanetriol, testosterone and human pituitary gonadotrophins (HPG) in body fluids of non-pregnant subjects. The section on HPG is concerned mainly with follicle-stimulating hormone (FSH) and luteinising hormone (LH) ; the lactogenic hormone, prolactin, which is generally classified as a gonadotrophin, is not considered because, as mentioned in Chapter I, the precise role of this substance in reproductive processes in the human female remains obscure. The literature on assay methods for the hormones and metabolites discussed herein has recently been reviewed by Loraine and Bell (1966). The present chapter describes only the more important procedures along with techniques developed since that review was published.

OESTROGENS

1. General Considerations

The three most important oestrogens in the assessment of ovarian function in women are oestrone (3-hydroxy-estra-1,3,5(10)-triene,17-one), oestradiol (estra-1,3,5(10)-triene-3,17β-diol) and oestriol (estra-1,3,5(10)-triene-3,16α,17β-triol). These are commonly referred to as the *classical oestrogens* while the term *total oestrogens*, when applied to clinical investigations, generally denotes the sum of the values for the three classical

30

compounds. In Figure 13 are shown the structural formulae of the classical oestrogens together with that of 16-epioestriol, a metabolite of oestradiol and oestrone; the structure of the steroid nucleus together with the conventional nomenclature of rings and carbon atoms is also illustrated.

Much of the pioneer work on the isolation of the classical oestrogens from various tissues and from pregnancy urine was performed in the late 1920's and early 1930's by workers such as Doisy *et al.* (1929), Marrian (1930) and MacCorquodale *et al.* (1935). Since the early 1950's a large number of other oestrogens have either been isolated from or detected in human

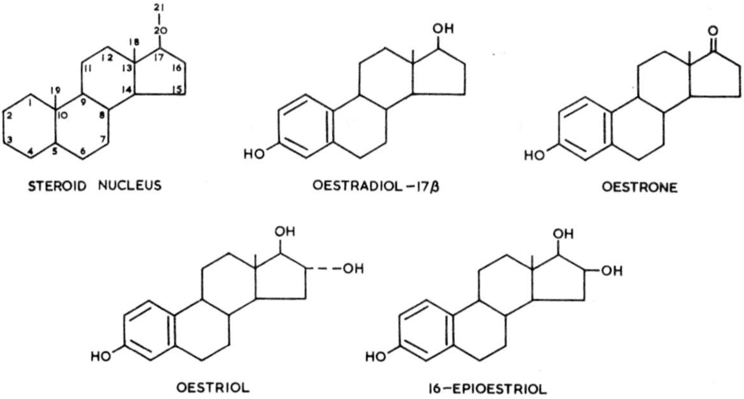

STEROID NUCLEUS   OESTRADIOL –17β   OESTRONE

OESTRIOL   16–EPIOESTRIOL

FIG. 13

Steroid nucleus and structural formulae of various oestrogens.

pregnancy urine, and the total number of such substances now known to be present exceeds twenty. For detailed information on the isolation of the more recently discovered oestrogens review articles by Breuer (1962) and by Dale and Greene (1965) should be consulted. At the time of writing the estimation of such compounds in body fluids has not been shown to provide valuable clinical information additional to that obtainable by measuring the three classical oestrogens, and accordingly, in the present chapter the discussion will be mainly concerned with the latter group of compounds.

In the non-pregnant human female oestrogens are secreted by the ovary and by the adrenal cortex. In the ovary both the theca interna and the stratum granulosum are capable of oestrogen production, and the hormones are elaborated by the corpus luteum as well as by the maturing Graafian follicle. Most investigators now believe that in women the principal ovarian oestrogens are oestrone and oestradiol (see Rabinowitz, 1956; Zander *et al.*, 1959; J. B. Brown, 1960). Evidence for the secretion of oestrogens by the adrenal cortex in human subjects is mainly indirect but is now reasonably strong. It is based, for example, on the detection of oestrogens in urine in postmenopausal and oöphorectomised women, on the increase in urinary oestrogen output when the adrenocorticotrophic hormone (ACTH) is administered to such subjects and on the fact that both male and female patients with certain types of adrenocortical tumours can excrete abnormally large quantities of oestrogens in their urine. In addition to being elaborated by the ovary and adrenal cortex oestrogens are also produced by the placenta during pregnancy and by the testes in male subjects.

Oestrogens occur in human urine as water soluble conjugates. Oestriol is conjugated mainly with glucuronic acid and excreted as oestriol glucuronide ; a small proportion is conjugated with sulphuric acid and excreted as a sulphate. Oestrone was formerly thought to occur in urine entirely as a sulphate until the work of Oneson and Cohen (1952) and others demonstrated that the steroid was also present in pregnancy urine in the form of a glucuronide. Oestradiol and the more recently discovered urinary oestrogens are excreted mainly as glucuronides.

2. Methods for the Estimation of the Classical Oestrogens in Urine *

Prior to the mid 1950's oestrogen assays in the urine of non-pregnant subjects were generally performed by biological techniques. Since then reliable chemical methods have become available and these have now almost completely replaced bio-assay procedures. The latter can now be regarded as of historical interest only, and for this reason they will not be further discussed in the present chapter. For details of such techniques articles by Pedersen-Bjergaard (1939), Emmens (1950, 1962), Claringbold (1954), L. Martin (1960, 1964) and Katzman (1965) should be consulted.

* See footnote, p. 69.

Chemical methods for the estimation of the classical oestrogens in urine fall into three main groups:

(a) Colorimetric methods.

(b) Fluorimetric methods.

(c) Gas chromatographic methods.

Isotopic methods and techniques depending on thin layer chromatography have also been proposed (see Beer and Gallagher, 1955 a b; Gallagher et al., 1958; Lisboa and Diczfalusy, 1962; Siiteri, 1963; Luisi et al., 1964). However, such procedures have so far been employed on a very limited scale in clinical practice, and further discussion of their advantages and limitations is not warranted in the present chapter.

Methods are also available for estimating the secretion rate of oestrogens in health and disease (see Fishman et al., 1962; Morse et al., 1963; Tait, 1963; Goering and Herrmann, 1966). Again, because these techniques have not been widely applied in clinical studies they will not be discussed herein. For the details of the procedures the reader is referred to the original articles.

(a) COLORIMETRIC METHODS.—These depend on the reaction originally described by Kober in 1931 which consists of heating the oestrogens with a mixture of phenol and sulphuric acid, diluting with water and reheating; a pink colour with an adsorption maximum at a wavelength of 520 mμ. is obtained. The historical aspects of the Kober reaction have recently been reviewed by Marrian (1966). A large number of colorimetric methods based on this reaction have been described of which the following will be discussed:

(i) The method of J. B. Brown (1955).

(ii) The method of J. B. Brown et al. (1957).

(iii) The method of Bauld (1956).

(iv) The method of Ittrich (1958).

(v) The method of Salokangas and Bulbrook (1961).

(vi) The method of Palmer (1964).

(vii) The method of Eechaute and Demeester (1965).

(i) *The Method of J. B. Brown (1955)*.—This has been by far the most widely used method for the quantitative determination of oestrogens in the urine of non-pregnant subjects. It has the following steps:

(α) Acid hydrolysis in order to liberate the free oestrogens from their conjugates.

D

33

(β) Ether extraction.

(γ) Carbonate wash of the ether extract.

(δ) Partition between a benzene-petroleum ether mixture and water and alkali.

(ε) A phase-change procedure for the phenolic fraction depending on methylation of the phenol group.

(ζ) Separation of the oestrogen methyl ethers by adsorption chromatography on alumina columns.

(η) Colorimetric determination by the Kober reaction.

(θ) Spectrophotometric correction for interfering chromogenic material using the formula described by Allen (1950)*.

The reliability critera of this method have been reviewed by its originator (J. B. Brown, 1960) and by Loraine and Bell (1966, 1967). Recovery experiments in which known amounts of oestriol, oestrone and oestradiol were added to urine have indicated that the overall yield for the method lies between 60 and 70 per cent; the precision of the technique is satisfactory. The lower limit of sensitivity is approximately 3 μg. per 24 hours for each of the three classical oestrogens. The specificity of the method has been shown to be acceptable on the basis of experiments involving counter-current distribution (Diczfalusy, 1955) and isotopic techniques (Gallagher *et al.*, 1958). The procedure is exacting and time-consuming, one technician performing four complete determinations in a period of two days. However, in skilled hands the technique is suitable for widespread application and has yielded much valuable information in clinical studies.

(ii) *The Method of J. B. Brown* et al. (*1957*).—This is a modification of the original method in which additional steps are inserted between steps δ and ε. These are:

(α) Saponification of the oestriol fraction in water and of the oestrone/oestradiol fraction by boiling with N NaOH.

(β) Extraction of the oestriol fraction with ether and of the oestrone/oestradiol fraction with benzene.

(γ) Extraction of the two fractions with NaOH prior to methylation.

---

* The Allen correction depends on the assumption that the contaminating colours have linear wavelength/adsorption curves in the region of the adsorption maximum of the oestrogen Kober colours.

These additional purification steps reduce the amount of chromogenic impurities in the final extract by approximately one half and diminish or eliminate interference by various drugs. The modification is to be preferred in urine samples containing small amounts of endogenous oestrogens, *e.g.* those derived from postmenopausal or oöphorectomised women, and is essential in urines obtained from patients receiving cortisone and other drugs which are known to interfere with the original method. The accuracy and precision of the modified technique are similar to those of the original method, but specificity and sensitivity are somewhat improved.

(iii) *The Method of Bauld (1956).*—This has been employed in clinical studies on a much more limited scale than that of J. B. Brown (1955). It has the following steps:

(α) Acid hydrolysis.

(β) Ether extraction.

(γ) Separation of oestriol from oestrone and oestradiol by partition between benzene and water.

(δ) Purification of oestriol by saponification and by column partition chromatography.

(ε) Separation and purification of oestrone and oestradiol by column partition chromatography and by saponification.

(ζ) Colorimetric determination of the purified fractions using a modified Kober reaction.

(η) Spectrophotometric correction for interfering chromogenic material by means of Allen's formula.

Bauld's method differs from that of J. B. Brown in employing partition chromatography on celite columns rather than adsorption chromatography on alumina columns. The oestrogens obtained in Bauld's method are in the free form and are therefore biologically active. According to Marrian (1955) the methods of Bauld and J. B. Brown are comparable in terms of their reliability criteria. When parallel assays by the two methods are conducted on urine samples from men and from normally menstruating and postmenopausal women the results obtained are in reasonably good agreement.

(iv) *The Method of Ittrich (1958).*—Ittrich's main contribution to this field was to increase the sensitivity and specificity of the Kober reaction by extracting the chromogen with chloroform, tetrachloroethane or tetrabromoethane each containing 2 per cent p-nitrophenol. Ittrich also described a method for the determination of " total oestrogens " during the menstrual cycle. This has the following steps:

(α) Acid hydrolysis.

(β) Extraction of the oestrogens with ether.

(γ) Washing of the ether extract with an alkaline buffer solution.

(δ) Re-extraction of the oestrogens into ether and subsequent evaporation of the ether.

(ϵ) Modified Kober reaction followed either by colorimetry or fluorimetry.

Although the reliability criteria of this technique are reasonably satisfactory, the method has not been widely used in clinical studies. Ittrich (1958) has also described methods for the estimation of oestrogens in mid and late pregnancy, but these are not relevant to the present chapter.

(v) *The Method of Salokangas and Bulbrook (1961)*.—In this procedure the purification step of Ittrich (1958) is incorporated into the method of J. B. Brown et al. (1957), the final Kober colour being measured in micro cells. The technique can detect as little as 0·5 µg. of each of the classical oestrogens in a 24 hour urine sample; accuracy and precision are comparable to those of the method of J. B. Brown et al. (1957).

(vi) *The Method of Palmer (1964)*.—This is based on the method of J. B. Brown (1955) and measures oestriol only. It involves acid hydrolysis, ether extraction, methylation, alumina chromatography and the Kober reaction. The lower limit of sensitivity of the technique is 1·3 µg. oestriol in a 24 hour urine sample. Accuracy, precision and sensitivity are claimed to be satisfactory. The procedure is reasonably practicable, one technician performing 10 estimations in a single day.

(vii) *The Method of Eechaute and Demeester (1965)*.—This is essentially a modification of the method of Beling (1963) and has the following steps:

(α) Enzymic hydrolysis using β-glucuronidase and sulphatase.

(β) Gel filtration on Sephadex.

(γ) Ether extraction.

36

(δ) Washing of the extract with alkali and water.

(ε) Evaporation of the ether extract.

(ζ) Performance of the Kober reaction with subsequent extraction of the colour complex as described by Ittrich (1960).

(η) Fluorimetric determination.

The reliability criteria of the technique have been carefully studied by its originators. Accuracy as determined by recovery experiments employing added oestrogens was approximately 95 per cent. Precision (s)*, estimated according to Snedecor (1956), was 0·5 for a series of 30 urine samples ranging in titre from 0 to 40 μg. total oestrogens per 24 hours. The figure for s must be regarded as satisfactory, as were the sensitivity and specificity of the procedure. The originators claim a high degree of practicability for the technique and state that it can be used routinely in clinical studies.

(b) FLUORIMETRIC METHODS.—Such procedures depend on the fact that an intense yellowish-green fluorescence develops when an oestrogen is heated with sulphuric acid or phorphoric acid. The fluorescence produced is proportional to the quantity of oestrogen present, and its intensity can be measured in a fluorimeter. The fluorescence reaction for oestrogens is more sensitive but less specific than the Kober reaction. This lack of specificity arises mainly from the fact that extracts prepared from urine contain substances other than oestrogens which are capable of producing fluorescence.

There are two main methods in this group—those of Preedy and Aitken (1961 a b) and of Ladany and Finkelstein (1963). The former employs sulphuric and the later phosphoric acid in the fluorescence reaction.

(i) *The Method of Preedy and Aitken (1961 a b).*—This has the following steps:

(α) Acid hydrolysis.

(β) Ether extraction.

(γ) Extraction of the ether with saturated sodium bicarbonate followed by evaporation.

---

* Precision (s) can be calculated by determining the mean difference between duplicate determinations in a series of at least 20 different samples of blood or urine. The standard deviation of the mean difference then provides an estimate of s.

(δ) Partition between toluene and N NaOH.

(ε) Neutralisation of the N NaOH and extraction with ether.

(ζ) Partition chromatography on celite columns.

(η) Evaporation and fluorimetric analysis of each fraction.

The accuracy of the procedure as determined by recovery experiments is approximately 80 per cent, and a high degree of specificity is achieved by the fractional elution method employed. Using a single chromatographic procedure, the method is capable of measuring as little as 1·0 µg. oestrone, 1·8 µg. oestradiol and 3·0 µg. oestriol in a 24 hour urine sample; if two chromatographic procedures are used, levels as low as 0·2 µg. per 24 hour urine sample for each of the classical oestrogens can be determined. The main disadvantage of the procedure is its very laborious nature. The chromatography steps cannot be completed under a period of 36 hours, and some 80 determinations of fluorescence are necessary for each urine sample assayed.

(ii) *The Method of Ladany and Finkelstein (1963).*—This involves:

(α) Enzyme hydrolysis with β-glucuronidase and sulphatase.

(β) Ether extraction.

(γ) Washing of the ether extract with alkali and water.

(δ) Partition between benzene-petroleum ether and water.

(ε) Separation and isolation of the oestrogens by thin layer and paper chromatography.

(ζ) Fluorimetric reaction using phosphoric acid.

The technique is claimed to be capable of measuring 1·0 µg. of each of the three classical oestrogens in a 24 hour urine sample; other reliability criteria have not been reported in detail by the originators. The technique is time-consuming and laborious and has been little used in clinical studies.

(*c*) GAS CHROMATOGRAPHIC METHODS.—Gas liquid chromatography has been shown to be of great value in the separation of pure steroids, including the oestrogens (Vanden-Heuvel *et al.*, 1960, 1961; Luukkainen *et al.*, 1961, 1962; Wotiz and

H. F. Martin, 1961). However, the successful application of techniques of this type to the estimation of oestrogens in body fluids depends primarily on the purity of the extract applied to the column. Several methods involving gas liquid chromatography have been described for the quantitative determination of oestrogens in the urine of pregnant women (Fishman and J. B. Brown, 1962; Wotiz, 1962, 1963a; Wotiz and H. F. Martin, 1962; Wotiz and Chattoraj, 1964; Yousem, 1964). However, only the techniques of Menini (1965) and Cagnazzo *et al.* (1965) are suitable for use in non-pregnant subjects.

(i) *The Method of Menini (1965).*—The main steps are as follows:

(α) Treatment of the unextracted urine by sodium borohydride in order to reduce oestrone to oestradiol.

(β) Acid hydrolysis.

(γ) Ether extraction.

(δ) Partition between a benzene-petroleum ether mixture and water and alkali.

(ε) Saponification step according to the specifications of J. B. Brown *et al.* (1957).

(ζ) Partition between benzene, light petroleum, ethanol and aqueous alkali.

(η) Methylation as described by J. B. Brown (1955).

(θ) Chromatography of the oestrogen methyl ethers on alumina columns.

(ι) Acetylation of the methyl ethers of oestradiol and oestriol.

(κ) Further alumina column chromatography.

(λ) Final determination by gas liquid chromatography.

Recovery experiments for oestradiol and oestriol using this procedure gave figures ranging from 68 to 77 per cent. The main disadvantage of the technique is its laborious nature, making it unsuitable for widespread clinical application. It may, however, prove of value in studies of selected patients.

(ii) *The Method of Cagnazzo* et al. *(1965).*—This involves enzyme hydrolysis with subsequent extraction and purification in a manner similar to that employed in the method of J. B. Brown (1955). The oestrogens are then saponified and applied to the column in the form of the trimethylsilyl ethers. Detailed reliability criteria of the procedure have not yet been reported; however, the method, like that of Menini (1965), is laborious and time-consuming and is almost certainly unsuitable for routine clinical application.

3. Method for the Estimation of 16-Epioestriol in Urine

Studies on the excretion of the urinary oestrogen metabolite, 16-epioestriol, during the menstrual cycle are now available. The method of choice for the quantitative determination of this steroid is that of Nocke and Breuer (1963), and the technique can readily be incorporated into the method of J. B. Brown et al. (1957) for the classical oestrogens. The basis of the procedure depends on the fact that 16-epioestriol can be separated from oestriol by forming the acetonide of the former compound. The acetonide of 16-epioestriol is then purified using an alumina column, and the final determination is made by the Kober reaction. The technique can measure with reasonable accuracy 1·7 µg. 16-epioestriol in a 24 hour urine sample.

4. Methods for the Estimation of the Classical Oestrogens in Blood

The oestrogens occur in blood in a variety of forms which have been designated " free ", " protein-bound " and " conjugated ". No method is at present capable of measuring the three forms of each oestrogen separately in the 10 to 20 ml. of blood generally available from an individual subject, and consequently, all measure total amounts of each oestrogen.

Techniques for the estimation of oestrogens in human blood fall into three main categories:

(a) Colorimetric.
(b) Fluorimetric.
(c) Isotopic.

(a) COLORIMETRIC METHODS.—The most important technique in this group is probably that of Roy and J. B. Brown (1960) which is suitable for studies during pregnancy and which is very similar to that described by J. B. Brown (1955) for urine. The main differences in the method for blood are the use of smaller quantities of alumina for chromatography and of micro cells for the final determination. By the latter modification the sensitivity of the Kober reaction is increased some tenfold. The reliability criteria of the method of Roy and J. B. Brown (1960) have been reviewed by its originators and by J. B. Brown (1960). Recoveries of oestrogens added to blood are less satisfactory than with the original Brown method for urine. If the steroids are added after hydrolysis, the amounts recovered range from 50 to 70 per cent; if added before hydrolysis, the corresponding figures are some 5 to 10 per cent lower. With levels below 5 μg. per 100 ml. blood, the figure for s (see p. 37) ranges from 0·06 to 0·22 μg. per 100 ml. for each of the three classical oestrogens; s becomes larger with increasing oestrogen concentration. The method was considered by its originators to be reasonably satisfactory in terms of specificity. With respect to sensitivity, the lowest amounts which can be measured with confidence are 0·15 μg. oestradiol, 0·3 μg. oestrone and 0·3 μg. oestriol per 100 ml. blood.

The technique of Roy and J. B. Brown (1960) was subsequently modified by Roy (1962), who incorporated the fluorescence reaction of Ittrich (1958) into the original method and made the final determination by fluorimetry. Recovery experiments indicated that the accuracy of the modified procedure was comparable to that of the original method, while the sensitivity was increased approximately tenfold. The increase in sensitivity made it possible to apply the technique to blood samples obtained from non-pregnant individuals (see p. 100).

Total oestrogens in non-pregnant plasma have also been determined by the method of Oertel (1961), which involves column or paper chromatography followed by the Ittrich modification of the Kober reaction. The reliability criteria of this technique have not been reported in detail.

(b) FLUORIMETRIC METHODS.—The procedure of Preedy and Aitken (1961 b) is very similar to that described by the same authors for urine. It is claimed to be capable of measuring as little as 0·05 μg. oestrone, 0·05 μg. oestradiol and 0·1 μg. oestriol per 100 ml. plasma. As with the urinary method its main limitation is its very laborious nature.

Schrepfer and Nicholas (1965) have recently described a method for the determination of plasma oestrogens which, like the technique of Roy (1962), is essentially a modification of the procedure of J. B. Brown (1955) for urine. Enzyme hydrolysis is employed, and the final determination is made by fluorimetry using sulphuric acid. The reliability criteria of the procedure have not yet been described in detail by the originators.

(*c*) ISOTOPIC METHODS.—One of the more important in this group is that of Svendsen (1960) which measures oestrone and oestradiol. It utilises S-35 and I-131 as isotopes, and its steps include extraction, purification, esterification of oestrone and oestradiol by *p*-iodobenzenesulphonyl chloride, purification of the esters by paper chromatography and counting of the radioactivity. The reliability criteria of the procedure have been extensively studied. The mean percentage recovery for oestrone was 65, and for oestradiol 64; precision and specificity were satisfactory. The procedure, although laborious, is extremely sensitive, being capable of measuring approximately 5 nanograms (ng.) oestrone and 5 ng. oestradiol per 100 ml. plasma.

Another isotopic method estimating oestrone and oestradiol only is that of Ichii *et al.* (1963). In this procedure the plasma is extracted with chloroform and ether, purified by paper chromatography and the final determination is made by fluorimetry. Accuracy as judged by recovery experiments was approximately 65 per cent. The method is very sensitive and can measure as little as 2 ng. oestrone or oestradiol per 100 ml. plasma.

PROGESTERONE

1. General Considerations

The structural formulae of progesterone (pregn-4-ene-3,20-dione) and of its main urinary metabolite, pregnanediol (5β-pregnane-3α,20α-diol), are shown in Figure 14. In the non-pregnant woman one of the main sources of progesterone production is the ovary, and it is believed that the hormone is secreted both by the granulosa and theca lutein cells (see Brambell, 1956). Progesterone has also been isolated from human follicular fluid by Zander *et al.* (1958) who demonstrated that its concentration in the human Graafian follicle was high immediately prior to ovulation, and that the progesterone content of the corpus luteum paralleled the functional activity of the tissue, being at its maximum on days 21 and 22 of the menstrual cycle. The other important source of progesterone production in the non-pregnant human female is the adrenal cortex. Evidence for the elaboration of the hormone by the gland is now reasonably secure and has recently been summarised by Loraine and Bell (1966). In pregnancy progesterone is secreted mainly by the placenta.

Progesterone can be measured in blood obtained from pregnant women and also from non-pregnant subjects. The hormone has recently been isolated from the urine of pregnant women by Ismail and Harkness (1965), but at the time of writing reliable figures for the excretion of the progesterone in normal and abnormal pregnancy are not available.

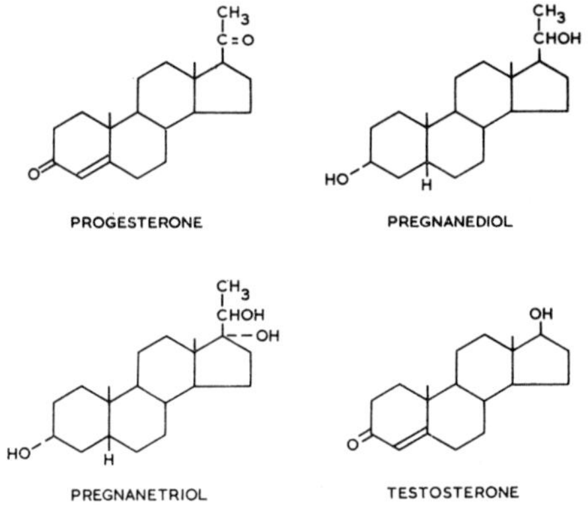

PROGESTERONE   PREGNANEDIOL

PREGNANETRIOL   TESTOSTERONE

FIG. 14

Structural formulae of progesterone, pregnanediol, pregnanetriol and testosterone.

2. Methods for the Estimation of Progesterone in Blood

Biological methods for the estimation of progesterone in body fluids are laborious and time-consuming and should no longer be used in clinical studies. Such techniques will not be described in the present chapter, and the reader is referred to review articles by Miyake (1962) and Loraine and Bell (1966) for the appropriate details. Chemical methods of assay of progesterone are now the procedures of choice and these fall naturally into three groups:

(a) Spectrophotometric and fluorimetric methods.
(b) Gas chromatographic methods.
(c) Isotopic methods.

43

(a) Spectrophotometric and Fluorimetric Methods.—
Such techniques have been described by various investigators,
including Zander and Simmer (1954), Short (1958), Sommerville and Deshpande (1958), Oertel *et al.* (1959), Touchstone
and Murawec (1960) and Heap (1964). The procedure which
has been most widely employed in clinical studies is probably
that of Short (1958). This is essentially a modification of the
original technique of Zander and Simmer (1954) and has the
following steps:

(i) Treatment of the plasma with NaOH.
(ii) Extraction of progesterone with ether.
(iii) Re-extraction of the dried ether extract with ethanol.
(iv) Separation by paper chromatography.
(v) Final determination using ultraviolet spectroscopy.

The accuracy of this method estimated on the basis of
recovery experiments was 73 per cent; sensitivity and specificity were reasonably satisfactory as was practicability.

(b) Gas Chromatographic Methods.—Procedures of this
type have been described by various investigators, including
Kumar *et al.* (1964), Collins and Sommerville (1964) and
Luisi *et al.* (1965); however, at the time of writing these have
been little used in clinical studies. In the method of Collins
and Sommerville (1964) progesterone is extracted from plasma
by ether following treatment with alkali; the extract is then
subjected to two-dimensional thin layer chromatography, the
final determination being made by gas liquid chromatography.
The procedure is claimed to be capable of detecting $0 \cdot 01$ μg. of
progesterone, and recoveries of added hormone are stated to be
greater than 80 per cent.

The method of Luisi *et al.* (1965) involves extraction with
ether, partition between methanol and heptane, separation by
thin layer chromatography and final determination by gas
liquid chromatography. Accuracy, based on recovery experiments with male plasma, was 90 per cent. Reproducibility and
specificity were claimed to be satisfactory, while the method is
capable of measuring as little as $0 \cdot 2$ μg. progesterone per 100 ml.
plasma. As with most methods involving gas liquid chromatography the technique is laborious and is unsuitable for routine
clinical use.

(c) ISOTOPIC METHODS.—Such procedures have been developed by Woolever and Goldfien (1963), Riondel et al. (1965) and Molen and Groen (1965). Only the method of Woolever and Goldfien (1963) will be described as this has been used to a greater extent clinically than other techniques. Its main steps are as follows:

(i) Addition to plasma of pure progesterone labelled with C-14.
(ii) Extraction of plasma with ethyl acetate and chloroform.
(iii) Isolation of progesterone by paper chromatography.
(iv) Reduction of the eluate from the paper by means of sodium borohydride labelled with tritium.
(v) Isolation of the borohydride derivative.
(vi) Separate counting of C-14 and tritium.

Counting of the C-14 provides an estimate of the recovery of the labelled progesterone added and thus enables an appropriate correction to be made for losses occurring during the extraction procedure. Counting of the tritium provides an estimate of the total progesterone present in the extract, and the difference between these two results is the amount of progesterone present in the unknown sample. The method, although laborious, is reasonably sensitive, being capable of detecting as little as 0·1 μg. of the hormone; reproducibility is claimed to be satisfactory.

PREGNANEDIOL

1. General Considerations

From the quantitative point of view this steroid is by far the most important metabolic reduction product of progesterone (see Fotherby, 1964 for review). As first demonstrated by Venning and Browne (1936), pregnanediol is excreted in the urine conjugated with glucuronic acid at position three of the steroid molecule. Radioactivity studies with tritium labelled progesterone have shown that small and variable amounts of the parent hormone, ranging from 6 to 27 per cent, are excreted as pregnanediol. It is therefore obvious that urinary pregnanediol determinations cannot provide an accurate quantitative assessment of endogenous progesterone production. Nevertheless, in spite of this fact, clinically useful information can often be obtained by performing pregnanediol assays in urine.

2. Methods for the Estimation of Pregnanediol in Urine

The steroid is not biologically active and must therefore be determined by chemical methods. Such procedures can be divided into three main categories.

(a) Colorimetric methods.

(b) Gas chromatographic methods.

(c) Isotopic methods.

Gravimetric methods such as those described by Venning (1937, 1938) and by Astwood and Jones (1941) in which the final product is weighed, are now of historical interest only and will not be further discussed. In all assay methods currently in use urinary pregnanediol is determined in the free rather than the conjugated form.

(a) COLORIMETRIC METHODS.—These have as their end point a colour reaction involving sulphuric acid. Four such techniques will be described.

(i) The method of Klopper et al. (1955).

(ii) The method of Goldzieher and Nakamura (1962).

(iii) The method of Oertel and Groot (1965).

(iv) The method of Sulimovici et al. (1965).

(i) *The Method of Klopper* et al. *(1955)*.—Of all the assay methods for pregnanediol which have been developed this has been by far the most widely used in clinical studies. Its main steps are as follows:

(α) Acid hydrolysis.

(β) Toluene extraction.

(γ) A permanganate oxidation step designed to remove from the pregnanediol fraction a contaminant which is probably a decomposition product of pregnanetriol.

(δ) Chromatography on alumina columns.

(ε) Acetylation of pregnanediol.

(ζ) Further chromatography on alumina columns.

(η) Colorimetry by means of a modified sulphuric acid reaction.

The accuracy of the procedure was tested by its originators in a series of recovery experiments. At concentrations of pregnanediol as low as 0·5 mg. per 24 hours the mean recovery of the added steroid was approximately 90 per cent; at higher concentrations the corresponding figures were even greater.

46

Klopper *et al.* (1955) and Coyle *et al.* (1956), using infra-red spectroscopy and mixed melting point determinations, showed that the specificity of the method was satisfactory. The procedure gives reproducible results down to levels between 1 and 2 mg. pregnanediol in a 24 hour urine sample; however, below these values its precision becomes unsatisfactory. The practicability of the method is acceptable, one technician readily performing some 20 determinations in one week. It must be emphasised that, although the procedure of Klopper *et al.* (1955) may eventually be superseded by more rapid and sensitive gas chromatographic methods, its widespread use in clinical practice over the past decade has enabled much valuable information to be accumulated.

(ii) *The Method of Goldzieher and Nakamura (1962)*.—This has the following steps:

(α) Enzymic hydrolysis by β-glucuronidase.

(β) Chloroform extraction.

(γ) Chromatography on silica gel columns.

(δ) Acetylation.

(ε) Further silica gel chromatography.

(ζ) Colorimetry by means of a modified sulphuric acid reaction.

The method estimates pregnanetriol as well as pregnanediol. Accuracy is claimed to be satisfactory, recoveries averaging 100 per cent. The technique is stated to be highly specific and to be capable of measuring 0·2 mg. pregnanediol in a 24 hour urine sample.

(iii) *The Method of Oertel and Groot (1965)*.—As with the method of Goldzieher and Nakamura (1962) this procedure measures both pregnanediol and pregnanetriol. It involves enzyme hydrolysis with β-glucuronidase, benzene extraction, alkali wash, thin layer chromatography and a final colour reaction employing sulphuric acid. Recovery experiments gave average yields of 79 and 86 per cent for pregnanediol and pregnanetriol respectively. The lower limit of sensitivity of the technique was 0·15 mg. per 24 hours for pregnanediol and 0·05 mg. per 24 hours for pregnanetriol.

(iv) *The Method of Sulimovici* et al. *(1965)*.—This measures allopregnanediol in addition to pregnanediol. Its main steps

47

are acid hydrolysis, extraction with diethyl ether and ethyl alcohol, washing with alkali, thin layer chromatography and finally a sulphuric acid colour reaction. Accuracy was approximately 90 per cent, while practicability compared favourably with that of other techniques, each estimation being completed in only four hours. The chief disadvantage of the method is its low degree of sensitivity, the lower limit being approximately 1 mg. pregnanediol in a 24 hour urine sample. The technique in its present form is unsuitable for use in the follicular phase of the cycle, but is satisfactory in the luteal phase and during pregnancy.

Sulimovici *et al.* (1965) have compared the reliability criteria of various assay methods for pregnanediol. This comparison is shown in Table 2.

TABLE 2

COMPARISON OF VARIOUS METHODS FOR THE ESTIMATION OF PREGNANEDIOL

(After Sulimovici *et al.*, 1965)

Reference	Accuracy %	Precision mg./litre	Sensitivity mg./24 hours	Time taken for one determination hours	Number of determinations per week
Borth (1952)	87	±0·4	0·8	3	20–30
Klopper *et al.* (1955)	94	±0·1	0·5	8	20
Eberlein and Bongiovanni (1958)	98	±0·1	0·3	15	16–24
Lipp (1960)	94	±1·5	0·002	2 days	16
Sulimovici *et al.* (1965)	92	±0·6	1·0–1·2	4	40–50

(*b*) GAS CHROMATOGRAPHIC METHODS.—A number of investigators, including Cooper *et al.* (1962), Patti *et al.* (1963), Turner *et al.* (1963), Wotiz (1963 *b*), Lau and Jones (1964), Panicucci and Taponeco (1965) and Chattoraj and Scommegna (1967) have described such procedures. At present information on their clinical application in non-pregnant conditions is very limited indeed, and for this reason only one representative method—that of Lau and Jones (1964)—will be described. The main steps in this procedure are as follows:

(α) Acid hydrolysis.

(β) Toluene extraction.

(γ) Thin layer chromatography on silica gel.

(δ) Elution of pregnanediol by ethyl alcohol.

(ε) Final determination using gas liquid chromatography.

The accuracy of this procedure was found to be satisfactory, recoveries ranging from 80 to 90 per cent. Sensitivity and specificity were not discussed; however, in the somewhat similar method of Wotiz (1963 b) which involves acetylation of the pregnanediol prior to gas liquid chromatography, a lower limit of sensitivity of 50 μg. of the steroid in a 24 hour urine sample was claimed.

(c) ISOTOPIC METHOD.—Such a technique has recently been described by Ehrlich (1965). It has the following steps:

(i) Addition of tritium-labelled pregnanediol as an internal standard.

(ii) Hydrolysis with β-glucuronidase.

(iii) Benzene extraction.

(iv) Thin layer chromatography.

(v) Elution and acetylation of pregnanediol labelled with C-14.

(vi) Further thin layer chromatography.

(vii) Final counting of C-14 and tritium.

According to Ehrlich (1965) accuracy, specificity and sensitivity are satisfactory. The major advantage of the technique is its high degree of sensitivity, assays being possible on as little as 1 ml. urine. The main disadvantage of the procedure is its laborious nature.

3. Methods for the Estimation of Pregnanediol in Blood

Two main methods have been described for the quantitative determination of pregnanediol in blood—those of Sommerville and Deshpande (1958) and Oertel et al. (1960). The method of Sommerville and Deshpande (1958) involves incubation of plasma with β-glucuronidase, treatment with alkali, extraction with organic solvents, chromatography on alumina columns and final colorimetric determination. Recoveries of added pregnanediol range from 85 to 95 per cent.

E   49

In the method of Oertel *et al.* (1960) plasma is deproteinised prior to hydrolysis either with acid or enzyme. Purification is effected by extraction with organic solvents and by paper chromatography; the final determination is made colorimetrically using a sulphuric acid reaction. Recoveries of pregnanediol added to blood before hydrolysis range from 75 to 85 per cent.

PREGNANETRIOL

This steroid, the structural formula of which is shown in Figure 14, is one of the main metabolites of 17α-hydroxyprogesterone and 17α-hydroxypregnenolone (Axelrod and Goldzieher, 1960; D. K. Fukushima *et al.*, 1961, 1963). It is mainly secreted by the adrenal cortex (see Heard *et al.*, 1956) but, as shown by Zander (1958), is probably also elaborated by the ovaries in women during reproductive life. Radioactivity studies in normal subjects using C-14 labelled 17α-hydroxyprogesterone have demonstrated that approximately 30 per cent of this steroid appears in urine as pregnanetriol (D. K. Fukushima *et al.*, 1962). The latter is excreted conjugated with glucuronic acid as pregnanetriol glucuronide.

Methods for the Estimation of Pregnanetriol in Urine

Several procedures have been developed including those of Stern (1957), Herrmann and Silverman (1957), Bongiovanni and Eberlein (1958), Cox (1959), Fotherby and Love (1960) and Harkness and Love (1966). In the present section only the techniques of Fotherby and Love (1960) and Harkness and Love (1966) will be described.

(*a*) THE METHOD OF FOTHERBY AND LOVE (1960).—The main steps are as follows:

    (i) Enzymic hydrolysis with β-glucuronidase.
    (ii) Extraction with benzene.
    (iii) Washing with alkali and water.
    (iv) Chromatography on an alumina column.
    (v) Final determination using a sulphuric acid colour reaction.

The reliability criteria of the procedure have been studied in detail by its originators. Recoveries were acceptable ranging from 84 to 89 per cent; the lower limit of sensitivity was 50 µg. pregnanetriol in a 24 hour urine sample. Precision and specificity were claimed to be satisfactory as was practicability, one technician readily performing 12 estimations in a single working day.

(*b*) THE METHOD OF HARKNESS AND LOVE (1966).—This is essentially a modification of the previously described method, the first four steps of the two procedures being identical. Following alumina chromatography sodium metaperiodate is added to the eluate, and the aetiocholanolone so formed is measured by the Zimmermann reaction. The method is claimed to be more specific than its predecessor, especially when applied to pregnancy urine; it is also somewhat more sensitive being capable of detecting as little as 30 µg. of the steroid in a 24 hour urine sample. Accuracy and precision are very similar in the two methods.

TESTOSTERONE

1. General Considerations

The structural formula of the male sex hormone, testosterone is shown in Figure 14. In women this steroid is secreted both by the ovaries and the adrenals (Ismail and Harkness, 1966 *a* ; Horton, 1966 ; Horton *et al.*, 1966). In addition the ovary secretes relatively large quantities of the C-19 steroid androstenedione (Δ^4-androstene-3,17-dione) which is believed to be a precursor of testosterone (Horton *et al.*, 1966). Testosterone is excreted in urine conjugated with glucuronic acid as a glucuronide; its biosynthesis and metabolism have been intensively studied in recent years and have been reviewed by Werbin *et al.* (1957), Fieser and Fieser (1959) and Dorfman *et al.* (1963).

Assays of testosterone can be performed either by biological or by chemical methods and can be conducted on urine or blood. As with the oestrogens and progesterone bio-assay methods for testosterone are now of historical interest only and for this reason will not be considered herein. A comprehensive review article on this subject is that of Dorfman (1962).

2. Methods for the Estimation of Testosterone in Urine

Many such methods have been described in recent years (see Futterweit *et al.*, 1963; Vermeulen and Verplancke, 1963;

Camacho and Migeon, 1963; Sandberg *et al.*, 1964; Ibayashi *et al.*, 1964; Rosner *et al.*, 1965; Ismail and Harkness, 1966 *b*; Horn *et al.*, 1966). They can be divided into three main groups:

    (*a*) Colorimetric methods.

    (*b*) Fluorimetric methods.

    (*c*) Gas chromatographic methods.

In the ensuing discussion one example in each of the first two categories and two in the third will be described.

(*a*) COLORIMETRIC METHOD.

The Method of Vermeulen and Verplancke (1963).—This involves:

    (i) Addition of a known amount of the C-14 labelled testosterone to urine.

    (ii) Hydrolysis by β-glucuronidase.

    (iii) Ether extraction.

    (iv) Alumina and thin layer chromatography.

    (v) Final determination using a micro Zimmermann reaction.

    (vi) Counting of radioactivity and correction for losses during the procedure.

The specificity of the method is claimed to be satisfactory, and the procedure can detect as little as 4 μg. of the hormone in a 24 hour urine sample. Its maximum error is 10 per cent for values above 20 μg. per 24 hours and 20 per cent for values between 10 and 20 μg. per 24 hours.

(*b*) FLUORIMETRIC METHOD

The Method of Horn et al. *(1966).*—This depends on the enzymatic conversion of testosterone to oestradiol and has the following steps:

    (i) Addition of a known amount of C-14 labelled testosterone to urine.

    (ii) Enzymatic hydrolysis by β-glucuronidase and sulphatase.

    (iii) Ether extraction.

    (iv) Washing with alkali and water.

    (v) Thin layer chromatography.

    (vi) Paper chromatography.

    (vii) Conversion of testosterone to oestradiol using a placental aromatizing enzyme system (" Aromatase ": Mann Research Laboratories, New York).

(viii) Paper chromatography.

(ix) Estimation of oestradiol by fluorimetry.

(x) Assessment of accuracy by counting of C-14.

The mean percentage recovery of added testosterone was 46 when assessed by counting radioactivity and 40 when calculated by fluorimetry. The co-efficient of variation (standard deviation expressed as a percentage of mean) ranged from 1 to 10 per cent in a series of triplicate estimations. The major disadvantage of this technique is its laborious nature, and this will preclude its widespread use in clinical practice.

(c) GAS CHROMATOGRAPHIC METHODS

(i) *The Method of Ibayashi* et al. (*1964*).—This has the following steps:

(α) Addition of a known amount of tritiated testosterone to urine.

(β) Hydrolysis by β-glucuronidase.

(γ) Extraction with ether.

(δ) Thin layer chromatography.

(ε) Acetylation.

(ζ) Further thin layer chromatography.

(η) Final determination by gas liquid chromatography.

(θ) Counting of radioactivity for assessment of losses during the procedure.

The technique is capable of detecting 5 μg. testosterone in a 24 hour urine sample. Specificity and precision are claimed to be satisfactory.

(ii) *The Method of Ismail and Harkness* (*1966 b*).—This involves:

(α) Acid hydrolysis.

(β) Ether extraction.

(γ) Separation of ketonic from non-ketonic fractions by the Girard-T reagent. In this step the resin Amberlite IRC-50 is used as a catalyst.

(δ) Chromatography on alumina columns and on paper.

(ε) Elution of testosterone from paper by ethanol.

(η) Final determination using gas liquid chromatography.

The reliability criteria of the method have been studied in detail by its originators. Accuracy was tested by recovery experiments involving both unlabelled and C-14 labelled testosterone; yields of approximately 80 per cent were achieved. Precision was estimated by calculating s (see p. 37); in male urine this figure was 3·2 µg. for a mean value of 50 µg. per 24 hours, and this must be regarded as satisfactory. Specificity was probably superior to that of other methods, especially as regards the separation of testosterone from epitestosterone. Sensitivity was also of a high degree, the method being capable of measuring with accuracy 0·5 µg. testosterone in a 24 hour urine sample. The practicability of the technique is comparable to that of the method of J. B. Brown (1955) for urinary oestrogens, six determinations being readily completed by one technician in two working days. Recently Ismail et al. (1968) have developed a method which permits the separate estimation of testosterone, epi-testosterone and androstenedione in the same urine sample. The application of this technique to clinical problems will be awaited with interest.

3. Methods for the Estimation of Testosterone in Blood†

As in the case of urine a large number of such procedures have been described in recent years (Finkelstein et al., 1961; Riondel et al., 1963; Brownie et al., 1964; Hudson et al., 1963; Burger et al., 1964; Rivarola and Migeon, 1966; Saez et al., 1967; Bardin and Lipsett, 1967). They are of three main types—fluorimetric, gas chromatographic and isotopic.

The *fluorimetric* group includes the technique of Finkelstein et al. (1961) which depends on the enzymatic conversion of testosterone to oestradiol, and is very similar to that recently described by Horn et al. (1966) for urine (see p. 52). One of the most widely used procedures in the *gas chromatographic* group is that of Brownie et al. (1964) which involves:

(α) Addition of tritium labelled testosterone to plasma.

(β) Extraction with diethyl ether.

(γ) Thin layer chromatography.

(δ) Acetylation.

(ϵ) Further thin layer chromatography.

(ζ) Final determination by gas liquid chromatography.

(η) Counting of tritium to assess losses during the procedure.

The precision and sensitivity of the method are claimed

† See footnote, p. 69.

to be satisfactory; however, specificity is doubtful since epitestosterone cannot be completely separated from testosterone.

Under the heading of *isotopic* methods three procedures will be described:

(*a*) THE METHOD OF HUDSON *et al.* (1963).—This is a double isotopic technique involving both C-14 and tritium labelling of testosterone. Purification of the extract is effected by paper chromatography prior to the final determination by gas liquid chromatography. The precision of the method is satisfactory, the co-efficient of variation ranging from 10 to 15 per cent. The lower limit of sensitivity is 0·05 μg. testosterone per 100 ml. plasma. The method has subsequently been somewhat simplified by Burger *et al.* (1964) who substituted thin layer chromatography for one of the paper chromatographic steps in the original procedure.

(*b*) THE METHOD OF RIONDEL *et al.* (1963).—The main steps in this procedure are as follows:

(i) Addition of tritium labelled testosterone to plasma.
(ii) Extraction of plasma with ether.
(iii) Preparation of the S-35 labelled thiosemicarbazide of both the tritiated progesterone and the progesterone present in the plasma sample.
(vi) Purification of the thiosemicarbazide derivative by thin layer and paper chromatography.
(v) Further thin layer and paper chromatography.
(vi) Separate counting of tritium and S-35.

The originators noted that recoveries of tritiated testosterone were low; precision was satisfactory, the co-efficient of variation on two pools of plasma from normal men being 6·0 and 5·5 per cent respectively. Specificity was reasonably satisfactory although the separation of epitestosterone from testosterone was not complete. The procedure is very sensitive and is capable of measuring as little as 0·02 μg. testosterone per 100 ml. plasma.

(*c*) THE METHOD OF RIVAROLA AND MIGEON (1966).—This double isotopic procedure determines androstenedione as well as testosterone. It has the following steps:

(i) Extraction with ether.

(ii) Column chromatography on florisil (magnesium tri-silicate).

(iii) Paper chromatography to separate testosterone from androstenedione.

(iv) Reduction of androstenedione to testosterone using sodium borohydride.

(v) Paper chromatography.

(vi) Acetylation of testosterone with ^{14}C-acetic anhydride.

(vii) Thin layer chromatography.

(viii) Further paper chromatography.

(ix) Reduction of testosterone to 3β-hydroxyandrost-4-ene-17β acetate by sodium borohydride.

(x) Final paper chromatography.

(xi) Counting of radioactivity.

The overall recovery for testosterone varied between 30 and 40 per cent and for androstenedione between 10 and 25 per cent. Specificity was claimed to be satisfactory, as was the co-efficient of variation (7·6 per cent for testosterone and 13·1 per cent for androstenedione). The main disadvantage of the method is its very laborious nature, making it quite unsuitable for widespread clinical use.

HUMAN PITUITARY GONADOTROPHINS (HPG)*

This section deals mainly with bio-assay methods for the separate estimation of follicle-stimulating hormone (FSH) and luteinising hormone (LH). Tests measuring a mixture of FSH and LH activities—so-called " total gonadotrophic activity " —are also considered as are immunological methods for the two hormones. The discussion concentrates predominantly but not exclusively on techniques which have been employed in clinical studies, procedures which are now of historical interest only being omitted. A limited amount of information is incorporated on reference preparations available for the comparative assay of HPG and on methods for the extraction of gonadotrophic hormones from urine and blood. For a fuller

* This term is used in a general sense to denote the gonadotrophic activity present in body fluids. Unless otherwise stated such activity is both follicle-stimulating and luteinising in character.

consideration of some of the topics considered in this section the reader is referred to review articles by Loraine (1956), Loraine and Bell (1966), Bell (1967 a) and Apostolakis and Loraine (1967).

1. Reference Materials

A large number of reference materials have been used for the assay of HPG in body fluids (see Loraine and Bell, 1966; Apostolakis and Loraine, 1967, for details). The two most important of these are the First and Second International Reference Preparations for Human Menopausal Gonadotrophin.

(a) FIRST INTERNATIONAL REFERENCE PREPARATION FOR HUMAN MENOPAUSAL GONADOTROPHIN (FIRST IRP-HMG).— This material was formerly known as HMG-24. It was prepared by Dekanski (Organon, Newhouse, Scotland) by an extraction method involving kaolin adsorption and elution, fractional acetone precipitation and purification of the crude kaolin-acetone extract by tricalcium phosphate. One HMG unit was defined as the gonadotrophic activity contained in 1 mg. of the First IRP-HMG (see Loraine and J. B. Brown, 1959; Bull. Wld. Hlth. Org., 1960; Borth et al., 1961 a).

(b) SECOND INTERNATIONAL REFERENCE PREPARATION FOR HUMAN MENOPAUSAL GONADOTROPHIN (SECOND IRP-HMG). This material was formerly known as Pergonal-23. It was prepared by Donini (Serono, Rome) from postmenopausal urine by a method involving kaolin adsorption followed by chromatography on permutit columns. Each ampoule of the Second IRP-HMG contains approximately 10 mg. of the freeze-dried material consisting of equal amounts of the hormone and lactose. Various investigators, including Rosemberg and Engel (1961) and Schmidt-Elmendorff et al. (1962), have shown that the Second IRP-HMG has a considerably higher specific activity than the First IRP-HMG when assayed by a variety of bio-assay methods. In 1965 the Expert Committee on Biological Standardisation assigned to each ampoule of the Second IRP-HMG 40 i.u. of human urinary FSH and 40 i.u. of human urinary LH activity.

2. Extraction Methods for HPG

For estimations in both blood and urine, gonadotrophic activity must be extracted and concentrated prior to bio-assay. Some of the more widely used extraction methods will be briefly discussed, the subject having been reviewed in more detail elsewhere (see Loraine and Bell, 1966).

(a) EXTRACTION OF HPG FROM URINE.—Two types of procedure will be described:

(i) Methods involving kaolin adsorption and acetone precipitation.

(ii) The method involving tannic acid precipitation.

(i) *Kaolin-acetone Methods.*—Three main variants of the technique have been developed.

(α) *The Method of Loraine and J. B. Brown (1959).*—In this procedure HPG is adsorbed onto kaolin at pH 4 and eluted therefrom by 5N NaOH at pH 11 to 11·5; the active material is then precipitated at pH 4 to 5 with five volumes of acetone. The precipitate is collected and washed with absolute ethanol and ether before being dried over calcium chloride.

The accuracy of the method was tested in a series of recovery experiments in which the reference material HMG-20A was added to urine; the mean percentage recovery was 76. When repeated determinations were carried out on a pooled sample of postmenopausal urine, the reproducibility of the technique was found to be satisfactory.

(β) *The Method of Albert (1955, 1956, 1966).*—In this procedure the pH of a 24 or 48 hour urine sample is adjusted to 4·5 prior to adsorption of the HPG onto kaolin. Elution is performed by 2M NH_4OH using an automatic self-regulating filter apparatus. The eluate is adjusted to pH 5·5 and the HPG is precipitated with two volumes of acetone.

(γ) *The Method of Borth* et al. *(1961 b).*—This is essentially a modification of method β. The self-regulating filter apparatus is not used, and instead the urine is rapidly filtered through a Büchner funnel. Filtration of the urine is hastened by the addition of the filter aid hyflo supercel to the kaolin.

Crude kaolin extracts have been purified by Albert *et al.* (1961 *b c d*, 1962) using ammonium acetate and ethanol, by Loraine and J. B. Brown (1959) using tricalcium phosphate and by Hipkin (1967) employing Sephadex. All of these steps result in the production of materials of higher specific activity than the original crude extracts. The first two reduce toxicity, but are generally associated with a loss of variable amounts of biological activity.

(ii) *Tannic Acid Precipitation.*—The technique of Johnsen (1958) is essentially a modification of that originally described by Levin and Tyndale (1936). In Johnsen's procedure the gonadotrophins are precipitated with tannic acid and the precipitate is washed to remove inert material. The hormones are subsequently eluted with 10 per cent ammonium acetate in 40 per cent ethanol, after which the biologically active material is precipitated with ethanol. In the experience of its originator, the method was satisfactory in terms of accuracy and reproducibility.

Extracts prepared by tannic acid precipitation are less toxic to experimental animals than those obtained by the majority of other extraction methods (see Borth and Menzi, 1964 ; McArthur *et al.*, 1967). The accuracy of the method has recently been reinvestigated by Herbst *et al.* (1967) who conducted recovery experiments involving the addition of the Second IRP-HMG to pools of normal male urine. It was found that approximately 100 per cent of the LH activity but only 50 per cent of the FSH activity was recovered.

(*b*) EXTRACTION OF HPG FROM BLOOD.—Two main techniques have been proposed, those of Apostolakis (1959) and of Keller and Rosemberg (1965).

(i) *The Method of Apostolakis (1959).*—In this procedure plasma is adjusted to pH 5 with 0·2N HCl. Five volumes of acetone are added slowly, and the suspension is left to stand in a refrigerator at 4°C. for at least one hour. After centrifugation the supernatant fluid is discarded, the precipitate washed with absolute ethanol and ethyl ether and dried over calcium chloride. The dried precipitate is removed, ground to a fine powder and stored at 4°C. prior to bio-assay.

According to Apostolakis (1959) little or no biological activity is lost during the extraction procedure. The method is simple and rapid, being suitable for widespread clinical application. Its precision depends on the bio-assay method used, but with the mouse uterus test as end point the figure for the index of precision (λ)* is generally satisfactory. With the extraction procedure proposed concentrations as low as 3 to 5 HMG units per 100 ml. plasma (First IRP-HMG) can be detected (see Apostolakis and Loraine, 1967).

(ii) *The Method of Keller and Rosemberg (1965).*—The main steps in this technique involve precipitation of the plasma proteins with ethanol, extraction of the precipitate with ammonium acetate in absolute ethanol, centrifugation of superantant fluid with subsequent precipitation with absolute ethanol saturated with ammonium acetate, and collection of precipitate by centrifugation followed by washing and drying.

The method is claimed by its originators to achieve approximately a tenfold concentration of HPG activity. With the mouse uterus test as end point the overall sensitivity of the procedure is superior to that of Apostolakis (1959), thus making it preferable for HPG estimations in patients in whom the plasma concentration is relatively low. On the other hand, the accuracy of the method in terms of the yield obtained is probably inferior to that of Apostolakis (1959), as is its practicability.

3. Methods for the Estimation of FSH

(*a*) BIOLOGICAL

(i) *Ovarian Augmentation Test in Intact Rats.*—This procedure, which was first described by Steelman and Pohley (1953), depends on the ability of human chorionic gonadotrophin (HCG) to augment the action of FSH on the rat ovary. Intact immature animals are injected three times per day for three days with the test material, which is administered simultaneously with HCG; the autopsy is performed 72 hours after the first injection, at which time the paired ovaries are weighed. A total dosage of 20 or 40 i.u. HCG per animal has been generally found to produce a satisfactory augmentation of ovarian weight. The test is reasonably precise, the λ figure

* In assays depending on graded effects the "index of precision" (λ) (Gaddum, 1933) is calculated by dividing the standard deviation of the responses (usually termed s) by the slope of the line connecting the response with the logarithm of the dose (usually termed b), i.e. $\lambda = \dfrac{s}{b}$. The precision of an assay is high when s is small and b is large.

usually ranging from 0·10 to 0·20 (Albert *et al.*, 1961 *a b*; Parlow and Reichert, 1963 *a*; Rosemberg *et al.*, 1964 *a*). Specificity appears to be satisfactory (Simpson, 1961), but the main disadvantage of the method from the point of view of clinical studies, is its relatively low degree of sensitivity.

(ii) *Ovarian Augmentation Test in Intact Mice.*—This technique (P. S. Brown, 1955) employs mice instead of rats but is otherwise similar to the method of Steelman and Pohley (1953). It has a high degree of precision when a suitable strain of animal is used (P. S. Brown and Wells, 1966; P. S. Brown, 1967 *a*; Bell, 1967 *b*; Herbst *et al.*, 1967). The procedure is considerably more sensitive than that employing rats and at present is probably the method of choice for investigations in patients.

(iii) *Uterine Weight Increase in Hypophysectomised Immature Mice.*—This technique, which was recently described by Lamond and Bindon (1966), depends on the ability of HCG to augment the effect of FSH on the mouse uterus. FSH and HCG are given subcutaneously at separate sites five hours after hypophysectomy, and the animals are killed two days later. The procedure is more sensitive than the mouse ovarian weight augmentation test; it is also reasonably precise as indicated by figures for λ ranging from 0·07 to 0·29. Lamond and Bindon (1966) noted that the injection of pituitary LH at the same time as FSH and HCG did not influence the results and concluded that the method was highly specific. It would appear that its specificity is greatly superior to that of a somewhat similar method described by Igarashi and McCann (1964) in which intact rather than hypophysectomised mice were employed (see Mukerji, 1963; P. S. Brown, 1967 *b*). According to Stevens (1967) the method of Lamond and Bindon (1966) can be used to estimate FSH in urine in normally menstruating women. It is however obvious that the applicability of the procedure to clinical problems will be limited because of the necessity for using hypophysectomised animals.

(*b*) IMMUNOLOGICAL.—Assay methods depending on haemagglutination-inhibition and on radio-immunological assay have recently been described (Wolf, 1966 ; Franchimont, 1966 ; Faiman and Ryan, 1967 ; Midgley, 1967 ; Saxena *et al.*, 1967). At the time of writing some of the reliability criteria of these techniques have not been extensively studied, and in particular a detailed correlation with biological methods has not yet been reported in the case of samples obtained from the blood and urine of individual subjects.

4. Methods for the Estimation of LH

(a) BIOLOGICAL.—Under this heading three procedures will be described. These are:

(i) The test depending on the enlargement of the ventral lobe of the prostate in the hypophysectomised immature male rat (Greep *et al.*, 1941, 1942).

(ii) The ovarian ascorbic acid depletion (OAAD) test in intact immature female rats (Karg, 1957, Parlow, 1958, 1961).

(iii) The ovarian cholesterol depletion (OCD) test in intact immature female rats (Bell *et al.*, 1964).

(i) *Ventral Prostatic Weight Test in Rats.*—This was originally described by Greep *et al.* (1941, 1942) and its reliability criteria have been examined by numerous investigators, including Loraine and J. B. Brown (1954), Segaloff *et al.* (1955), Diczfalusy and Loraine (1958) and Van Rees *et al.* (1961). In the experience of Loraine and J. B. Brown (1954) the method was reasonably precise, the average figure for λ being 0·20. Subsequent investigators, including Parlow and Reichert (1963 *b*), Albert *et al.* (1965 *a*) and Rosemberg *et al.* (1965), have found a less satisfactory degree of precision.

There are conflicting views in the literature regarding the effect of FSH on prostatic weight. According to Parlow and Reichert (1963 *b*) large dosages of FSH can influence the effect of LH on the prostate; Rosemberg *et al.* (1965) were unable to confirm this observation. The reason for these divergent findings is not at present clear but may be related to the fact that the two groups of investigators used different preparations of FSH. According to Albert *et al.* (1965 *a b c*) tannation of gonadotrophin preparations will enhance LH potency when estimated by the ventral prostatic weight test. Parlow (1963) has claimed that the presence of serum will also affect the response in the experimental animals.

The ventral prostatic weight method has been used to assay

human urinary LH by various workers, including J. B. Brown *et al.* (1958), Kovacic and Loraine (1961) and Taymor (1964). The sensitivity of the technique is not sufficient for routine clinical application, especially in low-titre urines, and the use of the method should probably now be restricted to purified materials.

(ii) *Ovarian Ascorbic Acid Depletion Test.*—This method depends on alterations in the level of ovarian ascorbic acid following the i.v. administration of LH to intact immature female rats which have been pre-treated with pregnant mare's serum gonado-trophin (PMSG) and HCG (see Parlow 1958, 1961). Since the description of the original method many modifications have been proposed including those of Schmidt-Elmendorff and Loraine (1962), Mukerji *et al.* (1962), McCann and Taleisnik (1960), Sakiz and Guillemin (1963), Hutchinson and Worden (1964), Persky and Norton (1964) and Bell *et al.* (1965). The two major modifications are probably the administration of the standard and unknown preparations by the i.p. rather than by the i.v. route (Bell *et al.*, 1965) and the use of each animal in two separate assays (Parlow, 1961; Sakiz and Guillemin, 1963; Persky and Norton, 1964; Hershberger *et al.*, 1965).

In the experience of Rosemberg *et al.* (1964 *b*), who used rats of the Sprague-Dawley strain, the precision of the OAAD method was generally satisfactory for quantitative work. In rats of the Wistar strain precision appears to be somewhat less satisfactory, figures for λ usually ranging from 0·25 to 0·35 (Visutakul *et al.*, 1966 *a b*; Herbst *et al.*, 1967). The specificity of the OAAD method for LH has recently been questioned by Rosemberg *et al.* (1965) who found that the administration of large dosages of FSH together with LH produced a depletion of ascorbic acid greater than that which would have been anticipated due to the LH content of the material under test. Parlow and Reichert (1963 *b*) could not confirm this finding and stated that purified FSH extracts given at varying dose levels did not affect the response to LH in the OAAD test. The differing results obtained by these two groups of investigators are hard to explain, but, as with similar studies on the ventral prostatic weight test (see p. 62), may be due to the fact that different FSH preparations were employed. According to Albert *et al.* (1965 *a b c*) the LH potency of extracts assayed by the OAAD method is not affected by tannation.

One of the main disadvantages of the OAAD test is that relatively crude extracts of human urine given either i.v. or i.p. tend to produce toxic reactions in the experimental animals and thus invalidate the assays (Schmidt-Elmendorff and Loraine, 1962; Herbst *et al.*, 1967). The toxicity of extracts is somewhat reduced when the tannic acid method of Johnsen (1958) rather than the kaolin-acetone method of Loraine and J. B. Brown (1959) is used (see Bell *et al.*, 1967). In assays performed by M. Fukushima *et al.* (1964) urine samples were extracted by the method of Albert (1955, 1956) and purified by the inclusion of a step involving extraction with ammonium acetate. Under these conditions the toxicity of extracts was abolished (Stevens, 1964) but information is not available on the recovery rate of the overall procedure.

In the animal strain used by M. Fukushima *et al.* (1964) the OAAD method, although precise, was relatively insensitive. For this reason these workers were forced to conduct three-point rather than four-point assays when estimating LH activity in urinary extracts derived from normally menstruating women. In the opinion of the present authors three-point assays by the OAAD method should be avoided if at all possible; when such a design is used slope differences cannot be tested and invalid assays may be included. The relatively high incidence of lack of parallelism between the dose-response curves of standard and unknown preparations when the OAAD test is used has been emphasised by Visutakul *et al.* (1966 *a b*) and by Herbst *et al.* (1967).

(iii) *Ovarian Cholesterol Depletion (OCD) Test.*—The end point in this technique is the decrease in ovarian cholesterol in intact immature rats pre-treated with PMSG and HCG (Bell *et al.*, 1964). The characteristics of the dose-response curve for LH using the OCD method have been studied by Skosey and Goldstein (1966) and by Bell (1967 *a c*), and the curve has been shown to be non-monotonic in type. The main advantage of the OCD test is its unique sensitivity, the procedure being some five million times more sensitive than the OAAD method. The specificity and practicability of the OCD method are reasonably satisfactory, but its precision is relatively low, the mean λ figure in a series of 85 assays reported by Bell *et al.* (1966) being 0·36. As emphasised by Bell (1967 *a*) the major difficulty in relation to the OCD method is its strain and colony dependence. For this reason the assay is difficult to reproduce unless a suitable colony of rats is selected and unless the conditions for the pre-treatment of the animals are investigated with great care.

Because of the unique sensitivity of the OCD method it is possible in assays conducted on body fluids to administer diluted rather than concentrated material to the experimental animals. The procedure may well become of considerable value in clinical studies provided that the problem of colony dependence can be overcome.

(b) IMMUNOLOGICAL.—Two main types of method have been employed—haemagglutination-inhibition tests and radio-immunological assays.

(i) *Haemagglutination-inhibition Tests.*—Wide and his colleagues (Wide, 1966; Wide et al., 1961; Wide and Gemzell, 1962) have described an assay method for LH in which the hormone cross-reacts with HCG in a haemagglutination-inhibition reaction between red blood cells coated with HCG and an antiserum prepared against HCG in rabbits. When applied to urine this technique yielded results much higher than those obtained by biological assay and probably provides a marked overestimate of true potency. Goss and Taymor (1962), who used an antiserum to HCG and latex particles coated with the hormone, also employed a haemagglutination-inhibition system to measure LH activity in pituitary extracts and human urine. They noted good agreement between their immunological method and the hypophysectomised rat prostate test when purified pituitary extracts were assayed; however, when parallel estimates by the two methods were performed on urinary extracts the results diverged considerably (see also Taymor, 1967).

(ii) *Radio-immunological Assays.*—Bagshawe and his associates (Wilde et al., 1965, 1967; Bagshawe et al., 1966) have described a radio-immunological assay method for LH in blood and urine similar in principle to the technique developed by Hales and Randle (1963) for insulin. In this procedure the antigen is HCG. The antiserum is prepared in rabbits and the antigen is labelled with I-131; the test depends on an immunological cross-reaction between HCG and pituitary LH. Details have not yet been provided of the results obtained when this method is compared with a bio-assay for LH. Until such information is available the specificity of the procedure must remain in doubt.

Recently Midgley (1966), Franchimont (1966) and Odell *et al.* (1967) have described further radio-immunological assay methods for LH involving cross-reactions with HCG. In the report of Midgley (1966) a small series of comparisons were made between his method and the OAAD test on purified material derived from urine and from pituitary tissue. Good agreement between the radio-immunological method and the bio-assay technique was claimed, but further work will be required to establish the validity and specificity of the former technique.

5. Methods for the Estimation of "Total Gonadotrophic Activity."

A great number of such procedures have been described most of which are now of historical interest only. For details of these methods the reader should consult review articles by Loraine (1956, 1958), Loraine and Bell (1966) and Apostolakis and Loraine (1967). The present section will be confined to consideration of two methods, both of which continue to be used in clinical practice. These are:

      (*a*) The mouse uterus test.
      (*b*) The rat ovarian weight test.

(*a*) THE MOUSE UTERUS TEST.—The majority of centres still use the assay design recommended over 20 years ago by Klinefelter *et al.* (1943) in which intact immature mice are injected subcutaneously once or twice per day for three days and are killed 72 hours after the first injection. The end point of the procedure is the increase in uterine weight, and the assay is generally conducted using mice on the first day after weaning. Early statements by Klinefelter *et al.* (1943) and by others led to the erroneous belief that the mouse uterus test was specific for FSH. However, it is now generally agreed that the procedure estimates a mixture of FSH and LH activities, and the term " total gonadotrophic activity " has been employed to describe the biological activity measured. Studies by Riley

(1961) and by P. S. Brown and Billewicz (1962) have clearly shown that both FSH and LH can influence the response of the mouse uterus. P. S. Brown and Billewicz (1962) demonstrated that the same uterine weight could be produced by FSH alone or by combinations of gonadotrophins containing different FSH/LH ratios, and from these observations it is obvious that any alteration in the FSH/LH ratio of a given extract cannot be accurately measured by the mouse uterus test. The precision of the method has been found to be satisfactory by various investigators (Loraine and J. B. Brown, 1954, 1956; Schmidt-Elmendorff et al., 1962; Borth and Menzi, 1964) and its practicability is superior to that of other bio-assay methods for HPG. Despite its limitations in respect to specificity valuable information in relation to pituitary activity in health and disease can be obtained by the use of this method, and it is likely that the procedure will continue to be employed in clinical studies for many years to come.

(b) RAT OVARIAN WEIGHT TEST.—This has been widely employed by Albert and his colleagues (see Albert, 1959, 1961; Albert and Rosemberg, 1959). Intact immature rats weighing 38 to 50 g. and aged from 21 to 23 days are injected subcutaneously once per day for four days; they are killed approximately 96 hours after the first injection at which time the ovaries are weighed. The main advantage of the test is its good precision, the average figure for λ being generally less than 0·10. Its main disadvantage is the low degree of sensitivity, the method being some seven times less sensitive than the mouse uterus test (Albert and Rosemberg, 1959). The relative lack of sensitivity makes the rat ovarian weight test of limited value for clinical work, especially when assays are conducted on blood and urine samples of low gonadotrophic potency.

SUMMARY AND CONCLUSIONS

1. Oestrogens

Many methods have been described for the extraction and purification of the three classical urinary oestrogens. Such procedures can have as their end points colorimetry, fluorimetry or gas liquid chromatography. Of the three types of end point that depending on colorimetry has been the most widely used in clinical studies.

For the estimation of the classical oestrogens in the urine of women during reproductive life the method of J. B. Brown (1955) is recommended. In low-titre urines the procedure of choice is probably that of J. B. Brown et al. (1957).

Methods for the estimation of oestrogens in blood can depend on colorimetry, fluorimetry or isotope dilution. For the measurement of these steroids in non-pregnant subjects the isotopic method of Svendsen (1960) is valuable because of its high sensitivity.

2. Progesterone, Pregnanediol and Pregnanetriol

Chemical methods for the estimation of progesterone in blood can be divided into spectrophotometric, fluorimetric, gas chromatographic and isotopic groups. One of the widely used procedures in clinical practice has been that of Short (1958) in which the final determination is made by ultraviolet spectroscopy.

For the quantitative determination of pregnanediol in urine the favoured technique has been that of Klopper et al. (1955). The widespread application of gas chromatographic procedures for pregnanediol to studies in non-pregnant subjects will be awaited with interest.

The method of Harkness and Love (1966) is recommended for the estimation of pregnanetriol in urine. The main advantage of this technique over previously described procedures is its relatively high sensitivity.

3. Testosterone

For the estimation of urinary testosterone in clinical practice the method of choice is probably that of Ismail and Harkness (1966 b). This procedure enables testosterone to be separated completely from the closely related compound 17-epitestosterone.

Various types of method have been described for the estimation of testosterone in blood, but at the time of writing such techniques have not been widely used in clinical practice.

4. HPG

The method recommended for the estimation of FSH in clinical work is that depending on the augmentation of ovarian weight in intact immature mice (P. S. Brown, 1955).

The ventral prostatic weight and ovarian ascorbic acid depletion methods in rats have been used clinically for the estimation of urinary LH. Neither of these procedures is entirely satisfactory, the former being somewhat insensitive and the latter imprecise.

Immunological assay methods for FSH and LH have not yet reached a stage at which they can be applied with confidence to clinical problems.

The mouse uterus test remains the method of choice for the estimation of " total gonadotrophic activity " in body fluids.

* Since this chapter was written Brown *et al.* (1968) have described a further method for the quantitative determination of urinary oestrogens. In this procedure a semi-automatic extractor is employed and this instrument greatly increases the practicability of the technique as compared with existing methods. In urines derived from non-pregnant subjects the final determination depends on the Kober reaction followed by fluorimetry. The application of this new procedure to clinical problems will be awaited with considerable interest.

† Very recently Horton *et al.* (1967) have described a new method for the quantitative determination of testosterone in the plasma of male subjects. The technique, which is similar to that used in the radio-immunological assay of protein and polypeptide hormones, involves the displacement of tritium-labelled testosterone from a specific binding protein by testosterone present in the plasma sample. The separation of the bound from the free testosterone is effected by absorption on charcoal particles coated with dextran. The technique has a high degree of practicability, and when compared with isotopic methods on the same plasma sample, gives comparable results. Further clinical applications of this procedure should provide interesting information.

REFERENCES

ALBERT, A. (1955). *Proc. Mayo Clin.* **30**, 552.
ALBERT, A. (1956). *Recent Prog. Hormone Res.* **12**, 227.
ALBERT, A. (1959). *Fertility Sterility* **10**, 60.
ALBERT, A. (1961). In *Human Pituitary Gonadotropins*, p. 53. Ed. Albert, A. Springfield: Thomas.
ALBERT, A. (1966). *Acta Endocrinol. Suppl.* 106.
ALBERT, A. & ROSEMBERG, E. (1959). *J. Clin. Endocrinol. Metab.* **19**, 518.
ALBERT, A., BENNETT, D., CARL, G., ROSEMBERG, E., KELLER, P. & LEWIS, W, B. (1965 *b*). *Endocrinology*, **76**, 259.
ALBERT, A., DERNER, I., LEIFERMAN, J., STELLMACHER, V. & BARNUM, J. (1961 *d*). *J. Clin. Endocrinol. Metab.* **21**, 839.
ALBERT, A., DERNER, I., ROSEMBERG, E. & LEWIS, W. B. (1965 *a*). *Endocrinology*, **76**, 139.
ALBERT, A., DERNER, I., STELLMACHER, V., LEIFERMAN, J. & BARNUM, J. (1961 *a*). *J. Clin. Endocrinol. Metab.* **21**, 1260.
ALBERT, A., DERNER, I., STELLMACHER, V., LEIFERMAN, J. & BARNUM, J. (1962). *J. Clin. Endocrinol. Metab.* **22**, 996.
ALBERT, A., GENTNER, D., ROSEMBERG, E. & FERRECHIO, G. (1965 *c*). *Endocrinology*, **77**, 226.
ALBERT, A., KOBI, J., LEIFERMAN, J. & DERNER, I. (1961 *b*). *J. Clin. Endocrinol. Metab.* **21**, 1.
ALBERT, A., STELLMACHER, V. & LEIFERMAN, J. (1961 *c*). *J. Clin. Endocrinol. Metab.* **21**, 856.
ALLEN, W. M. (1950), *J. Clin. Endocrinol. Metab.* **10**, 71.
APOSTOLAKIS, M. (1959) *J. Endocrinol.* **19**, 377.

APOSTOLAKIS, M. & LORAINE, J. A. (1967). In *Hormones in Blood*, Second ed. Vol. 1, p. 273 Eds. Gray, C. H., and Bacharach, A. L. New York: Academic Press.
ASTWOOD, E. B. & JONES, G. E. S. (1941). *J. Biol. Chem.* **137**, 397.
AXELROD, L. R. & GOLDZIEHER, J. W. (1960). *J. Clin. Endocrinol. Metab.* **20**, 238.
BAGSHAWE, K. D., WILDE, C. E. & ORR, A. H. (1966). *Lancet, i*, 1118.
BARDIN, C. W. & LIPSETT, M. B. (1967). *Steroids*, **9**, 71.
BAULD, W. S. (1956). *Biochem. J.* **63**, 488.
BEER, C. T. & GALLAGHER, T. F. (1955 a). *J. Biol. Chem.* **214**, 335.
BEER, C. T. & GALLAGHER, T. F. (1955 b). *J. Biol. Chem.* **214**, 351.
BELING, C. G. (1963). *Acta Endocrinol. Suppl.* 79.
BELL, E. T. (1967 a). *Vitamins Hormones*, **24**, 63.
BELL, E. T. (1967 b). In *Recent Research on Gonadotrophic Hormones*, p. 9. Eds. Bell, E. T., and Loraine, J. A. Edinburgh: Livingstone.
BELL, E. T. (1967 c). In *Recent Research on Gonadotrophic Hormones*, p. 33. Eds. Bell, E. T., and Loraine, J. A. Edinburgh: Livingstone.
BELL, E. T., HERBST, A. L., KRISHNAMURTI, M., LORAINE, J. A., MEARS, E., JACKSON, M. C. N. & GARCIA, C-R. (1967). *Acta Endocrinol.* **54**, 96.
BELL, E. T., MUKERJI, S. & LORAINE, J. A. (1964). *J. Endocrinol.* **28**, 321.
BELL, E. T., MUKERJI, S., LORAINE, J. A. & LUNN, S. F. (1966). *Acta Endocrinol.* **51**, 578.
BELL, E. T., LORAINE, J. A., MUKERJI, S. & VISUTAKUL, P. (1965). *J. Endocrinol.* **32**, 1.
BONGIOVANNI, A. M. & EBERLEIN, W. R. (1958). *Anal. Chem.* **30**, 388.
BORTH, R. (1952). *Ciba Found. Colloq. Endocrinol.* **2**, 45.
BORTH, R. & MENZI, A. (1964). *Acta Endocrinol. Suppl.* 90, p. 17.
BORTH, R., LUNENFELD B. & MENZI, A. (1961 a). In *Human Pituitary Gonadotropins*, p. 153. Ed Albert, A. Springfield: Thomas.
BORTH, R., LUNENFELD, B. & MENZI, A. (1961 b). In *Human Pituitary Gonadotropins*, p. 13. Ed. Albert, A. Springfield: Thomas.
BRAMBELL, F. W. R. (1956). In *Marshall's Physiology of Reproduction*, Vol. 1, p. 397. Third ed. Ed. Parkes, A. S. London: Longmans Green.
BREUER, H. (1962). *Vitamins Hormones*, **20**, 285.
BROWN, J. B. (1955). *Biochem. J.* **60**, 185.
BROWN, J. B. (1960). *Advan. Clin. Chem.* **3**, 157.
BROWN, J. B., BULBROOK, R. D. & GREENWOOD, F. C. (1957). J. *Endocrinol.* **16**, 49.
BROWN, J. B., KLOPPER, A. & LORAINE, J. A. (1958). *J. Endocrinol.* **17**, 401.
BROWN, J. B., MACLEOD, S. C., MACNAUGHTON, C., SMITH, M. A. & SMYTH, B. (1968). *J. Endocrinol, submitted for publication.*
BROWN, P. S. (1955). *J. Endocrinol.* **13**, 59.
BROWN, P. S. (1967 a). In *Recent Research on Gonadotrophic Hormones*, p. 7. Eds. Bell, E. T. and Loraine, J. A. Edinburgh: Livingstone.
BROWN, P. S. (1967 b). In *Recent Research on Gonadotrophic Hormones*, p. 13. Eds. Bell, E. T. and Loraine, J. A. Edinburgh: Livingstone.
BROWN, P. S. & BILLEWICZ, W. Z. (1962). *J. Endocrinol.* **24**, 65.
BROWN, P. S. & WELLS, M. (1966). *J. Endocrinol.* **35**, 199.
BROWNIE, A. C., MOLEN, H. J. van der, NISHIZAWA, E. & EIK-NES, K. B. (1964). *J. Clin. Endocrinol. Metab.* **24**, 1091.
Bulletin World Health Organisation (1960), **22**, 563.
BURGER, H. G., KENT, J. R. & KELLIE, A. E. (1964). *J. Clin. Endocrinol. Metab.* **24**, 432.
CAGNAZZO, G., ROS, A. & BIGNARDI, G. (1965). *J. Chromatog.* **19**, 185.
CAMACHO, A. M. & MIGEON, C. J. (1963). *J. Clin. Endocrinol. Metab.* **23**, 301.
CHATTORAJ, S. C. & SCOMMEGNA, A. (1967). *Steroids*, **9**, 329.
CLARINGBOLD, P. J. (1954). *J. Endocrinol.* **11**, 36.
COLLINS, W. P. & SOMMERVILLE, I. F. (1964). *Nature*, **203**, 836.
COOPER, J. A., ABBOTT, J. P., ROSENGREEN, B. K. & CLAGGETT, W. R. (1962). *Am. J. Clin. Pathol.* **38**, 388.
COX, R. I. (1959). *J. Biol. Chem.* **234**, 1693.
COYLE, M. G., MITCHELL, F. L. & RUSSELL, C. S. (1956). *J. Obstet, Gynaecol. Brit. Empire*, **63**, 560.

HORMONAL METHODS

DALE, E. & GREENE, J. W. Jr. (1965). *Am. J. Med. Sci.* **250,** 700.
DICZFALUSY, E. (1955). *Acta Endocrinol.* **20,** 216.
DICZFALUSY, E. & LORAINE, J. A. (1958). *J Endocrinol.* **17,** 425.
DOISY, E. A., VELER, C. D. & THAYER, S. A. (1929). *Am. J. Physiol.* **90,** 329.
DORFMAN, R. I. (1962). In *Methods in Hormone Research,* Vol. 2, p. 275. Ed. Dorfman, R. I. New York: Academic Press.
DORFMAN, R. I., FORCHIELLI, E. & GUT, M. (1963). *Rec. Prog. Hormone Res.* **19,** 251 Verlag. *In press.*
EBERLEIN, W. R. & BONGIOVANNI, A. M. (1958). *J. Clin. Endocrinol. Metab.* **18,** 300.
EECHAUTE, W. & DEMEESTER, G. (1965). *J. Clin. Endocrinol. Metab.* **25,** 480.
EHRLICH, E. N. (1965). *J. Lab. Clin. Med.* **65,** 869.
EMMENS, C. W. (1950). In *Hormone Assay,* Ch. 16. New York: Academic Press.
EMMENS, C. W. (1962). In *Methods in Hormone Research,* Vol. 2, p. 59. Ed. Dorfman, R. I. New York: Academic Press.
FAIMAN, C. & RYAN, R. J. (1967). *J. Clin. Endocrinol. Metab.* **27,** 444.
FIESER, L. F. & FIESER, M. (1959). *Steroids.* New York: Reinhold.
FINKELSTEIN, M., FORCHIELLI, E. & DORFMAN, R. I. (1961). *J. Clin. Endocrinol. Metab.* **21,** 98.
FISHMAN, J. & BROWN, J. B. (1962). *J. Chromatog.* **8,** 21.
FISHMAN, J., BROWN, J. B., HELLMAN, L., ZUMOFF, B. & GALLAGHER, T. F. (1962). *J. Biol. Chem.* **237,** 1489.
FOTHERBY, K. (1964). *Vitamins Hormones,* **22,** 153.
FOTHERBY, K. & LOVE, D. N. (1960). *J. Endocrinol.* **20,** 157.
FRANCHIMONT, P. (1966). *Le Dosage des Hormones Hypophysaires Somatotrope et Gonodotropes et son Application en Clinique.* Brussels: Editions Arscia S.A.
FUKUSHIMA, D. K., BRADLOW, H. L., HELLMAN, L. & GALLAGHER, T. F. (1962). In *The Human Adrenal Cortex,* p. 371. Eds. Currie, A. R., Symington, T., and Grant, J. K. Edinburgh: Livingstone.
FUKUSHIMA, D. K., BRADLOW, H. L., HELLMAN, L. & GALLAGHER, T. F. (1963). *J Clin. Endocrinol. Metab.* **23,** 266.
FUKUSHIMA, D. K., BRADLOW, H. L., HELLMAN, L., ZUMOFF, B. & GALLAGHER, T. F. (1961). *J. Clin. Endocrinol. Metab.* **21,** 765.
FUKUSHIMA, M., STEVENS, V. C., GANTT, C. L. & VORYS, N. (1964). *J. Clin. Endocrinol. Metab.* **24,** 205.
FUTTERWEIT, W., McNIVEN, N. L., NARCUS, L., LANTOS, C., DROSDOWSKY, M. & DORFMAN, R. I. (1963). *Steroids,* **1,** 628.
GADDUM, J. H. (1933). *Spec. Rep. Ser. Med. Res. Coun. Lond.* No. 183.
GALLAGHER, T. F. KRAYCHY, S., FISHMAN, J., BROWN, J. B. & MARRIAN, G. F. (1958). *J. Biol. Chem.* **233,** 1093.
GOERING, R. W. & HERRMANN, W. L. (1966). *J. Clin. Endocrinol. Metab.* **26,** 65.
GOLDZIEHER, J. W. & NAKAMURA, Y. (1962). *Acta Endocrinol.* **41,** 371.
GOSS, D. A. & TAYMOR, M. L. (1962). *Endocrinology,* **71,** 321.
GREEP, R. O., VAN DYKE, H. B. & CHOW, B. F. (1941). *Proc. Soc. Exp. Biol. Med.* **46,** 644.
GREEP, R. O., VAN DYKE, H. B. & CHOW, B. F. (1942). *Endocrinology,* **30,** 635.
HALES, C. N. & RANDLE, P. J. (1963). *Biochem. J.* **88,** 137.
HARKNESS, R. A. & LOVE, D. N. (1966). *Acta Endocrinol.* **51,** 526.
HEAP, R. B. (1964). *J. Endocrinol.* **30,** 293.
HEARD, R. D. H., BLIGH, E. G., CANN, M. C., JELLINCK, P. H., O'DONNELL, V. J., RAO, B. J. & WEBB, J. L. (1956). *Recent Prog. Hormone Res.* **12,** 45.
HERBST, A. L., BELL, E. T. & LORAINE, J. A. (1967). *Endocrinology.* **80,** 378.
HERRMANN, W. & SILVERMAN, L. (1957). *Proc. Soc. Exp. Biol. Med.* **94,** 426.
HERSHBERGER, L. G., HANSEN, L. M., & THOMPSON, C. R. (1965). *Endocrinology,* **77,** 1143.
HIPKIN, L. J. (1967). *J. Endocrinol.* **38,** 39.
HORN, H., STATTER, M. & FINKELSTEIN, M. (1966). *Steroids,* **7,** 118.
HORTON, R. (1966). *Recent Prog. Hormone Res.* **22,** 279.
HORTON, R., KATO, T. & SHERINO R. (1967). *Steroids* **10,** 245.
HORTON, R., ROMANOFF, E. & WALKER, J. (1966). *J. Clin. Endocrinol. Metab.* **26,** 1267.

71

HUDSON, B., COGHLAN, J., DULMANIS, A., WINTOUR, M. & EKKEL, I. (1963). *Australian J. Exp. Biol. Med. Sci.* **41**, 235.
HUTCHINSON, J. S. M. & WORDEN, J. M. (1964). *J. Endocrinol.* **29**, 47.
IBAYASHI, H., NAKAMURA, M., MURAKAWA, S., ICHIKAWA, T., TANIOKA, T. & NAKAO, K. (1964). *Steroids*, **3**, 559.
ICHII, S., FORCHIELLI, E., PERLOFF, W. H. & DORFMAN, R. I. (1963). *Anal. Biochem.* **5**, 422.
IGARASHI, M. & McCANN, S. M. (1964). *Endocrinology*, **74**, 440.
ISMAIL, A. A. A., DAVIDSON, D. W., FARO, L. C. F. & LORAINE, J. A. (1968). *Proc. Workshop Conference on Testosterone* Hamburg 1967. Stuttgart: Thieme-Verlag. *In press.*
ISMAIL, A. A. A. & HARKNESS, R. A. (1965). *Biochem. J.* **98**, 15P.
ISMAIL, A. A. A. & HARKNESS, R. A. (1966 a). *J. Endocrinol.* **34**, xvii.
ISMAIL, A. A. A. & HARKNESS, R. A. (1966 b). *Biochem. J.* **99**, 717.
ITTRICH, G. (1958). *Hoppe-Seylers Z. Physiol. Chem.* **312**, 1.
ITTRICH, G. (1960). *Acta Endocrinol.* **35**, 34.
JOHNSEN, S. G. (1958). *Acta Endocrinol*, **28**, 69.
KARG, H. (1957). *Klin. Weschr.* 35, 643.
KATZMAN, P. A. (1965). *Endocrinology*, **76**, 131.
KELLER, P. J. & ROSEMBERG, E. (1965). *J. Clin. Endocrinol. Metab.* **25**, 1050.
KLINEFELTER, H. F. Jr., ALBRIGHT, F. & GRISWOLD, G. C. (1943). *J. Clin. Endocrinol. Metab.* **3**, 529.
KLOPPER, A., MICHIE, E. A. & BROWN, J. B. (1955). *J. Endocrinol.* **12**, 209.
KOBER, S. (1931). *Biochem. Z.* **239**, 209.
KOVACIC, N. & LORAINE, J. A. (1961). *Endocrinology*, **68**, 356.
KUMAR, D., WARD, E. F. & BARNES, A. C. (1964) *Am. J. Obstet. Gynecol.* **90**, 1360.
LADANY, S. & FINKELSTEIN, M. (1963). *Steroids*, **2**, 297.
LAMOND, D. R. & BINDON, B. M. (1966). *J. Endocrinol.* **34**, 365.
LAU, H. L. & JONES, G. E. S. (1964). *Am. J. Obstet. Gynecol.* **90**, 132.
LEVIN, L. & TYNDALE, H. H. (1936). *Proc. Soc. Exp. Biol. Med.* **34**, 516.
LIPP, G. (1960). *Acta Endocrinol.* **33**, 501.
LISBOA, B. P. & DICZFALUSY, E. (1962). *Acta Endocrinol.* **40**, 60.
LORAINE, J. A. (1956). *Vitamins Hormones*, **14**, 305.
LORAINE, J. A. (1958). *The Clinical Application of Hormone Assay*, First ed. Ch. 2. Edinburgh: Livingstone.
LORAINE, J. A. & BELL, E. T. (1966). *Hormone Assays and their Clinical Application*, Second ed. Edinburgh: Livingstone.
LORAINE, J. A. & BELL, E. T. (1967). In *Genital Abnormalities*. Eds. Rashad, M. N. and Morton W. R. M. Thomas: Springfield. *In Press.*
LORAINE, J. A. & BROWN, J. B. (1954). *Acta Endocrinol.* **17**, 250.
LORAINE, J. A. & BROWN, J. B. (1956). *J. Clin. Endocrinol. Metab.* **16**, 1180.
LORAINE, J. A. & BROWN, J. B. (1959). *J. Endocrinol.* **18**, 77.
LUISI, M., SAVI, C. & MARESCOTTI, V. (1964). *J. Chromatog.* **15**, 428.
LUISI, M., GAMBASSI, G., MARESCOTTI, V., SAVI, C. & POLVANI, F. (1965). *J. Chromatog.* **18**, 278.
LUUKKAINEN, T., VANDEN-HEUVEL, W. J. A., HAAHTI, E. O. A. & HORNING, E. C. (1961). *Biochim. Biophys. Acta*, **52**, 599.
LUUKKAINEN, T., VANDEN-HEUVEL, W. J. A. & HORNING, E. C. (1962). *Biochim. Biophys. Acta*, **62**, 153.
McARTHUR, J. W., HOWARD, A., SOMERVILLE, A., PERLEY, R. & KEYNES, C. (1967). *J. Clin. Endocrinol. Metab.* **27**, 534.
McCANN, S. M. & TALEISNIK, S. (1960). *Am. J. Physiol.* **199**, 847.
MacCORQUODALE, D. W., THAYER, S. A. & DOISY, E. A. (1935). *Proc. Soc. Exp. Biol. Med.* **32**, 1182.
MARRIAN, G. F. (1930). *Biochem. J.* **24**, 435.
MARRIAN, G. F. (1955). *Mem. Soc. Endocrinol.* **3**, 48.
MARRIAN, G. F. (1966). *J. Endocrinol.* **35**, vi.
MARTIN, L. (1960). *J. Endocrinol.* **20**, 187.
MARTIN, L. (1964). *J. Endocrinol.* **30**, 21.
MENINI, E. (1965). *Biochem. J.* **94**, 15P.

MIDGLEY, A. R. Jr. (1966). *Endocrinology*, **79**, 10.
MIDGLEY, A. R. (1967). *J. Clin. Endocrinol. Metab.* **27**, 295.
MIYAKE, T. (1962). In *Methods in Hormone Research*, Vol. 2, p. 127. Ed. Dorfman, R. I. New York: Academic Press.
MOLEN, H. J. van der & GROEN, D. (1965). *J. Clin. Endocrinol. Metab.* **25**, 1625.
MORSE, W. I., CLARK, A. F. & MACLEOD, S. C. (1963). *J. Endocrinol.* **26**, 25.
MUKERJI, S. (1963). Ph.D. Thesis, University of Edinburgh.
MUKERJI, S., BELL, E. T. & LORAINE, J. A. (1962). *Acta Endocrinol. Suppl.* **67**, p. 127.
NOCKE, W. & BREUER, H. (1963). *Acta Endocrinol.* **44**, 47.
ODELL, W. D., ROSS, G. T. & RAYFORD, P. C. (1967). *J. Clin. Investig.* **46**, 248.
OERTEL, G. W. (1961). *Clin. Chim. Acta*, **6**, 237.
OERTEL, G. W. & GROOT, K. (1965). *Clin. Chim. Acta*, **11**, 512.
OERTEL, G. W., BECKMANN, I. N. & EIK-NES, K. B. (1960). *Arch. Biochem.* **86**, 148.
OERTEL, G. W., WEISS, S. P. & EIK-NES, K. B. (1959). *J. Clin. Endocrinol. Metab.* **19**, 213.
ONESON, I. B. & COHEN, S. L. (1952). *Endocrinology*, **51**, 173.
PALMER, R. F. (1964). *J. Obstet. Gynaecol. Brit. Commonwealth*, **71**, 744.
PANICUCCI, F. & TAPONECO, G. (1965). *Folia Endocrinol. (Pisa)*, **18**, 188.
PARLOW, A. F. (1958). *Federation Proc.* **17**, 402.
PARLOW, A. F. (1961). In *Human Pituitary Gonadotropins*, p. 300. Ed. Albert, A. Springfield: Thomas.
PARLOW, A. F. (1963). *Endocrinology*, **73**, 456.
PARLOW, A. F. & REICHERT, L. E. Jr. (1963 a). *Endocrinology*, **73**, 740.
PARLOW, A. F. & REICHERT, L. E. Jr. (1963 b). *Endocrinology*, **73**, 377.
PATTI, A. A., BONANNO, P., FRAWLEY, T. F. & STEIN, A. A. (1963). *Acta Endocrinol. Suppl.* 77.
PEDERSEN-BJERGAARD, K. (1939). *Comparative Studies Concerning the Strength of Oestrogenic Substances*. London: Oxford University Press.
PERSKY, H. & NORTON, J. (1964). *J. Clin. Endocrinol. Metab.* **24**, 319.
PREEDY, J. R. K. & AITKEN, E. H. (1961 a). *J. Biol. Chem.* **236**, 1297.
PREEDY, J. R. K. & AITKEN, E. H. (1961 b). *J. Biol. Chem.* **236**, 1300.
RABINOWITZ, J. L. (1956). *Arch. Biochem.* **64**, 285.
RILEY, G. M. (1961). In *Human Pituitary Gonadotropins*, p. 133. Ed. Albert, A. Springfield: Thomas.
RIONDEL, A., TAIT, J. F., GUT, M., TAIT, S. A. S., JOACHIM, E. & LITTLE, B. (1963). *J. Clin. Endocrinol. Metab.* **23**, 620.
RIONDEL, A., TAIT, J. F., TAIT, S. A. S., GUT, M. & LITTLE, B. (1965). *J. Clin. Endocrinol. Metab.* **25**, 229.
RIVAROLA, M. A. & MIGEON, C. J. (1966). *Steroids*, **7**, 103.
ROSEMBERG, E. & ENGEL, I. (1961). *J. Clin. Endocrinol. Metab.* **21**, 603.
ROSEMBERG, E., KELLER, P., LEWIS, W. B., ALBERT, A., CARL, G. & BENNETT, D. (1965). *Endocrinology*, **76**, 1150.
ROSEMBERG, E., LEWIS, W. B. & SOLOD, E. A. (1964 a). *J. Clin. Endocrinol. Metab.* **24**, 673.
ROSEMBERG, E., SOLOD, E. A. & ALBERT, A. (1964 b). *J. Clin. Endocrinol. Metab.* **24**, 714.
ROSNER, J. M., CONTE, N. F., BRIGGS, J. H., CHAO, P. Y., SUDMAN, E. M. & FORSHAM, P. H. (1965). *J. Clin. Endocrinol. Metab.* **25**, 95.
ROY, E. J. (1962). *J. Endocrinol.* **25**, 361.
ROY, E. J. & BROWN, J. B. (1960). *J. Endocrinol.* **21**, 9.
SAEZ, J. M., SAEZ, S. & MIGEON, C. J. (1967). *Steroids*, **9**, 1.
SAKIZ, E. & GUILLEMIN, R. (1963). *Endocrinology*, **72**, 804.
SALOKANGAS, R. A. A. & BULBROOK, R. D. (1961). *J. Endocrinol.* **22**, 47.
SANDBERG, D. H., AHMAD, N., CLEVELAND, W. W. & SAVARD, K. (1964). *Steroids*, **4**, 557.
SAXENA, B. B., DEMURA, H. & DAVIS, M. A. (1967). *Federation Proc.* **26**, 391.
SCHMIDT-ELMENDORFF, H. & LORAINE J. A. (1962). *J. Endocrinol.* **23**, 413.
SCHMIDT-ELMENDORFF, H., LORAINE, J. A. & BELL, E. T. (1962). *J. Endocrinol.* **24**, 349.
SCHREPFER, R. & NICHOLAS, H. J. (1965). *Am. J. Obstet. Gynecol.* **92**, 755.

FERTILITY AND CONTRACEPTION

SEGALOFF, A., FLORES, A. & STEELMAN, S. L. (1955). *J. Clin. Endocrinol. Metab.* **15,** 847.
SHORT, R. V. (1958). *J. Endocrinol.* **16,** 415.
SIITERI, P. K. (1963). *Steroids,* **2,** 687.
SIMPSON, M. E. (1961). In *Human Pituitary Gonadotropins,* p. 276. Ed. Albert, A. Springfield: Thomas.
SKOSEY, J. L. & GOLDSTEIN, D. P. (1966). *Endocrinology,* **78,** 218.
SNEDECOR, G. W. (1956). *Statistical Methods,* Fifth ed. Iowa: State University Press.
SOMMERVILLE, I. F. & DESHPANDE, G. N. (1958). *J. Clin. Endocrinol. Metab.* **18,** 1223.
STEELMAN, S. L. & POHLEY, F. M. (1953). *Endocrinology,* **53,** 604.
STERN, M. I (1957). *J. Endocrinol.* **16,** 180.
STEVENS, V. C. (1964). Quoted by Bell, E. T. (1967 a). *Vitamins Hormones,* **24,** 63.
STEVENS, V. C. (1967). In *Recent Research on Gonadotrophic Hormones,* p. 17. Eds. Bell, E. T., and Loraine, J. A. Edinburgh: Livingstone.
SULIMOVICI, S., LUNENFELD, B. & SHELESNYAK, M. C. (1965). *Acta Endocrinol.* **49,** 97.
SVENDSEN, R. (1960). *Acta Endocrinol.* **35,** 161.
TAIT, J. F. (1963). *J. Clin. Endocrinol. Metab.* **23,** 1285.
TAYMOR, M. L. (1964).. *J. Clin. Endocrinol. Metab.* **24,** 803.
TAYMOR, M. L. (1967). In *Recent Research on Gonadotrophic Hormones,* p. 68. Eds. Bell, E. T., and Loraine, J. A. Edinburgh: Livingstone.
TOUCHSTONE, J. C. & MURAWEC, T. (1960). *Anal. Chem.* **32,** 822.
TURNER, D. A., JONES, G. E. S., SARLOS, I. J., BARNES, A. C. & COHEN, R. (1963). *Anal. Biochem.* **5,** 99.
VANDEN-HEUVEL, W. J. A., SJÖVALL, J. & HORNING, E. C. (1961). *Biochim. Biophys. Acta,* **48,** 596.
VANDEN-HEUVEL, W. J. A., SWEELEY, C. C. & HORNING, E. C. (1960). *Biochem. Biophys. Res. Commun.* **3,** 33.
VAN REES, G. P., WOLTHIUS, O. L. & DE JONGH, S. E. (1961). *Acta Physiol. Pharmacol. Neerl,* **10,** 197.
VENNING, E. H. (1937). *J. Biol. Chem.* **119,** 473.
VENNING, E. H. (1938). *J. Biol. Chem.* **126,** 595.
VENNING, E. H. & BROWNE, J. S. L. (1936). *Proc. Soc. Exp. Biol. Med.* **34,** 792.
VERMEULEN, A. & VERPLANCKE, J. C. M. (1963). *Steroids,* **2,** 453.
VISUTAKUL, P., BELL, E. T., LORAINE, J. A. & FISHER, R. B. (1966 a). *J. Endocrinol.* **36,** 15.
VISUTAKUL, P., BELL, E. T., LORAINE, J. A. & FISHER, R. B. (1966 b). *J. Endocrinol.* **36,** 23.
WERBIN, H., BERGENSTAL, D. M., GOULD, R. G. & LE ROY, G. V. (1957). *J. Clin. Endocrinol. Metab.* **17,** 337.
WIDE, L. (1966). In *Ovulation,* p. 283. Ed. Greenblatt, R. B. Philadelphia: Lippincott.
WIDE, L. & GEMZELL, C. A. (1962). *Acta Endocrinol.* **39,** 539.
WIDE, L., ROOS, P. & GEMZELL, C. A. (1961). *Acta Endocrinol.* **37,** 445.
WILDE, C. E., ORR, A. H. & BAGSHAWE, K. D. (1965). *Nature,* **205,** 191.
WILDE, C. E., ORR, A. H. & BAGSHAWE, K. D. (1967). *J. Endocrinol.* **37,** 23.
WOLF, A. (1966). *Nature,* **211,** 942.
WOOLEVER, C. A. & GOLDFIEN, A. (1963). *Intern. J. Appl. Radiation Isotopes,* **14,** 163.
WOTIZ, H. H. (1962). *Biochim. Biophys. Acta,* **63,** 180.
WOTIZ, H. H. (1963 a). *Biochim. Biophys. Acta,* **74,** 122.
WOTIZ, H. H. (1963 b). *Biochim. Biophys. Acta,* **69,** 415.
WOTIZ, H. H. & CHATTORAJ, S. C. (1964). *Anal. Chem.* **36,** 1466.
WOTIZ, H. H. & MARTIN, H. F. (1961). *J. Biol. Chem.* **236,** 1312.
WOTIZ, H. H. & MARTIN, H. F. (1962). *Anal. Biochem.* **3,** 97.
YOUSEM, H. L. (1964). *Am. J. Obstet. Gynecol.* **88,** 375.
ZANDER, J. (1958). *J. Biol. Chem.* **232,** 117.
ZANDER, J. & SIMMER, H. (1954). *Klin. Wochschr.* **32,** 529.
ZANDER, J., BRENDLE, E., MÜNSTERMANN, A-M.v., DICZFALUSY, E., MARTINSEN, B. & TILLINGER, K-G. (1959). *Acta Obstet. Gynaecol. Scand.* **38,** 724.
ZANDER, J., FORBES, T. R., MÜNSTERMANN, A-M.v. & NEHER, R. (1958). *J. Clin. Endocrinol. Metab.* **18,** 337.

CHAPTER IV

Hormone Levels during the Normal Menstrual Cycle

INTRODUCTION

THE aim of this chapter is to review the literature dealing with levels of hormones and their metabolites in the urine and blood of normally menstruating women. In the section on urine consideration is given to the oestrogens, pregnanediol, pregnanetriol, testosterone and HPG; endocrine interrelationships during the normal menstrual cycle as assessed by urinary assays are also discussed. The section on blood embraces the oestrogens, progesterone and its meta-bolites, testosterone and HPG. Information on hormone levels in the blood of women during reproductive life is much less extensive than in the case of urine, and, little or no attempt has been made to elucidate hormonal inter-relationships in blood.

Much of the data presented in this chapter has already been reviewed in a recent publication by Loraine and Bell (1966); the new information centres mainly on recent studies on levels of testosterone and HPG during the normal menstrual cycle. The chapter is included for the sake of completeness, and because a thorough understanding of hormone levels in normally menstruating women is an essential prerequisite to a consideration of the endocrinology of gynaecological disorders and to an appreciation of the effects produced by Clomiphene and gonadotrophic hormones on ovarian function.

URINARY EXCRETION OF HORMONES AND THEIR METABOLITES DURING THE NORMAL MENSTRUAL CYCLE

1. Oestrogens

The pattern of oestrogen excretion in normally menstruating women is now well established (see J. B. Brown, 1955 *a*; Borth *et al.*, 1957; J. B. Brown *et al.*, 1958; Ittrich, 1960; Loraine and Bell, 1963, 1967 *a b*; Nocke and Breuer, 1963). In the majority of the studies reported in recent years the chemical method of J. B. Brown (1955 *b*) has been employed (see p. 33), and the results in two subjects in whom this assay procedure was used are shown in Figures 15 and 16.

During the first seven to 10 days of a normal 28 day cycle excretion values for oestrone, oestradiol and oestriol are low, readings for each steroid often being below a level of 5 μg. per 24 hours. Values start to rise about the 7th day during the follicular phase and reach a well-defined maximum at or near midcycle. This maximum which has been termed the " ovulation peak " is thought to coincide with the rupture of the follicle (see also p. 20) After the ovulatory peak there occurs a rapid decrease in oestrogen excretion. This fall is succeeded by a second rise which takes place in the luteal phase at or about the 21st day of the cycle and is continued until shortly before the onset of menstrual bleeding. The second rise has been designated the " luteal maximum " and probably reflects the secretion of oestrogens by the corpus luteum. Immediately prior to menstruation excretion values for the three classical oestrogens fall rapidly, the lowest levels at any time during the cycle being encountered some days after the onset of bleeding.

Generally, values for the three classical oestrogens rise and fall together during the cycle. Urinary oestradiol is present

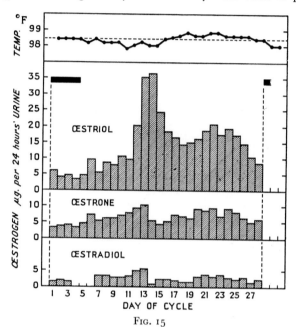

FIG. 15

Oestrogen excretion during the normal menstrual cycle
Basal temperature readings are also shown
■ = menstrual bleeding
(From J. B. Brown, 1955 a)

in smaller amounts than oestrone, the ratio oestrone/oestradiol being relatively constant at approximately two to one. Oestriol is usually excreted in larger quantities than oestrone, but a constant ratio for the amounts of the two steroids present in the urine is not found. At and immediately after the ovulatory peak alterations in the pattern of oestrone and oestradiol excretion occur simultaneously, but changes in oestriol output tend to lag some 24 hours behind; this is probably due to the fact that oestriol is a metabolic product of the other two oestrogens rather than a true ovarian hormone. At the time of the luteal maximum this lag in oestriol output is generally not observed.

In Figure 17 the method of Eechaute and Demeester (1965) (see p. 36) has been used to estimate the output of " total oestrogens " in a normally menstruating woman. It is apparent

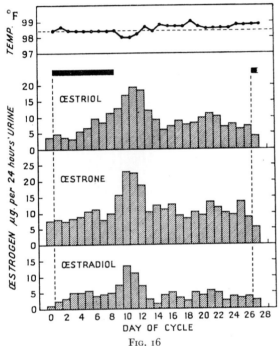

FIG. 16

Oestrogen excretion during the normal menstrual cycle
Basal temperature readings are also shown
■■■ = menstrual bleeding
(From J. B. Brown, 1955 *a*)

that the pattern of excretion is very similar to that shown in Figures 15 and 16 for the three classical oestrogens measured separately. Excretion values for 16-epioestriol together with those for the three classical oestrogens are shown in Figure 18. The method of estimation of 16-epioestriol was that of Nocke and Breuer (1963) (see p. 40). It will be noted that the highest reading for 16-epioestriol occurred at the time of ovulation on days 11 and 12 of a 27 day cycle, and that during the luteal phase excretion values for this steroid gradually decreased.

OESTROGEN ASSAYS IN RELATION TO THE TIME OF OVULATION

Bell and Loraine (1965) have correlated the time of ovulation as measured by urinary oestrogen assays with the length of the menstrual cycle. They studied a total of 45 cycles in 31 subjects, the series including 18 women who had received no hormonal medication and 13 subjects who had been treated

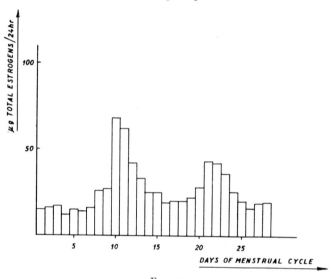

FIG. 17

" Total oestrogen " excretion during the normal menstrual cycle

(From Eschaute and Demeester, 1965)

previously with various compounds including progestogen-oestrogen mixtures as oral contraceptives, the retro-progestational compound, Duphaston (Phillips-Duphar) and the dithiocarbamoylhydrazine derivative, Compound 33,828 (Imperial Chemical Industries Ltd.). In the women receiving therapy the data were derived from the first and in some cases the second post-treatment cycle.

In Table 3 are shown the results obtained in this investigation. For the purposes of the study " midcycle " was defined

TABLE 3

RELATION OF OVULATION TO MIDCYCLE IN 45 MENSTRUAL CYCLES

(From Bell and Loraine, 1965)

Subject	−4	−3	−2	−1	Midcycle	+1	+2	+3	+4	+5	+6	Total
Normal	1	1	2	2	7	6	2	1			1	23
Long term treatment with progestogen-oestrogen mixtures ...	1	1	1		4	2	1			2		12
Short term treatment with various compounds		1	3	1	1	3		1				10
Total	2	3	6	3	12	11	3	2	0	2	1	45

as the length of the cycle divided by two, *e.g.* in a 28 day cycle " midcycle " was day 14. The date of occurrence of ovulation as judged by oestrogen excretion was also noted, and the figures in the top column of the table represent the difference between these two dates. Thus, " —4 " indicates that ovulation

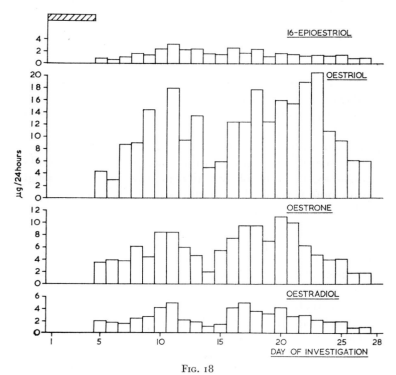

FIG. 18

Oestrogen excretion during the normal menstrual cycle
//// = menstrual bleeding
(From Nocke and Breuer, 1963)

took place four days before midcycle, i.e. on day 10 of a 28 day cycle. Similarly " +6 " indicates that ovulation occurred six days after midcycle, *i.e.* on day 20 of a 28 day cycle. The following points emerge from the table.

(*a*) In the normal untreated subjects ovulation occurred either at or within 24 hours of midcycle in 15 of the 23 cycles (65 per cent). Of the remaining eight cycles ovulation took place from two to four days before midcycle in four and from two to six days after midcycle in four.

(*b*) In subjects who had received long term therapy with progestogen-oestrogen mixtures as oral contraceptives ovulation occurred at or within 24 hours of midcycle in six out of 12 cycles (50 per cent). In the remainder ovulation was early in three and late in three.

(*c*) In the 10 cycles derived from women treated with other compounds ovulation occurred at or within 24 hours of midcycle in five (50 per cent), was early in four and late in one.

The main conclusion to emerge from this study was that the day on which ovulation occurred was very variable indeed, and that this event could take place as early as four days before or as late as six days after midcycle. It was also noteworthy that in women previously treated on a long term basis with progestogen-oestrogen mixtures or on a short term basis with other compounds, the time of ovulation in relation to cycle length was no more variable than in untreated subjects.

The findings of Bell and Loraine (1965) lend support to the view that any form of contraception employed whether by oral progestational agents or by other means should span a wide area of the cycle. By emphasising the great variability in the time of ovulation from one subject to another the data go far to explain the high failure rate when a contraceptive technique such as the "rhythm method" is used (see p. 131). Mention has already been made of the fact that the information in Table 3 was obtained by relating the time of ovulation to cycle length. It must also be stressed that when the results were analysed so that the midcycle oestrogen peak was related to other parameters such as the first day of the cycle or the first day of the succeeding cycle, the relationship between the time of ovulation and these indices was just as variable as that shown in Table 3.

2. Pregnanediol

The pattern of excretion of urinary pregnanediol during the normal menstrual cycle has been studied by numerous investigators over the past three decades and is now well established. Typical results obtained by the method of Klopper *et al.* (1955) are shown in Figures 19, 20 and 21.

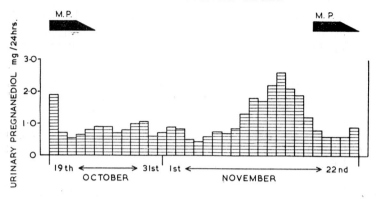

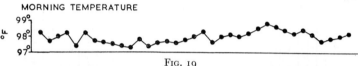

FIG. 19

**Pregnanediol excretion during the normal menstrual cycle—
juvenile type**

Basal temperature readings are also shown. M.P. = menstrual period
(From Klopper, 1957, *J. Obstet. Gynaecol. Brit. Empire*)

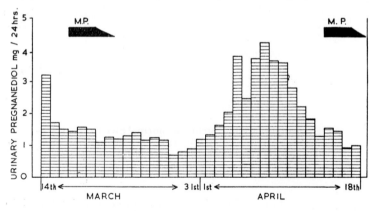

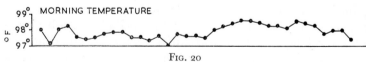

FIG. 20

**Pregnamediol excretion during the normal menstrual cycle
—adult type**

Basal temperature readings are also shown. M.P. = menstrual period.
(From Klopper, 1957, *J. Obstet. Gynaecol. Brit. Empire*)

In the follicular phase of the cycle pregnanediol output is usually at or below the level of 1 mg. per 24 hours; this material presumably represents mainly " adrenal pregnanediol " which is derived from precursors secreted by the adrenal cortex. Following ovulation a rise in pregnanediol excretion occurs, and during the luteal phase values generally lie between 2 and

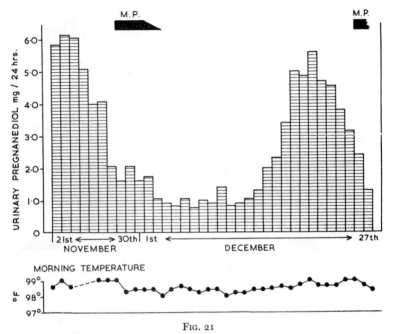

FIG. 21

Pregnanediol excretion during the normal menstrual cycle—adult type

Basal temperature readings are also shown. M.P. = menstrual period

(From Klopper, 1957, *J. Obstet. Gynaecol. Brit. Empire*)

5 mg. per 24 hours. At this time the pregnanediol found in urine is almost certainly derived from the progesterone secreted by the luteal tissue of the ovary. Pregnanediol output begins to fall several days before menstruation commences and continues to decline for the first two or three days after the onset of bleeding.

Klopper (1957) has emphasised that pregnanediol levels in normally menstruating women remain relatively constant from one subject to another during the follicular phase of the cycle but vary greatly in the luteal phase. This point is well illustrated in Figures 19 to 21 which indicate that luteal activity as judged by pregnanediol assays was low in one subject (Figure 19) and higher in the other two (Figures 20 and 21). It is also noteworthy that pregnanediol readings in the luteal phase in Figure 19 are not dissimilar to those in the follicular phase in Figure 20, and that the levels during menstruation in Figure 21 are in the same range as those in the luteal phase in Figure 19. These observations taken in conjunction clearly illustrate the great variation in pregnanediol output from one subject to another and emphasise the futility of placing any reliance for diagnostic purposes on isolated readings in individual subjects. A similar degree of variability in pregnanediol excretion during the menstrual cycle to that noted by Klopper (1957) has been observed by other investigators including J. B. Brown *et al.* (1958), Pickett and Sommerville (1962) and Loraine and Bell (1963, 1967 *a*).

3. Pregnanetriol

The output of pregnanetriol during the normal menstrual cycle has been studied by Fotherby (1960, 1962), Pickett and Sommerville (1962), Loraine and Bell (1963, 1967 *a*) and others. It is generally agreed that levels are low during the follicular phase, begin to rise about midcycle, are maximal in the luteal phase and fall before menstruation. Fotherby (1962) has noted that pregnanetriol excretion during the luteal phase reaches a peak and begins to decrease before the maximum level of pregnanediol is observed. He has also suggested that the increased amounts of pregnanetriol found in the urine in the luteal phase arise from a precursor of the steroid, probably 17α-hydroxyprogesterone, which is secreted by the ovary. Subsequently, D. K. Fukushima *et al.* (1963) have postulated that during the luteal phase urinary pregnanetriol can also be derived from 17α-hydroxypregnenolone. A typical curve of pregnanetriol excretion during the normal menstrual cycle is shown in Figure 22.

4. Testosterone

Assays of urinary testosterone in women have been performed by numerous investigators. Some of the results reported in the literature are shown in Table 4 which is taken from a paper by Ismail and Harkness (1966 a) and which includes data obtained both from normally menstruating and from postmenopausal subjects. The great variation in excretion values should be noted, and it is probable that some of this variation arises from methodological considerations.

The pattern of testosterone excretion during the normal menstrual cycle has been investigated by various workers including Hudson et al. (1963), Apostolakis et al. (1966) and Ismail and Harkness (1966 b). In all these studies chemical methods of assay have been used. It is now generally agreed

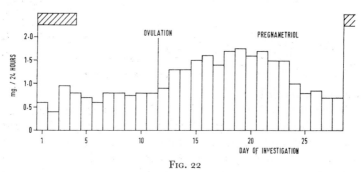

Mrs. E.W. : AGE 29 YEARS : PARA 2 + 0

FIG. 22

Pregnanetriol excretion during the normal menstrual cycle
//// = menstrual bleeding
(After Bell et al., 1962)

that levels are low during menstruation and that a two to threefold rise occurs during the luteal phase. Small peaks of testosterone output have also been reported during the follicular phase and at the time of ovulation.

Serial assays of testosterone together with pregnanediol in a typical ovulatory cycle described by Ismail et al. (1967) are shown in Figure 23. The marked rise in testosterone output during the luteal phase should be noted together with the fluctuating values for the hormone at midcycle and in the follicular phase. In Figure 24 is shown a similar study conducted by Apostolakis et al. (1966). Testosterone excretion was low during the follicular phase, values ranging from 5 to

10 µg. per 24 hours. At the time of ovulation an increase in the output of the hormone occurred, excretion values rising to 20 µg. per 24 hours. In the early luteal phase readings fell slightly; however, between the 26th and 30th days of the cycle levels were at their maximum reaching a figure of approximately 30 µg. per 24 hours. During menstruation testosterone output decreased sharply, falling to the low levels characteristic of the follicular phase.

TABLE 4

URINARY EXCRETION OF TESTOSTERONE IN NORMAL WOMEN

(After Ismail and Harkness, 1966 a)

Age of subjects years	Number	Testosterone µg./24 hours		Reference
		Mean	Range	
19–23	4	5·9	3·5– 7·5	Camacho and Migeon (1963)
23–37	6	6·1	2·8– 8·0	Futterweit et al. (1963)
18–63	4	8·3	5·0– 12·0	Vermeulen and Verplancke (1963)
21–32	4	12	7·0– 18·0	Brooks (1964)
20–72	10	<5·3	<5·0– 8·0	Ibayashi et al. (1964)
22–35	4	10	3·0– 18·0	Voigt et al. (1964)
21–68	18	48·9	2·9–196·7	Dulmanis et al. (1964)
29–35	2	4·8	4·1– 5·6	Zurbrügg et al. (1965)
20–40	20	19·0	6 – 57	Rosner et al. (1965)
22–59	16	7·1	4·3– 10·4	Lim and Dingman (1965)
20–55	15	6·5	2·1– 10·7	Ismail and Harkness (1966 a)

5. HPG

The output of HPG during the normal menstrual cycle will be considered under two headings:

(a) Excretion of " total gonadotrophic activity " as measured by the mouse uterus test.

(b) Separate excretion of FSH and LH measured by assays specific for these hormones.

(a) EXCRETION OF " TOTAL GONADOTROPHIC ACTIVITY ".—This has been studied by various investigators including Klinefelter et al. (1943), Pedersen-Bjergaard and Tønnesen (1948), J. B. Brown et al. (1958), P. S. Brown (1959), Johnsen

(1959) and Loraine and Bell (1963, 1967 a). In general, the results obtained have been less informative than those found when specific assay methods are used.

J. B. Brown et al. (1958) measured HPG excretion together with the output of oestrogens and pregnanediol in a series of nine ovulatory menstrual cycles. They found that the HPG peak at midcycle was by no means an invariable occurrence; when present it did not precede the oestrogen peak, but either

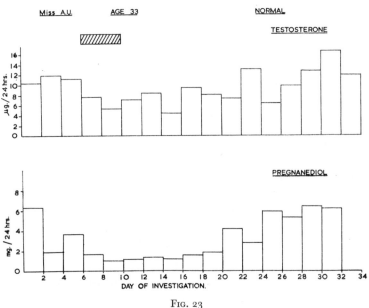

FIG. 23

Testosterone and pregnanediol excretion during the normal menstrual cycle

//// = menstrual bleeding

(From Ismail et al., 1968)

coincided with or postdated it by periods ranging from 48 to 72 hours. When these workers conducted parallel assays on the same urine sample for " total gonadotrophic activity " and for LH by the hypophysectomised rat prostate test they found that the results obtained agreed closely at all stages of the cycle. Loraine and Bell (1963) noted a peak of " total gonado-trophic activity " at midcycle in only three out of 11 menstrual cycles; in none of the subjects studied did the midcycle HPG peak precede that of the oestrogens. In the investigations of Johnsen (1959) and P. S. Brown (1959) HPG levels at midcycle were higher than at any other stage, although in a proportion of the subjects studied a definite peak at this time was not observed.

Loraine (1962) examined the effect of the age of the subject and the phase of the cycle on HPG excretion in both non-parous and parous women. For the purposes of the study he divided the cycle into four phases designated menstruation, follicular phase, ovulatory phase and luteal phase (see also

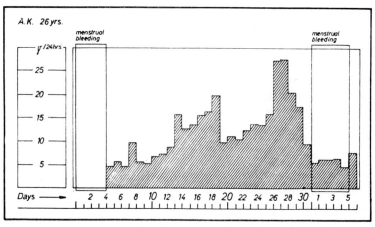

FIG. 24

Testerone excretion during the normal menstrual cycle

(From Apostolakis *et al.*, 1966)

p. 97). He found that in the non-parous women the factor of age was not significant, but that the mean HPG excretion in the ovulatory phase was significantly higher than that in the other three phases. He also noted that the mean HPG level for the four phases of the cycle was higher in the parous than in the non-parous women.

(*b*) SEPARATE EXCRETION OF FSH AND LH.—Publications on this subject in recent years include those of McArthur *et al.* (1958), P. S. Brown (1959), M. Fukushima *et al.* (1964), Rosemberg and Keller (1965), Becker and Albert (1965), Bell *et al.* (1966), Midgley (1966), Wolf (1966) and Stevens

(1967). In the majority of studies on FSH levels the assay methods used have been the rat or mouse ovarian augmentation tests; in one investigation (Wolf, 1966) an immunological technique depending on a haemagglutination-inhibition reaction was employed. Bioassays for LH have included the ventral prostatic weight test in rats and the rat ovarian ascorbic acid and cholesterol depletion methods; in addition, a variety of immunological methods have been used in attempts to measure urinary LH.

Bell *et al.* (1966) studied FSH and LH output in a series of seven normally menstruating subjects, all of whom showed evidence of ovulation as judged by urinary steroid assays. A notable feature of this investigation was the great variation in the pattern of FSH excretion from one woman to another. In some subjects levels did not alter throughout the cycle; in others readings were maximal at the time of ovulation while in others the highest levels occurred in the follicular phase. Variable patterns for FSH excretion have also been reported by Rosemberg and Keller (1965), Becker and Albert (1965) and Taymor (1967). On the other hand, M. Fukushima *et al.* (1964) claimed that the curve of FSH output during the cycle tended to be rather constant with high levels in the follicular and luteal phases and low readings at midcycle. However. subsequent work by the same group (see Stevens, 1967) has demonstrated that the pattern of FSH excretion in normally menstruating women is more variable than that previously reported by M. Fukushima *et al.* (1964).

Numerous workers including J. B. Brown *et al.* (1958), McArthur *et al.* (1958) and M. Fukushima *et al.* (1964) have reported that a peak of LH excretion at midcycle is a relatively constant occurrence, and that this peak is closely associated with ovulation as judged by urinary steroid assays or by basal temperature records. The data of Bell *et al.* (1966) suggest that the pattern of LH excretion in individual women may be more variable than had previously been supposed. Thus, in only one of their subjects did a marked increase in LH output occur within 48 hours of the midcycle peak of oestrogen excretion; in two, evidence of an LH peak was not clear-cut and in one LH levels were maximal seven days prior to the time of ovulation. Results of FSH and LH assays conducted by Stevens

(1967) in 64 normal menstrual cycles are shown in Figure 25. The characteristic peak of LH output at midcycle is noteworthy, while the pattern of FSH output is similar to that originally reported by M. Fukushima *et al.* (1964).

Urinary LH assays during the normal menstrual cycle by immunological methods have been performed by Wide and Gemzell (1962), Sato *et al.* (1965), Bagshawe *et al.* (1966), Wide (1966) and Midgley (1966). In general, a peak of LH output has been reported at or about midcycle in association with low levels of excretion during the follicular and luteal phases. The specificity of some of the methods employed in

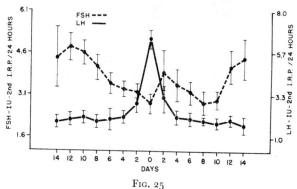

FIG. 25

Mean urinary FSH and LH levels and S.E. in 64 normal menstrual cycles

(From Stevens, 1967)

these studies is unsatisfactory, and the quantitative significance of the results obtained is doubtful (see Loraine and Bell, 1966; Apostolakis and Loraine, 1967). During the normal menstrual cycle Midgley (1966) reported a peak of LH excretion at the time of ovulation, the latter being assessed by basal temperature records. Further application of his radio-immunological technique to clinical problems will be awaited with interest.

6. Hormonal Interrelationships in Urine during the Normal Menstrual Cycle

Comprehensive studies of hormonal interrelationships during the normal menstrual cycle include those of J. B. Brown *et al.* (1958), Loraine and Bell (1963, 1967 a), Bell *et al.*

(1966) and Apostolakis *et al.* (1966). In all these investigations serial rather than isolated assays were performed, and a number of hormones and their metabolites were estimated in the same urine sample. Examples of the results obtained are shown in Figures 26, 27 and 28.

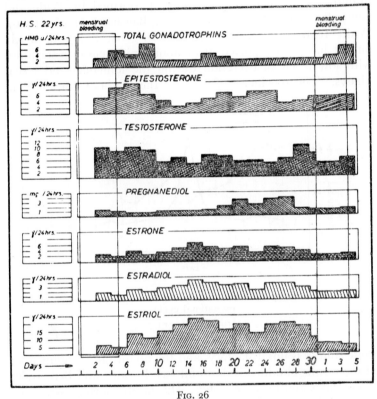

FIG. 26

Hormone excretion pattern during the normal menstrual cycle

(From Apostolakis *et al.*, 1966)

In Figure 26 excretion values for " total gonadotrophic activity ", testosterone, epitestosterone, pregnanediol and oestrogens are shown throughout a cycle in a normally menstruating woman aged 22 years. " Total gonadotrophic activity " was within the normal range for a woman during reproductive life; a midcycle peak of excretion was not

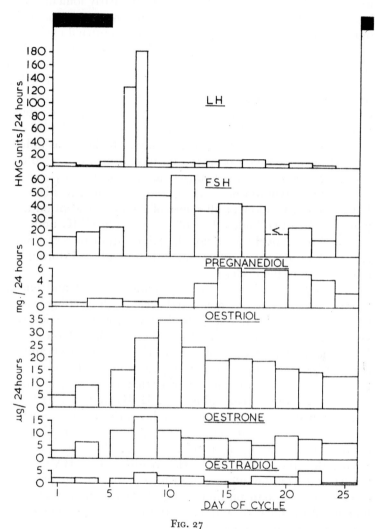

FIG. 27

Hormone excretion pattern during the normal menstrual cycle

■ = menstrual bleeding

(From Bell *et al.*, 1966)

observed. Epitestosterone levels showed no definite pattern throughout the cycle, while testosterone readings were at their maximum during menstruation and in the early follicular and late luteal phases. The pattern of oestrogen and pregnanediol output was typical of a normal ovulatory menstrual cycle.

In Figures 27 and 28 are shown results obtained by Bell *et al.* (1966) in two cycles in which HPG assays were conducted by methods specific for FSH and LH; results were expressed in terms of the First IRP-HMG (see p. 57), and estimations of oestrogens and pregnanediol were also performed. The subject in Figure 27 was aged 31 and had a history of regular 26 day cycles with bleeding lasting for five days. Ovulation as judged by oestrogen excretion occurred on days 8 or 9 of the 26 day cycle. Pregnanediol values started to rise on days 13 and 14, reaching a maximum on days 15 and 16 of the investigation. LH excretion was low at all stages of the cycle except on days 7 and 8 when two high values of 120 and 180 HMG units per 24 hours respectively were noted. FSH output rose gradually to a peak on days 11 and 12 and subsequently fell during the luteal phase of the cycle.

The subject shown in Figure 28 was aged 24 and had a history of regular 28 day menstrual cycles with bleeding lasting for five days. Ovulation as judged by oestrogen excretion was very late and did not occur until the 21st day of the cycle. Pregnanediol values did not start to rise until days 26 and 27 and reached their maximum on days 28 and 29. LH excretion throughout was generally much lower than in the subject shown in Figure 27, but a peak value of 72 HMG units per 24 hours was obtained on day 14, some seven days prior to ovulation. In spite of the fact that the so-called " rhythm " method of contraception was being used the subject became pregnant during the study, and the " LH " reading of 23 HMG units per 24 hours on day 28 may well have indicated the presence of HCG rather than pituitary LH. FSH excretion was at its maximum on days 10 and 11 of the cycle, subsequently fell, and rose again from days 24 to 27.

The most recent study of hormonal interrelationships in the urine of normally menstruating women is that of Loraine and Bell (1967 *a*) who conducted assays of " total gonado-trophic activity ", oestrogens, pregnanediol and pregnanetriol.

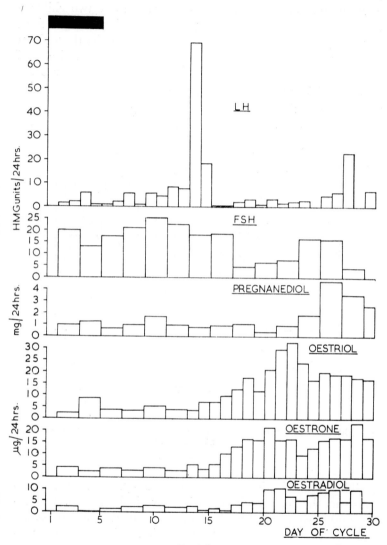

FIG. 28

Hormone excretion pattern during the normal menstrual cycle

■ = menstrual bleeding

(From Bell *et al.*, 1966)

95

Complete 24 hour urine samples were collected continuously throughout 18 normal cycles from 12 women, seven of whom were nulliparous, one had had one child, three two children and one three children. The age of the subjects ranged from 18 to 37 years; all continued their normal activities throughout the period of study and in none was there a previous history of menstrual abnormalities. Four women collected their urine throughout two or three cycles, these being either consecutive or separated by periods of up to two years.

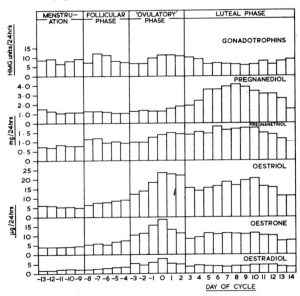

FIG. 29

Mean hormone excretion pattern during the normal menstrual cycle

(From Loraine and Bell, 1967 a)

The data obtained from these 18 cycles were used to construct the " composite cycle " shown in Figure 29. Oestrogen and pregnanediol assays were performed in all the cycles included in this figure while estimations of HPG and pregnanetriol were conducted in nine and five respectively.

The day of the midcycle peak of excretion of oestrone and oestradiol was designated day zero; the average length of the 18 cycles was $28 \cdot 1 \pm 2 \cdot 0$ days (S.D.). The composite cycle was divided into four phases designated *menstruation, follicular phase, ovulatory phase* and *luteal phase*. The ovulatory phase was considered to extend over six days; it included the day of the oestrone/oestradiol peak and incorporated data on three 48 hour pools of urine. The division of the cycle into the four phases resulted in the elimination of approximately 5 per cent of the readings from subjects in whom the follicular phase was longer than five days or the luteal phase longer than 12 days.

Figure 29 shows the characteristic midcycle peak of oestrogen excretion (day o) followed seven to 10 days later by the luteal phase rise in oestrogen output. In six of the cycles the peak of oestriol excretion occurred on the day after the oestrone/oestradiol peak while in the remainder maximum values for oestriol output coincided with those for oestrone and oestradiol. Urinary pregnanediol readings rose to a maximum on the 8th day after ovulation, while pregnanetriol values began to rise at the time of ovulation and reached their highest levels on the 6th to 10th days after the midcycle oestrogen peak.

A peak of HPG excretion was noted in only three cycles. In two it followed and in the third it coincided with the midcycle oestrogen peak. HPG output rose to a maximum of 11·5 HMG units per 24 hours on day o of the composite cycle. However, when the mean HPG values for the four phases of the cycle were compared this rise was not found to be significant. The marked difference between the pattern of HPG excretion as estimated by the· mouse uterus test in the composite cycle and that obtained when separate determinations of FSH and LH are made as in Figures 27 and 28 is apparent. It is now generally accepted that the results obtained with specific assays are more in keeping with the expected physiological events than those found with non-specific assays such as the mouse uterus test, and for this reason it appears unlikely that the latter group of methods will continue to be used in studies designed to elucidate hormonal interrelationships during the normal cycle.

Table 5 shows the mean and standard deviation for each of the six substances measured in the four phases of the cycle. It will be noted that variations in hormone excretion from one

H

97

individual to another were considerable and that in the case of the three groups of steroids estimated the standard deviations were highest in the ovulatory and luteal phases of the cycle.

TABLE 5

HORMONE EXCRETION DURING THE NORMAL MENSTRUAL CYCLE

(Mean ± standard deviation)

(From Loraine and Bell, 1967 a)

Phase of cycle	Oestradiol		Oestrone		Oestriol	
	Number of observations	µg./24 hr.	Number of observations	µg./24 hr.	Number of observations	µg./24 hr.
Menstruation	79	2·1±1·8	79	4·2±2·0	79	5·6± 2·6
Follicular ...	77	2·7±2·1	77	6·2±3·0	77	7·9± 5·0
" Ovulatory "	108	5·8±3·2	108	13·4±5·4	108	18·9±11·5
Luteal ...	202	4·2±2·7	202	10·4±5·0	202	16·3± 9·7

Phase of cycle	Pregnanediol		Pregnanetriol		HPG	
	Number of observations	mg./24 hr.	Number of observations	mg./24 hr.	Number of observations	HMG units /24 hr.
Menstruation	80	1·3±0·6	20	0·8±0·2	39	8·4±3·4
Follicular ...	75	1·3±0·6	25	1·0±0·3	37	9·1±6·0
" Ovulatory "	108	1·5±0·9	30	1·1±0·5	48	9·2±5·9
Luteal ...	196	3·2±1·5	57	1·5±0·5	84	8·0±2·2

HORMONE LEVELS IN BLOOD DURING THE NORMAL MENSTRUAL CYCLE

1. Oestrogens

Levels of these hormones in the blood of normally menstruating women have been estimated by various investigators including Svendsen and Sørensen (1964), Roy et al. (1965) and Ichii et al. (1963). The most detailed study so far reported is probably that of Svendsen and Sørensen (1964) who, using the method developed by Svendsen (1960), measured " free " oestrone and oestradiol throughout the menstrual cycle. Results obtained in one of their subjects are shown in Figure 30 which illustrates the rise in plasma concentrations of both oestrogens at midcycle. In the majority of the women investigated by Svendsen and Sørensen (1964) the concentration

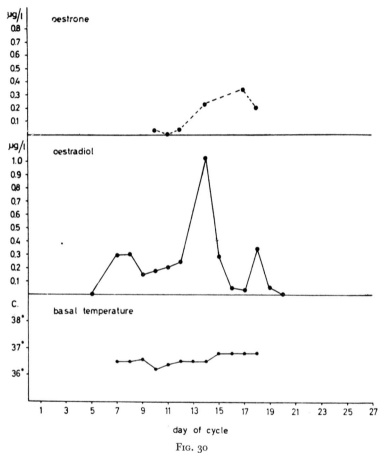

FIG. 30

Plasma levels of oestrone and oestradiol during the normal menstrual cycle

(From Svendsen and Sørensen, 1964)

of the two oestrogens during the follicular and luteal phases ranged from 0·01 to 0·03 µg. per 100 ml. plasma. In the middle third of the cycle at or about the time of ovulation higher readings up to a figure of 0·1 µg. per 100 ml. plasma were found.

The concentration of the three classical oestrogens in peripheral blood in women during the normal cycle has been studied by Roy *et al.* (1965) using the method of Roy (1962). During the follicular and luteal phases the concentration of all three oestrogens was generally below 0·025 μg. per 100 ml. blood, a figure regarded as the lower limit of sensitivity of the method. At midcycle, only the value for oestrone was above this limit, the mean level for this steroid being 0·07 μg. per 100 ml. blood.

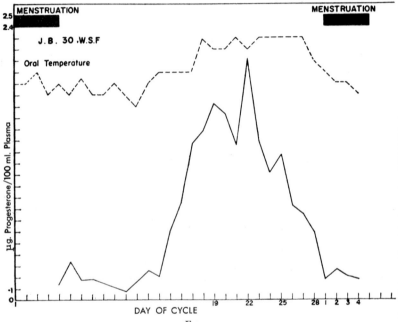

FIG. 31

Plasma levels of progesterone (μg. per 100 ml.) during the normal menstrual cycle

(From Woolever, 1963)

2. Progesterone and its Metabolites

The most detailed study of plasma progesterone levels in the normally menstruating woman remains that of Woolever (1963) who employed the assay method originally developed by Woolever and Goldfien (1963). Serial assays were made in five subjects, and a typical example of the results obtained is shown in Figure 31. It will be noted that levels were low during menstruation and in the follicular phase of the cycle; they rose markedly at midcycle in association with the increase in basal temperature and fell steeply in the latter part of the luteal phase. In the first half of the cycle plasma progesterone levels in Woolever's series ranged from o to 0·53 µg. per 100 ml.; the corresponding range in the luteal phase was from 0·6 to 2·1 µg. per 100 ml. plasma.

Molen *et al.* (1965), using a method involving gas liquid chromatography and isotopic dilution, have recently studied progesterone levels in pooled blood samples obtained from normally menstruating women; the results obtained were quantitatively similar to those reported by Woolever (1963). Runnebaum *et al.* (1965) have identified progesterone, 20α-hydroxypregn-4-ene-3-one, 20β-hydroxypregn-4-ene-3-one, 17α-hydroxyprogesterone and testosterone in pooled blood samples obtained from normally menstruating women during the luteal phase of the cycle. The mean concentrations from the 16th to the 25th day (µg. per 100 ml. plasma) were 0·69 for progesterone, 0·13 for 20α-hydroxypregn-4-ene-3-one, 0·04 for 20β-hydroxypregn-4-ene-3-one, 0·03 for 17α-hydroxy-progesterone and 0·04 for testosterone. Recently Runnebaum and Zander (1967) have measured plasma progesterone nine and four days before the time of ovulation in normally men-struating women and noted figures of 0·084 and 0·279 µg per 100 ml respectively. These results suggest that progesterone may be secreted by the ripening Graafian follicle in addition to the corpus luteum.

Very little information is currently available regarding levels of plasma pregnanediol during the normal menstrual cycle. In the study of Oertel *et al.* (1960) concentrations ranged from 10 to 20 µg. per 100 ml., the highest reading occurring on the 21st day of the cycle. Much further work in this field is required before the true pattern of plasma preg-nanediol levels in normally menstruating women is finally established.

3. Testosterone

One of the more detailed studies of plasma testosterone levels in menstruating women is that of Lobotsky *et al.* (1964) who, using the method of Riondel *et al.* (1963), noted that concentrations of the hormone were generally higher in the luteal than in the follicular phase of the cycle. These workers were unable to demonstrate any correlation between plasma testosterone levels on the one hand and the output of total urinary 17-oxosteroids on the other. As in the case of pregnanediol much remains to be learned regarding the relationship of plasma testosterone assays to the various phases of the cycle.

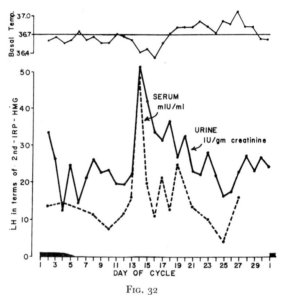

FIG. 32

Serum and urinary LH levels during the normal menstrual cycle

◢◣ = menstrual bleeding

(From Midgely, 1966)

4. HPG

Apostolakis (1959) has shown that HPG activity as estimated by the mouse uterus test is generally detectable in plasma at or about midcycle. He found values ranging from 11 to 19 HMG units (First IRP-HMG) per 100 ml. plasma between the 12th and 16th days in subjects with a history of regular 28 to 30 day cycles. During the follicular and luteal phases plasma HPG levels were low and generally did not exceed 4 HMG units per 100 ml. Keller and Rosemberg

(1965), using pooled plasma from normally menstruating women, reported a mean value of 1·3 mg. equivalents of the Second IRP per litre; the results of these investigators agree reasonably well with those of Apostolakis (1959). In a subsequent study reported by Keller (1966) plasma samples from normally menstruating women were pooled in three batches—from days 1 to 9, 10 to 19, and 20 to 30—of the cycle. He detected HPG activity in all three pools and found that the mean values obtained did not differ significantly. From the quantitative point of view his results were similar to those previously reported by Keller and Rosemberg (1965).

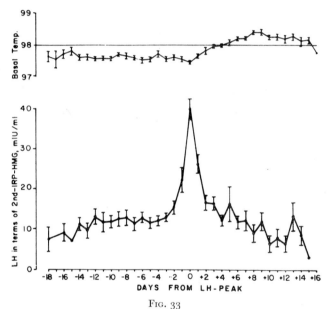

FIG. 33

Mean serum LH levels $\pm$ S.E. in 16 normal menstrual cycles
(From Midgley and Jaffe, 1966)

Valid estimates by bioassay of plasma FSH and LH levels in normally menstruating women are not yet available. According to Franchimont (1966) FSH can be estimated throughout the menstrual cycle by means of a recently developed radio-immunological assay; the validity of this claim requires to be substantiated, and, in particular, the reliability criteria of the assay method used must be thoroughly investigated with special reference to specificity.

Recent studies on serum LH levels in normally menstruating women include those of Midgley (1966) Midgley and Jaffe (1966) and Odell et al. (1967) all using radio-immunological procedures. In Figure 32 taken from Midgley's paper serum and urinary LH levels in one subject are shown. The LH peak at midcycle is obvious, as is the fact that the peak was of shorter duration in the serum than in the urine. In a further study Midgley and Jaffe (1966) have reported serum LH levels in 15 cycles from 10 normally menstruating women. The mean values are shown in Figure 33 which also demonstrates the marked LH peak at midcycle together with the low levels of the hormone in the follicular and luteal phases.

COMMENT

The last decade has seen great advances in our understanding of the endocrinology of the normal menstrual cycle, and many of the previously held views on this subject have either had to be discarded or considerably modified. Traditional as well as current hypotheses regarding the hormonal control of the cycle have recently been reviewed by Borth (1967) to whose article the reader is referred for further details. As emphasised previously, present concepts on hormonal interrelationships in the normal menstrual cycle have mainly been obtained from studies on urine rather than on blood.

There is now general agreement in the literature on the pattern of excretion of oestrogens, pregnanediol, pregnanetriol and LH in normally menstruating women. It is also established that urinary testosterone levels are generally higher in the luteal than in the follicular phase. The excretion of FSH varies greatly from one subject to another, and further work is necessary before the true pattern is established.

It is now recognized that in the majority of women both FSH and LH are excreted throughout the cycle. This observation indicates that older hypotheses purporting to show that FSH was only secreted prior to ovulation and LH at the time of and after this event are no longer tenable. Controversy still exists with respect to the role of the lactogenic hormone, prolactin, in the normal menstrual cycle. This substance has not yet been demonstrated with certainty in the blood or urine of women during reproductive life, suggesting that the traditional view implicating prolactin in the maintenance of the corpus luteum in human subjects must be accepted with considerable reserve.

SUMMARY AND CONCLUSIONS

The literature on levels of hormones and their metabolites in the urine and blood of normally menstruating women is reviewed. Particular attention is given to the values reported for oestrogens, pregnanediol, pregnanetriol, testosterone and HPG.

The curve of excretion of the three classical oestrogens during the normal menstrual cycle is now well established. Readings are low during and immediately prior to menstruation and in the follicular phase; peaks of excretion occur at or about the time of ovulation and in the luteal phase. The time of ovulation as judged by the midcycle urinary oestrogen peak varies greatly from one subject to another. Plasma oestrogen levels show a peak at midcycle and are low in the follicular and luteal phases.

Levels of plasma progesterone rise following the occurrence of ovulation. The pattern of pregnanediol output is well established, values showing a marked increase in the luteal phase of an ovulatory menstrual cycle. Urinary pregnanetriol levels also rise in the luteal phase of the cycle, the increase generally occurring immediately after ovulation.

Testosterone readings in urine are generally at their maximum during the second half of the ovulatory menstrual cycle. Smaller peaks of excretion of this hormone have also been noted in the follicular phase and at midcycle.

A peak of serum and urinary LH is a relatively constant finding at midcycle and is presumably connected with ovulation. The output of FSH varies greatly from one subject to another, and the true pattern of excretion of this hormone remains to be established.

Reliable information is now available on interrelationships between pituitary and ovarian function in normally menstruating women. In this connection it cannot be too strongly emphasised that in individual subjects meaningful results are likely to be obtained only if serial rather than isolated assays are performed.

REFERENCES

APOSTOLAKIS, M. (1959). *J. Endocrinol.* **19,** 377.
APOSTOLAKIS, M. & LORAINE, J. A. (1967). In *Hormones in Blood*, Second Ed. Vol. I, p. 273, Eds. Gray, C. H. and Bacharach, A. L. New York: Academic Press. *In press.*
APOSTOLAKIS, M., BECKER, H. & VOIGT, K. D. (1966). *Steroids,* **7,** 146.
BAGSHAWE, K. D., WILDE, C. E. & ORR, A. H. (1966). *Lancet, i,* 1118.
BECKER, K. L. & ALBERT, A. (1965). *J. Clin. Endocrinol. Metab.* **25,** 962.
BELL, E. T. & LORAINE, J. A. (1965). *Lancet, i,* 1029.
BELL, E. T., BROWN, J. B., FOTHERBY, K. & LORAINE, J. A. (1962). *Lancet, ii,* 528.
BELL, E. T., MUKERJI, S., LORAINE, J. A. & LUNN, S. F. (1966). *Acta Endocrinol.* **51,** 578.
BORTH, R. (1967). *Vitamins Hormones,* **24.** *In press.*
BORTH, R., LUNENFELD, B. & DE WATTEVILLE, H. (1957). *Fertility Sterility,* **8,** 233.
BROOKS, R. V. (1964). *Steroids* **4,** 117.
BROWN, J. B. (1955 a). *Lancet, i,* 320.
BROWN, J. B. (1955 b). *Biochem. J.* **60,** 185.
BROWN, J. B., KLOPPER, A. & LORAINE, J. A. (1958). *J. Endocrinol.* **17,** 401.
BROWN, P. S. (1959). *J. Endocrinol.* **18,** 46.
CAMACHO, A. M. & MIGEON, C. J. (1963). *J. Clin. Endocrinol. Metab.* **23,** 301.
DULMANIS, A., COGHLAN, J. P., WINTOUR, M. & HUDSON, B. (1964). *Australian J. Exp. Biol. Med. Sci.* **42,** 385.
EECHAUTE, W. & DEMEESTER, C. (1965). *J. Clin. Endocrinol. Metab.* **25,** 480.
FOTHERBY, K. (1960). *Brit. Med. J.* **1,** 1545.
FOTHERBY, K. (1962). *J. Endocrinol.* **25,** 19.
FRANCHIMONT, P. (1966). *Le Dosage des Hormones Hypophysaires Somatotrope et Gonadotropes et son Application en Clinique.* Brussels: Editions Arscia S.A.
FUKUSHIMA, D. K., BRADLOW, H. L., HELLMAN, L. & GALLAGHER, T. F. (1963). *J. Clin. Endocrinol. Metab.* **23,** 266.
FUKUSHIMA, M., STEVENS, V. C., GANTT, C. L. & VORYS, N. (1964). *J. Clin. Endocrinol. Metab.* **24,** 205.
FUTTERWEIT, W., MCNIVEN, N. L., NARCUS, L., LANTOS, C., DROSDOWSKY, M. & DORFMAN, R. I. (1963). *Steroids,* **1,** 628.
HUDSON, B., COGHLAN, J., DULMANIS, A., WINTOUR, M. & EKKEL, I. (1963). *Australian J. Exp. Biol. Med. Sci.* **41,** 235.
IBAYASHI, H., NAKAMURA, M., MURAKAWA, S., UCHIKAWA, T., TANIOKA, T. & NAKAO, K. (1964). *Steroids,* **3,** 559.
ICHII, S., FORCHIELLI, E., PERLOFF, W. H. & DORFMAN, R. I. (1963). *Anal. Biochem.* **5,** 422.
ISMAIL, A. A. A. & HARKNESS, R. A. (1966 a). *Biochem. J.* **99,** 717.
ISMAIL, A. A. A. & HARKNESS, R. A. (1966 b). *J. Endocrinol.* **34,** xvii.
ISMAIL, A. A. A., HARKNESS, R. A. & LORAINE, J. A. (1968). *Acta Endocrinol. In press.*
ITTRICH, G. (1960). *Acta Endocrinol.* **35,** 34.
JOHNSEN, S. G. (1959). *Acta Endocrinol.* **31,** 209.
KELLER, P. J. (1966). *Acta Endocrinol.* **52,** 341.
KELLER, P. J. & ROSEMBERG, E. (1965). *J. Clin. Endocrinol. Metab.* **25,** 1050.
KLINEFELTER, H. F., Jr., ALBRIGHT, F. & GRISWOLD, G. C. (1943). *J. Clin. Endocrinol. Metab.* **3,** 529.
KLOPPER, A. (1957). *J. Obstet. Gynaecol. Brit. Empire,* **64,** 504.
KLOPPER, A., MICHIE, E. A. & BROWN, J. B. (1955). *J. Endocrinol.* **12,** 209.
LIM, N. Y. & DINGMAN, J. F. (1965). *J. Clin. Endocrinol. Metab.* **25,** 563.
LOBOTSKY, J., WYSS, H. I., SEGRE, E. J. & LLOYD, C. W. (1964). *J. Clin. Endocrinol. Metab.* **24,** 1261.

LORAINE, J. A. (1962). *Rev. Iberica Endocrinol.* **9,** 7.
LORAINE, J. A. & BELL, E. T. (1963). *Lancet,* i, 1340.
LORAINE, J. A. & BELL, E. T. (1966). *Hormone Assays and their Clinical Application.* Second ed. Edinburgh: Livingstone.
LORAINE, J. A. & BELL, E. T. (1967 a). *Obstet. Gynecol. Surv.* **22,** 463.
LORAINE, J. A. & BELL, E. T. (1967 b). In *Genital Abnormalities.* Eds. Rashad, M. N. & Morton W. R. M. Thomas: Springfield. *In press.*
McARTHUR, J. W., WORCESTER, J. & INGERSOLL, F. M. (1958). *J. Clin. Endocrinol. Metab.* **18,** 1186.
MIDGLEY, A. R., Jr. (1966). *Endocrinology* **79,** 10.
MIDGLEY, A. R., Jr. & JAFFE, R. B. (1966). *J. Clin. Endocrinol. Metab.* **26,** 1375.
MOLEN, H. J. van der, RUNNEBAUM, B., NISHIZAWA, E. E., KRISTENSEN, E., KIRSCHBAUM, T., WIEST, W. G. & EIK-NES, K. B. (1965). *J. Clin. Endocrinol. Metab.* **25,** 170.
NOCKE, W. & BREUER, H. (1963). *Acta Endocrinol.* **44,** 47.
ODELL, W. D., ROSS, G. T. & RAYFORD, P. L. (1967). *J. Clin. Investig.* **46,** 248.
OERTEL, G. W., BECKMANN, I. N. & EIK-NES, K. B. (1960). *Arch. Biochem.* **86,** 148.
PEDERSEN-BJERGAARD, K. & TØNNESEN, M. (1948). *Acta Endocrinol.* **1,** 38.
PICKETT, M. T. & SOMMERVILLE, I. F. (1962). *Acta Endocrinol.* **41,** 135.
RIONDEL, A., TAIT, J. F., GUT, M., TAIT, S. A. S., JOACHIM, E. & LITTLE, B. (1963). *J. Clin. Endocrinol. Metab.* **23,** 620.
ROSEMBERG, E. & KELLER, P. J. (1965). *J. Clin. Endocrinol. Metab.* **25,** 1262.
ROSNER, J. M., CONTE, N. F., BRIGGS, J. H., CHAO, P. Y., SUDMAN, E. M. & FORSHAM, P. H. (1965). *J. Clin. Endocrinol. Metab.* **25,** 95.
ROY, E. J. (1962). *J. Endocrinol.* **25,** 361.
ROY, E. J., HARKNESS, R. A. & KERR, M. G. (1965). *J. Endocrinol.* **31,** 177.
RUNNEBAUM, B., MOLEN, H. J. VAN DER & ZANDER, J. (1965). *Steroids Suppl.* **2,** 189.
RUNNEBAUM, B. & ZANDER, J. (1967). *Acta Endocrinol.* **55,** 91.
SATO, T., GREENBLATT, R. B. & MAHESH, V. B. (1965). *Fertility Sterility,* **16,** 223.
STEVENS, V. C. (1967). In *Recent Research on Gonadotrophic Hormones,* p. 223. Eds. Bell, E. T. and Loraine, J. A. Edinburgh: Livingstone.
SVENDSEN, R. (1960). *Acta Endocrinol.* **35,** 161.
SVENDSEN, R. & SØRENSEN, B. (1964). *Acta Endocrinol.* **47,** 245.
TAYMOR, M. L. (1967). In *Recent Research on Gonadotrophic Hormones* p. 229. Eds. Bell, E. T. and Loraine, J. A. Edinburgh: Livingstone.
VERMEULEN, A. & VERPLANCKE, J. C. M. (1963). *Steroids,* **2,** 453.
VOIGT, K. D., VOLKWEIN, U. & TAMM, J. (1964). *Klin. Wochschr.* **42,** 642.
WIDE, L. (1966). In *Ovulation,* p. 283. Ed. Greenblatt, R. B. Lippincott: Philadelphia.
WIDE, L. & GEMZELL, C. A. (1962). *Acta Endocrinol.* **39,** 539.
WOLF, A. (1966). *Nature* **211,** 942.
WOOLEVER, C. A. (1963). *Am. J. Obstet. Gynecol.* **84,** 981.
WOOLEVER, C. A. & GOLDFIEN, A. (1963). *Intern. J. Appl. Radiation Isotopes* **14,** 163.
ZURBRÜGG, R. P., JACOBS, R. D. B. & GARDNER, L. I. (1965). *J. Clin. Endocrinol. Metab.* **25,** 315.

CHAPTER V

Other Hormonal Effects during the Normal Menstrual Cycle

INTRODUCTION

IN the previous chapter consideration was given to endocrine function in normally menstruating women, such activity being assessed by the estimation of hormones and their metabolites in body fluids. This chapter deals with other effects produced by the secretion of biologically active substances from the endocrine glands, especially the anterior pituitary and the ovaries. Four important indices of this type are discussed, namely effects on endometrial histology, vaginal cytology, cervical mucus and basal body temperature.

It is well recognised that, in addition to the four effects mentioned above, alterations in many other parameters take place during the menstrual cycle. These include changes in pulse and respiratory rate, blood pressure, breast development, oral cytology, skin pigmentation and permeability, gastric motility and the central nervous system ; in addition, there occur characteristic alterations in the formed elements of the blood and in the biochemical composition of blood and urine. However, none of the indices in this latter category is capable of providing data by means of which the menstrual cycle can be accurately dated, and, in view of this fact, a detailed discussion of such parameters is not merited within the terms of reference of this book.

The literature contains a number of review articles dealing with physiological changes characteristic of the normal menstrual cycle. Two of the more comprehensive of these are publications by Speck (1959) and Southam and Gonzaga (1965) to which the reader is referred for further information on some of the topics considered in the present chapter.

ENDOMETRIAL BIOPSIES

There has been little new work on endometrial patterns during the normal menstrual cycle since a number of classical monographs were published during the 1930's and 1940's (see Bartelmez, 1931 ; Rock and Bartlett, 1937 ; Hertig, 1946 ; Reynolds, 1947 ; Papanicolaou et al., 1948). More recent review articles and books dealing with the topic include contributions by Hamilton et al. (1963), Novak and Woodruff (1962), Browne and McClure Browne (1964) and Noyes (1966).

The system whereby an endometrial biopsy could be dated according to the time of the cycle was originally developed by Rock and Bartlett (1937) and was later modified by various investigators including Hertig (1946) and Noyes et al. (1950). Endometrial changes throughout the cycle are now well documented and for detailed information on this subject the appropriate monographs and textbooks should be consulted. The ensuing discussion will be confined to a description of representative endometrial patterns at four different times of the cycle, namely menstruation itself, the proliferative phase, the early secretory phase immediately after ovulation and the late secretory phase.

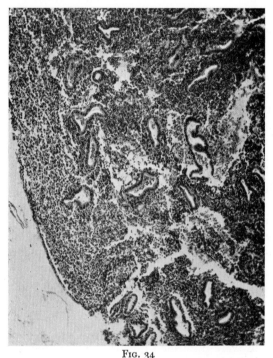

FIG. 34
Endometrial biopsy obtained during menstruation.
(From Browne and McClure Browne, 1964.)

In Figure 34 are shown the histological changes in an endometrium obtained from a subject during menstruation. The main feature is disintegration of the lining of the uterus, and in women with regular cycles of normal length this process lasts from the first to the fourth or fifth day of the cycle. During this time the greater part of the endometrium is sloughed off including most of the superficial, " functional " or spongy zone. Repair occurs rapidly, regeneration being generally complete within 48 hours of the cessation of menstruation. The process of repair consists essentially of an outgrowth of epithelium from the lower basal layers of the endometrium.

An example of an endometrium obtained during the proliferative phase of the cycle is shown in Figure 35. This phase starts immediately after menstruation has ceased and

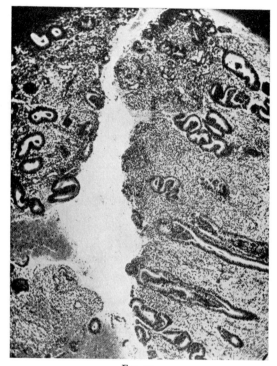

FIG. 35
Endometrial biopsy obtained during the proliferative phase.
(From Browne and McClure Browne, 1964.)

lasts until the occurrence of ovulation at or about midcycle. During it the vascularity of the endometrium increases while the cells constituting the glandular epithelium become longer and more sinuous. In the earlier part of the phase the nuclei of the cells lining the glands show the presence of numerous mitotic figures ; by its end the number of mitotic figures has decreased considerably, and there is some stromal oedema. As a consequence of these changes the endometrium becomes thicker.

One of the earliest signs that ovulation has taken place is the appearance of the subnuclear vacuole in the cells of the columnar epithelium ; this change is well illustrated in Figure 36. The vacuole is produced by the migration of the nucleus towards the lumen of the gland, resulting in the formation of a clear zone below the nucleus. For the first time

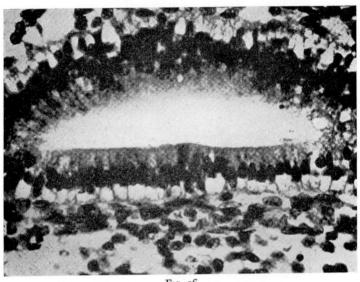

FIG. 36

Endometrial biopsy obtained immediately following ovulation and showing subnuclear vacuolation.

(From Novak and Woodruff, 1962.)

during the cycle the influence of progesterone becomes important, and as a consequence of the action of this hormone, the glands become increasingly convoluted and tortuous.

A typical endometrium obtained on the 20th day of the cycle during the secretory phase is shown in Figure 37. The main features to note are the marked tortuosity of the glands together with the secretory nature of the epithelium.

Recently a detailed description of the changes in the endometrium during the secretory phase of the normal cycle has been given by Noyes (1966). On the sixth day of the phase the main characteristics are the presence of large glands distended with intraluminal secretion, the absence of the sub-nuclear vacuole and the appearance of stromal oedema. By day 7 stromal oedema has become more pronounced ; this reaches its maximum on day 8 and thereafter is replaced by the so-called predecidua. The first change characteristic of the

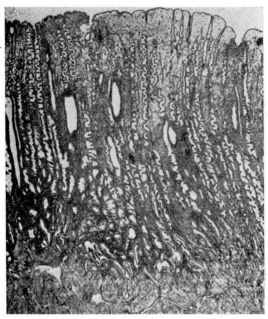

FIG. 37
Endometrial biopsy obtained during the secretory phase.
(From Novak and Woodruff, 1962.)

predecidua takes place around the spiral arterioles which by day 10 show the presence of the predecidual " cuffs " by then several cell layers thick. Day 11 sees the appearance of predecidual cells under the surface epithelium, together with the coalescence of the peri-arteriolar cuffs ; by day 12 the predecidua is virtually solid. On day 13 leucocytes can be detected in the endometrium and red blood cells make their appearance in the stroma. These changes occur immediately prior to menstruation which frequently commences on the 14th day of the secretory phase. Figure 38 is taken from a paper by Noyes (1966) and presents some of the morphological changes

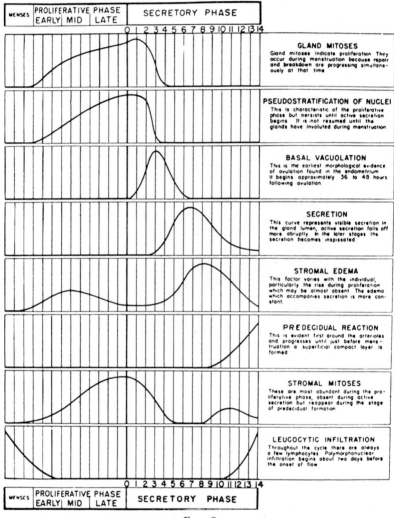

FIG. 38

Some morphological changes in the endometrium during the menstrual cycle.

(From Noyes, 1966.)

occurring during the normal menstrual cycle. The figure is constructed on the assumption that the length of the cycle is 28 days.

CERVICAL MUCUS

Cervical mucus is the secretion of the glands of the cervix uteri. It is a viscous fluid, which is alkaline in pH, and varies in quantity at different stages of the cycle. The fluid is most copious at ovulation at which time it becomes clear, less viscous, acellular and more readily penetrable by spermatozoa. Changes in the cervical mucus are mainly under the control of the oestrogenic hormones and are absent in women in whom ovarian function is lacking.

For many years alterations in cervical mucus have been used clinically in the investigation of patients with problems of infertility (see Zondek, 1957 ; Israel, 1959 for reviews). The five indices most widely employed have been *weight, viscosity, arborisation (ferning), protein content* and *chloride content,* and it is with these parameters that the present section is concerned.

1. Weight

Various investigators including Viergiver and Pommerenke (1944) and more recently McArthur (1967) have studied changes in cervical mucus weight during the menstrual cycle. Figure 39, taken from a paper by Viergiver and Pommerenke (1944), illustrates the relationship between the weight of the

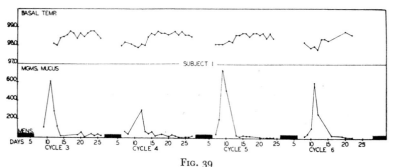

Fig. 39

Relationship between cervical mucus weight and basal body temperature in four menstrual cycles in the same subject.

(From Viergiver and Pommerenke, 1944.)

cervical mucus and basal body temperature readings in four ovulatory menstrual cycles. It will be noted that mucus weight was at its maximum at or about the time of ovulation, the highest figure being encountered just before the rise in basal body temperature. At the time of writing the consensus of opinion is that changes in cervical mucus weight provide a more reliable indication of the occurrence of ovulation than do alterations in other characteristics of the mucus such as " *spinnbarkeit* " and arborisation.

2. Viscosity

Clift (1945) has carefully reviewed the changes taking place in the viscosity of the cervical mucus at different stages of the cycle, and for those especially interested in this subject his paper should be consulted. Three indices are generally included under the heading of viscosity, viz. " *spinnbarkeit* ", *elastic recoil* and " *tack* ".

(*a*) " SPINNBARKEIT ". The English equivalent for this term is " stringiness " and by it is meant the capacity of the mucus to be drawn into threads. The phenomenon is well illustrated in Figure 40. " Spinnbarkeit " is at its maximum at the time of ovulation and is absent during pregnancy.

(*b*) ELASTIC RECOIL. This property is measured by means of an instrument known as a menstroscope (see Figure 41). The menstroscope consists of a graduated glass tube 10 cm. in length and calibrated in mm. One end of the tube fits on to a syringe, a small side tube being interposed between the end of the instrument and the syringe. The side tube is kept closed by the finger and the mucus is drawn up the capillary until it reaches the 7 cm. mark. The column of mucus is now forced down the tube until the meniscus reaches the mark at 4 cm. At this point the finger is rapidly removed from the side tube ; this releases the pressure on the column of mucus, and, because of the elasticity of the latter, the meniscus is forced along the tube. The amount of recoil can then be measured in mm.

Clift (1945) has investigated in detail the relationship of elastic recoil of the cervical mucus to the stage of the menstrual cycle. He noted a characteristic pattern in normal subjects, recoil rising to a maximum at or about midcycle.

(c) " TACK ". This is a form of stickiness present only in pregnancy. It is measured by rapidly removing a cover slip from a blob of cervical mucus placed on a glass slide. When this is done the mucus does not form long threads as in the non-pregnant subject ; instead the entire surface of the blob

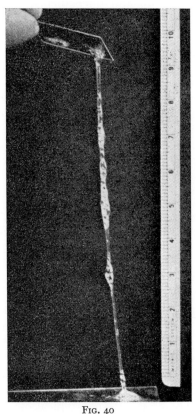

FIG. 40

Diagram illustrating "spinnbarkeit" in relation to cervical mucus.

(From Cohen, 1966.)

adheres to the cover slip and separates with difficulty from the slide. A pregnancy test depending on the altered properties of the cervical mucus in which " tack " is present but elastic recoil and spinnbarkeit are absent has been proposed but has not found wide acceptance.

3. Arborisation

In 1946 Papanicolaou noted that crystallisation of cervical mucus sometimes occurred when the latter was dried on a slide and that this effect was absent during pregnancy. Subsequently Rydberg (1949) described this crystallisation as resembling fern leaves, and since then the phenomenon has been referred to as cervical mucus ferning or arborisation. Da Paz (1951) and others have demonstrated that ferning is associated with the occurrence of ovulation, is produced by the administration of oestrogens and is inhibited by progesterone therapy.

A satisfactory description of the fern test has been provided by Riley (1959). Typical ferning is characterised by frond-like patterns of crystallisation, these being shown in Figure 42a. Such patterns are most conspicuous for a period ranging from 4 to 7 days at or about the time of ovulation. During the

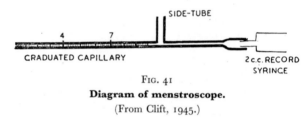

FIG. 41

Diagram of menstroscope.

(From Clift, 1945.)

early follicular phase partial ferning may be observed (see Figure 42b) ; at these times non-crystallising mucus is present together with cellular material. Lack of crystallisation of the cervical mucus is characterised by the absence of any fern-like structures, by the presence of numerous mucosal cells and sometimes by the appearance of craters formed by the collapse of air bubbles. Such a pattern is typical of patients in whom ovarian function is lacking.

4. Protein Content

Studies on the protein content of the cervical mucus have been performed by various investigators among whom are Neuhaus and his colleagues (Moghissi and Neuhaus, 1962, 1966 ; Moghissi *et al.*, 1960 ; Neuhaus and Moghissi, 1962), Heinen (1962) and Schumacher *et al.* (1965). A recent publication in this field is that of Moghissi and Neuhaus (1966)

who separated the proteins by electrophoresis using the dilute
agar gel method of Zak *et al.* (1960) and estimated albumen,
globulin and indigenous mucoids throughout the normal
menstrual cycle. They noted that prior to ovulation there
occurred a marked decrease in albumen content, this being
associated with a rise in mucoid concentration ; shortly after
ovulation these changes were reversed. No marked variations

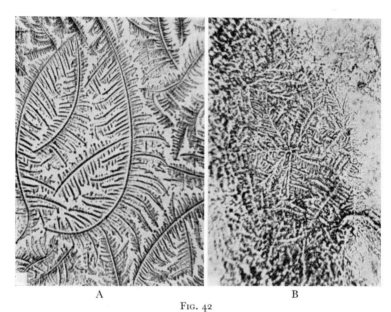

A   B

FIG. 42

**Cervical mucus arborisation during the normal menstrual
cycle.**

Left of diagram (a) at approximately midcycle ; right of diagram
(b) during the early follicular phase. (From Riley, 1959.)

in the globulin content of the cervical mucus were observed
during the cycle. In Figure 43 are shown typical results of the
studies conducted by Moghissi and Neuhaus (1966).

Alterations in the albumen and mucoid content of cervical
mucus are believed to result from the secretion of oestrogens
and progesterone from the ovaries. Such changes vary greatly
from one individual to another and have not been found to be
useful in determining the precise time of ovulation.

5. Sodium Chloride Content

Important recent papers on this subject are those of McSweeney and Sbarra (1964, 1965) and Herzberg *et al.* (1964). Slightly different methods for the estimation of chloride content were used by the two groups. The technique of McSweeney and Sbarra (1964, 1965) involved taking a smear of cervical mucus directly from the canal and rubbing the smear onto a test paper previously impregnated with silver nitrate and potassium chromate. In the presence of chloride ions a precipitate of silver chromate appeared as a white or buff coloured spot; for the final determination the colour

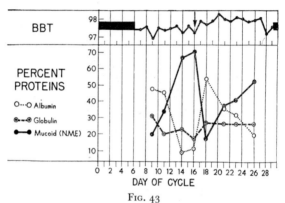

Fɪɢ. 43

Protein content of cervical mucus during the menstrual cycle.

(From Moghissi and Neuhaus, 1966.)

produced was compared with that of a set of standards. In the method of Herzberg *et al.* (1964) the sodium chloride content of the fresh or dried cervical mucus was measured by titration with mercuric nitrate.

In the experience of Herzberg *et al.* (1964) the chloride content of fresh mucus does not change throughout the cycle. However, if dried mucus is used alternations do occur, a sharp peak in chloride content being found at or about the time of ovulation. Figure 44 illustrates results obtained in a single subject studied during three consecutive cycles in which the highest chloride levels were associated with the lowest point of the temperature record.

In Figure 45 are shown comparable data obtained by McSweeney and Sbarra (1964). It will be noted that the pattern of chloride content is somewhat different to that reported by Herzberg *et al.* (1964) there being a tendency for the chloride content to increase before ovulation and to fall immediately after this event.

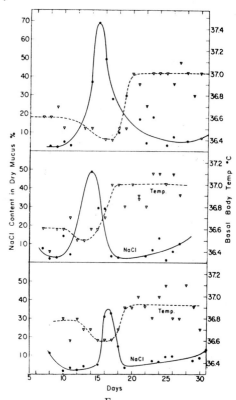

FIG. 44

Sodium chloride content of cervical mucus and basal body temperature readings in three consecutive cycles.
(From Herzberg *et al.*, 1964.)

VAGINAL CYTOLOGY

The literature contains numerous reviews dealing with changes in vaginal cytology during the menstrual cycle. Among the more comprehensive of these are articles by De Allende and Orías (1950), Riley (1959), Frost (1962),

Rakoff (1966) and Hughes and Dodds (1968). Much of the present section is based on a recent paper by Rakoff (1966).

An account will first be given of the cell types in the vaginal smear, together with the cytological indices used. Subsequently alterations in vaginal cytology characteristic of the normal menstrual cycle will be described ; a short section is also included on changes in vaginal cytology in patients with

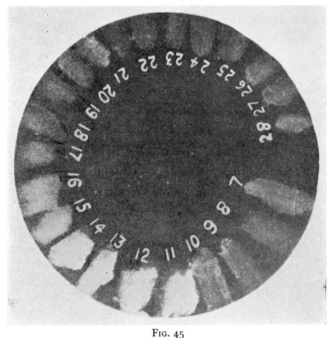

FIG. 45
**Sodium chloride content of cervical mucus from day 7 to 28
of the menstrual cycle.**
(From McSweeney and Sbarra, 1964.)

carcinoma of the cervix. No review of this subject would be complete without emphasising the great importance of technical factors both in taking and in staining such smears (see Frost, 1962 ; Rakoff, 1966 ; Hughes and Dodds, 1967, for details).

1. Cell Types in the Vaginal Smear
Three main types are of importance designated respectively *parabasal*, *intermediate* and *superficial* cells.

(*a*) *Parabasal cells* are small and round and contain nuclei which are relatively large in relation to their cytoplasm. The cytoplasm itself is generally cyanophilic.

(*b*) *Intermediate cells* are ovoid or polygonal in shape being smaller than the superficial cells (*c*). Their nuclei are vesicular and their cytoplasm generally cyanophilic.

(*c*) *Superficial cells* are flattened and polygonal in shape, with relatively small nuclei. Those with pyknotic nuclei are known as *cornified or karyopyknotic* cells. They generally show an eosinophilic cytoplasm. Cells with vesicular nuclei are termed *precornified* ; their cytoplasm is usually cyanophilic.

2. Cytological Indices

(*a*) THE MATURATION INDEX. This is essentially a differential count of parabasal, intermediate and superficial cells. Usually one hundred cells are counted on a random basis and a percentage is calculated of the various types seen. The maturation index, as its name implies, provides a measurement of the degree of development of the vaginal mucosa. It is of especial value in estimating the oestrogenic activity of body fluids and in assessing ovarian function in health and disease.

(*b*) THE KARYOPYKNOTIC INDEX. This can be estimated when the vaginal smear is made up predominantly of pre-cornified and cornified cells. Under such circumstances the percentage of superficial cells with pyknotic nuclei irrespective of the staining reaction of the cytoplasm is believed to provide an accurate assessment of the degree of oestrogenic activity in body fluids. In normally menstruating women serial estimations of the karyopyknotic index have proved of value in demonstrating the increase in oestrogenic activity which occurs during the follicular phase of the cycle and which culminates in a peak at or about midcycle.

(*c*) THE EOSINOPHILIC INDEX. The proportion of superficial cells showing eosinophilic staining of their cytoplasm is directly proportional to the degree of oestrogenic activity of body fluids and has been used to measure such activity. The index is maximal at or about the time of ovulation. Care is necessary in interpreting calculations of the eosinophilic index because of the well recognised fact that such cytoplasmic changes may be nonspecific in nature and may be caused by the presence of inflammatory changes or even by purely mechanical factors such as the drying of the smear on the slide.

(d) REGRESSIVE CHANGES. These are seen during the luteal phase of the cycle and are essentially nonspecific in character. Quantitative assessment of such changes is a matter of considerable difficulty. Several parameters have been suggested including the " folded cell index ", which is a count of the proportion of cells showing definite folding, and the " clustered cell index " which attempts to estimate the number of large clusters of cells. Frequently regressive changes are designated on a purely subjective basis as " slight ", " moderate " or " marked ".

3. Cytological Changes during the Menstrual Cycle

These have been carefully documented by many investigators, and the present account is based on the excellent description of De Allende and Orías (1950). Examples of typical smears from early follicular, ovulatory and luteal phases are shown in Figures 46 to 48.

(a) EARLY FOLLICULAR PHASE (Figure 46). The smear was taken on the 9th day of the cycle. The cells are somewhat dispersed and have smooth edges. Some 12 per cent are cornified, the remainder being mainly intermediate in type. The number of leucocytes is small.

(b) OVULATORY PHASE (Figure 47). This is a characteristic " follicular " smear obtained on the 15th day of the cycle. There are many large, smooth, well-separated, cornified cells (73 per cent) ; a moderate degree of leucocytosis is present.

(c) LUTEAL PHASE (Figure 48). This smear was obtained on day 25 and shows clumped cells with folded edges and a wrinkled cytoplasm. Eighteen per cent of the cells are cornified, the remainder being mainly intermediate in type.

A summary of the changes illustrated in Figures 46 to 48 is given in Figure 49.

4. Vaginal Cytology in Relation to Carcinoma of the Uterus

In 1943 Papanicolaou and Traut suggested that alterations in vaginal cytology might be of value in the diagnosis of

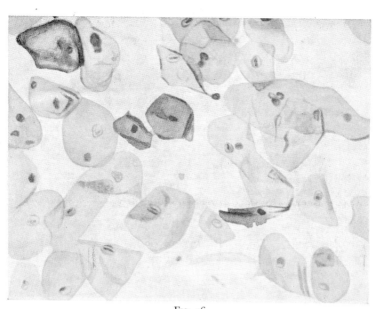

Fig. 46
Vaginal cytology during the early follicular phase.
(From De Allende and Orías, 1950.)

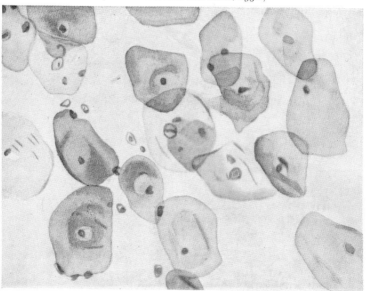

Fig. 47
Vaginal cytology at the time of ovulation.
(From De Allende and Orías, 1950.)

[To face page 124

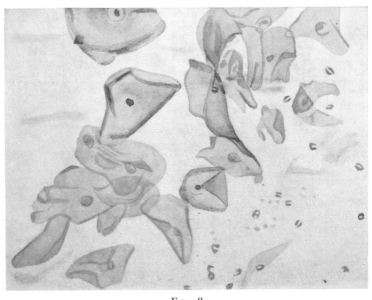

FIG. 48

Vaginal cytology during the luteal phase.
(From De Allende and Orías, 1950.)

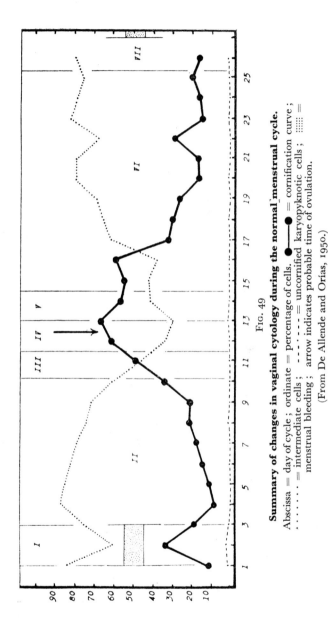

Summary of changes in vaginal cytology during the normal menstrual cycle.

Abscissa = day of cycle; ordinate = percentage of cells. ——— = cornification curve;
•••••• = intermediate cells; - - - - - = uncornified karyopyknotic cells; ⫶⫶⫶⫶ =
menstrual bleeding; arrow indicates probable time of ovulation.

(From De Allende and Orías, 1950.)

Fig. 49

carcinoma of the cervix in women. In the intervening years this suggestion has been amply confirmed by numerous investigators. A consideration of the cytological changes occurring in carcinoma of the cervix and uterus is outside the scope of this book, and for relevant information the reader should consult review articles by Gates and Warren (1950), Papanicolaou (1954) and Riley (1959). The classification of vaginal smears originally proposed by Papanicolaou remains of great value and is as follows :

Class I   Normal cells only.

Class II   Atypical cells which are not carcinomatous in type.

Class III Cells sufficiently " suspicious " to suggest malignant disease.

Class IV   Abnormal cells characteristic of malignant disease.

Class V   Many cells showing marked deviation from normality and leaving little doubt that a malignant change has occurred.

URINARY CYTOLOGY

Detailed studies of urinary cytology during the normal menstrual cycle have been published by del Castillo *et al.* (1948, 1949), Castellanos and Sturgis (1958, 1963) and Vincze *et al.* (1959). One of the most comprehensive accounts of this subject is that of Castellanos and Sturgis (1963) on which the present section is mainly based.

All investigators agree that the technique of collection of the sample is of prime importance in studies of urinary cytology. It is recommended that an aliquot of a first morning urine sample should be used and that the specimen should be brought to the laboratory within six hours ; in the event of delay alcohol should be added to the urine as a preservative. The specimen is centrifuged, the supernatant fluid decanted and the sediment is smeared on a slide, onto which a thin layer of albumen has previously been placed. When the smear is almost dry it is fixed in an alcohol-ether solution and is then stained by Shorr's technique. The latter stains epithelial cells, the characteristics of which are the same as those already described for the vagina (see p. 122) ; in addition, the crystals, bacteria, leucocytes and mucus present in urinary sediments are stained.

The typical cytological pattern obtained from urinary sediment during the normal menstrual cycle is shown in Figure 50. The most prominent changes are in the cornified cells, the percentage of which starts to rise on day 6 and reaches a peak on the 14th day of the cycle ; this peak is thought to be related to the occurrence of ovulation. During the luteal phase the count of cornified cells drops, the percentage being at its minimum prior to the onset of the next menstruation. It must be emphasised that the results in Figure 50 are illustrative of a so-called " classical cycle " and in many other subjects studied in a similar manner the percentage of cornified cells does not show such a distinctive pattern.

During the follicular phase of the cycle the cytoplasm of the cells tends to be smooth and the cells themselves are evenly distributed over the slide. Two or three days following the presumed date of ovulation the cells begin to show clumping, and at this time their edges become folded and their cytoplasm wrinkled. The majority of the intermediate cells increase in length and the characteristic " tadpole " cells make their appearance, these being analogous to the " navicular " cells of the vaginal smear originally described by Papanicolaou et al. (1948). In contrast to the findings when vaginal smears are taken, leucocytic infiltration is not a characteristic feature of urinary sediment obtained during the luteal phase of the cycle.

It is generally accepted that a single urinary smear cannot provide evidence that ovulation has occurred. At present, the consensus of opinion is that the minimum requirement in this respect is the collection of a series of at least five smears taken a few days apart but concentrated mainly at midcycle.

BASAL BODY TEMPERATURE

The biphasic changes in the body temperature which occur during the normal menstrual cycle were known in the nineteenth century (see Von Fricke, 1838 ; Goodman, 1878 ; Reinl, 1887 ; Giles, 1897), and in 1904 Van de Velde suggested that ovulation took place at the time of the decrease in temperature

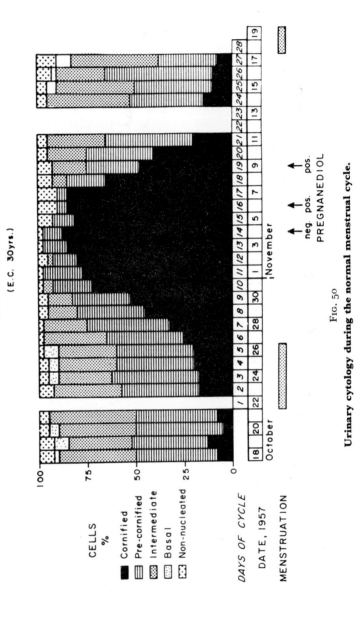

Fig. 50

Urinary cytology during the normal menstrual cycle.

(From Castellanos and Sturgis, 1958.)

which preceded the raised luteal phase plateau. The literature on the subject of basal temperature is now very extensive indeed, and important review articles include those of Siegler (1945), Tompkins (1944, 1945), Geller (1960, 1961 *a b*) and Southam and Gonzaga (1965). It is generally agreed that the characteristic changes in temperature are most marked when the latter is taken under basal conditions, and that readings based on rectal, oral and vaginal temperatures are equally reliable (see Halbrecht, 1947). Recently, Adducci *et al.* (1965) have suggested that cranial temperature readings may provide a more accurate assessment of body temperature than either oral or rectal measurements.

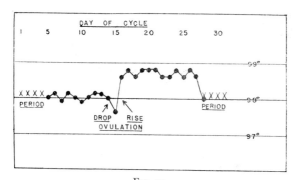

FIG. 51

Idealised basal body temperature record during the normal menstrual cycle.

(From Tomkins, 1945, *J. Obstet. Gynaecol. Brit. Empire.*)

In Figure 51 is shown an idealised basal temperature chart illustrating the changes which occur during a 28 day cycle. It will be noted that levels are relatively low following menstruation, that a slight drop in temperature occurs some fourteen days before the next menstrual period and that the drop is followed by an abrupt rise, high levels being maintained until the next menstrual period when a marked decrease occurs. There is now general agreement that the major factor responsible for the increase in basal temperature at midcycle is the ovarian hormone, progesterone (see Southam and Gonzaga, 1965 for references). The length of the basal temperature plateau is generally 14 days ; however, considerable variations occur from one subject to another, and a range of from nine to seventeen days has been reported by Geller (1961 *b*). Tompkins (1945) and others have stated that, irrespective of the length of the whole cycle, the temperature shift occurs

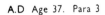

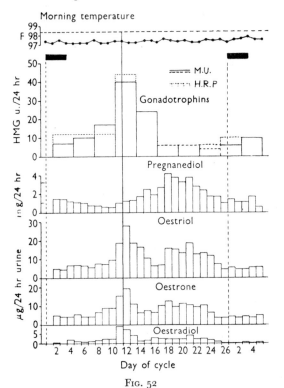

FIG. 52

Hormone excretion pattern during the normal menstrual cycle.

M.U. = mouse uterus test;   H.R.P. = Hypophysectomized rat prostate test;   ▰▰▰ = menstrual bleeding.

(From J. B. Brown *et al.*, 1958.)

approximately fourteen days before the next menstruation, and that the length of the luteal phase is relatively constant. The observation is not in agreement with findings of Bell and Loraine (1965) who estimated the time of ovulation by the midcycle peak of urinary oestrogen excretion (see also p. 79).

These investigators found that, when this parameter was used, not only was the time of ovulation very variable from one woman to another but that the length of the luteal phase also showed considerable variation, ranging from nine to seventeen days in individual subjects.

The relationship of the exact time of ovulation to the pattern of basal temperature readings remains controversial. For example, it has been suggested that ovulation may take place, (a) just before the drop in temperature, (b) precisely at the temperature nadir, (c) at the time of the temperature rise, or (d) immediately following the rise (see Speck, 1959 for references). In view of the fact that the corpus luteum represents the main source of ovarian progesterone (see p. 42), the most tenable hypothesis would appear to be that ovulation occurs just before the rise in basal temperature produced by this hormone.

Although in a reasonably high proportion of subjects basal temperature records can furnish evidence as to whether a given cycle is ovulatory or anovulatory in type, it must be emphasised that in individual cases the information provided by this method may sometimes be misleading. This point is well illustrated by the results presented in Figures 52 and 119. In the woman shown in Figure 52 ovulation, judged by the pattern of urinary oestrogen and pregnanediol excretion, certainly occurred ; however, in spite of this, the basal temperature chart was monophasic. Conversely, in the subject shown in Figure 119 (see p. 290) who was treated with the oral contraceptive, norethisterone acetate, a biphasic temperature chart was encountered in the second treatment cycle although this was certainly anovulatory on the basis of urinary steroid assays.

As is well known basal temperature records form the basis of the so-called " rhythm method " of contraception favoured by the Roman Catholic Church. P. F. E. Brown (1965) has recently reported studies with this technique. According to him the infertile phase of the cycle generally commences after the basal temperature reading has been elevated for three days during the luteal phase. The results in one of his subjects are shown in Figure 53 in whom there was a 28 day cycle with the preovulatory phase extending from days 1 to 13. The

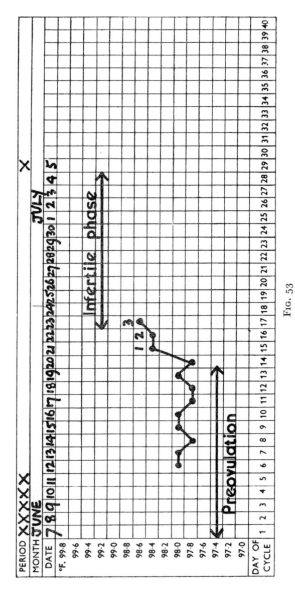

FIG. 53

Basal body temperature readings in a normally menstruating woman showing the post-ovulatory rise and infertile phase.

(From P. F. E. Brown, 1965.)

post-ovulatory rise in basal body temperature commenced on day 15, and it was accordingly assumed that the infertile or " safe " period of the cycle extended from day 17 to 28. A comprehensive account of the calculations necessary in estimating the duration of the " safe " period has been given by Kleinman (1964). In Chapter XI the efficacy of various contraceptive techniques is compared, and it is emphasised that the rhythm method is inferior to many others including those depending on oral contraception and on the intra-uterine device. The limitations of the rhythm method have recently been stressed by Parkes (1965).

BODY WEIGHT

It is well recognised that changes in body weight can occur during the normal menstrual cycle, and research on this subject has been performed by numerous investigators including Thorn *et al.* (1938), Bruce and Russell (1962), Taggart (1962), Robinson and Watson (1965) and Watson and Robinson (1965). The reason for the fluctuations in body weight in menstruating women remains obscure. Thorn *et al.* (1938) believed that premenstrual weight gain was a result of retention of water, sodium and chloride. On the other hand, Klein and Carey (1957) in a careful investigation, failed to find any change either in sodium balance or in body weight during the cycle.

Probably the most detailed study of this subject is that of Watson and Robinson (1965). These workers measured body weights daily for a period of 68 days in 28 normally menstruating women all of whom were living under comparable conditions. For the purposes of their investigation the cycle was divided into eight parts i.e. the first and second halves of menstruation, the first and second halves of the follicular phase including the presumed day of ovulation, and four parts during the luteal phase. Watson and Robinson (1965) found that body weight readings increased steadily throughout the second half of the premenstrual phase, reaching their maximum during the first half of menstruation ; thereafter they fell rapidly to the low levels characteristic of the follicular phase. They observed that ovulation, based on basal temperature records, was associated with a small rise in body weight, the increase occurring just after this event had taken place. In women in whom two or more consecutive cycles were studied only minor variations in body weight from cycle to cycle were observed. Figure 54 presents the results obtained by Watson and Robinson (1965). The parameter used was the ratio δ/σ where δ is the average deviation of body weight for each part of the cycle from the mean body weight for that cycle, and σ is the standard deviation. It is apparent that the ratio was positive during the first half of menstruation, fell during the second half, and remained negative until the third quarter of the luteal phase, when it again rose and became positive.

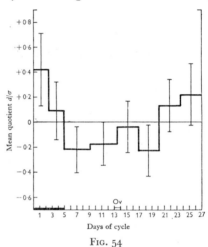

FIG. 54

Body weight changes during the normal menstrual cycle.

■■ = menstrual bleeding; Ov = ovulation (see also text). (From Watson and Robinson, 1965.)

INORGANIC CONSTITUENTS OF BLOOD

A comprehensive review of this complex subject has been given by Southam and Gonzaga (1965) to whose article the reader is referred for further details. It is claimed that levels of serum calcium rise at the time of ovulation and are somewhat lower premenstrually. On the other hand, blood concentrations of inorganic phosphorus and phosphate tend to be higher during menstruation. Consistent changes in blood copper and in serum sodium, chloride and potassium have not been noted during the normal menstrual cycle. A recent study of serum iron levels in normally menstruating women is that of Zilva and Patston (1966). These investigators found that such levels started to fall some two or three days premenstrually and continued to decrease during menstruation itself ; readings rose

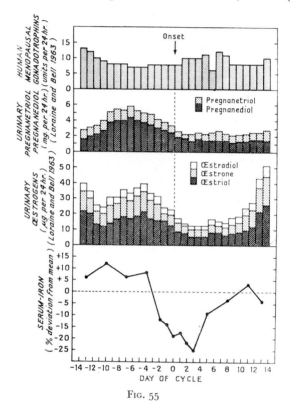

FIG. 55

Serum iron levels and hormone excretion pattern during the normal menstrual cycle.

Arrow = first day of menstruation.

(From Zilva and Patston, 1966.)

again during the follicular phase and were maximal in the early luteal phase. Relationships between serum iron levels on the one hand and those of urinary oestrogens, pregnanediol, pregnanetriol, and HPG on the other are presented in Figure 55. Zilva and Patston (1966) consider that the variations in

135

serum iron are probably hormonal in origin and do not result from haemorrhage or from alterations in the state of hydration of the subject.

SUMMARY AND CONCLUSIONS

Hormonal effects during the normal menstrual cycle are considered, special attention being given to endometrial histology, vaginal cytology, cervical mucus and basal body temperature.

Representative endometrial patterns at various stages of the cycle are described and it is emphasised that the cycle can be accurately dated in this way.

Changes in cervical mucus are considered under the headings of weight, viscosity, arborisation, and protein and sodium chloride content. Alterations in all these indices occur at or about the time of ovulation.

The cell types found in the vaginal smear together with the maturation, karyopyknotic and eosinophilic indices are described. Changes in vaginal and urinary cytology during the normal menstrual cycle are discussed, it being emphasised that the time of ovulation is associated with a marked increase in the number of cornified cells.

The pattern of basal body temperature readings during the cycle has been reviewed, and it is concluded that the rhythm method of contraception has serious limitations.

Body weight tends to rise premenstrually reaching its maximum during the first half of menstruation. Readings are low in the follicular phase of the cycle and rise slightly at or about midcycle.

REFERENCES

ADDUCCI, A. J., WEIDENKOPS, T. E. & GARWACKI, D. J. (1965). I.E.E.E. Trans. Biomed. Eng. 12, 2.

BARTELMEZ, G. W. (1931). Am. J. Obstet. Gynecol. 21, 623.

BELL, E. T. & LORAINE, J. A. (1965). Lancet, i, 1029.

BROWN, J. B., KLOPPER, A. & LORAINE, J. A. (1958). J. Endocrinol. 17, 401.

BROWN, P. F. E. (1965). Practitioner, 194, 525.

BROWNE, F. J. & McCLURE BROWNE, J. C (1964). Post Graduate Obstetrics and Gynecology, 3rd ed. London : Butterworths.

BRUCE, J. & RUSSELL, G. F. M. (1962). Lancet, ii, 267.

CASTELLANOS, H. & STURGIS, S. H. (1958). J. Clin. Endocrinol. Metab. 18, 1369.

CASTELLANOS, H. & STURGIS, S. H. (1963). In Progress in Gynecology, vol. 4, p. 98. Eds. Meigs, J. V. and Sturgis, S H. London : Heinemann.

DEL CASTILLO, E. B., ARGONZ, J. & GALLI-MAININI, C. (1948). *J. Clin. Endocrinol. Metab.* **8,** 76.
DEL CASTILLO, E. B., ARGONZ, J. & GALLI-MAININI, C. (1949). *J. Clin. Endocrinol. Metab.* **9,** 1362.
CLIFT, A. F. (1945). *Proc. Roy. Soc. Med.* **39,** 1.
COHEN, M. R. (1966). In *Ovulation*, p. 291. Ed. Greenblatt, R. B. Philadelphia : Lippincott.
DE ALLENDE, I. L. C. & ORÍAS, O. (1950). *Cytology of the Human Vagina.* New York : Hoeber-Harper.
FROST, J. K. (1962). In *Gynecologic and Obstetric Pathology*, p. 594, 5th ed. Eds. Novak, E. R. and Woodruff, J. D. Philadelphia : Saunders.
GATES, O. & WARREN, S (1950). *A Handbook for the Diagnosis of Cancer of the Uterus by the use of Vaginal Smears.* Cambridge : Harvard University Press.
GELLER, S. (1960). *La Temperature Guide de la Femme.* Paris.
GELLER, S. (1961 a). *La Courbe Thermique*, Paris.
GELLER, S. (1961 b). *Rev. Franc. Etudes Clin. Biol.* **6,** 706.
GILES, A. E. (1897). *Trans. Obstet. Soc. London,* **39,** 115.
GOODMAN, J. (1878). *Am. J. Obstet. Gynecol.* **11,** 673.
HALBRECHT, I. (1947). *J. Obstet. Gynaecol. Brit. Empire,* **54,** 848.
HAMILTON, W. J., BOYD, J. D. & MOSSMAN, H. W. (1963). *Human Embryology,* Third ed. Cambridge : Heffer.
HEINEN, G (1962) *Geburtsh. Frauenheilk,* **22,** 983.
HERTIG, A. T. (1946). In *Proc. Conf. on Diagnosis in Sterility.* Springfield : Thomas.
HERZBERG, M., JÖEL, C. A. & KATCHALSKY, A. (1964). *Fertility Sterility,* **15,** 684.
HUGHES, H. E. & DODDS, T. C. (1968). Handbook of Diagnostic Cytology. Edinburgh : Livingstone. *In press.*
ISRAEL, S. L. (1959). *Diagnosis and Treatment of Menstrual Disorders and Sterility.* New York : Hoeber.
KLEIN, L. & CAREY, J. (1957). *Am. J. Obstet. Gynecol.* **74,** 956.
KLEINMAN, R. L. (1964). *Medical Handbook on Contraception,* London : International Planned Parenthood Federation.
McARTHUR, J. W. (1967). In *Recent Research on Gonadotrophic Hormones*, p. 282. Eds. Bell, E. T. and Loraine, J. A. Edinburgh : Livingstone.
McSWEENEY, D. J. & SBARRA, A. J. (1964). *Am. J. Obstet. Gynecol.* **88,** 705.
McSWEENEY, D. J. & SBARRA, A. J. (1965). *Obstet. Gynecol.* **26,** 201.
MOGHISSI, K. S. & NEUHAUS, O. W. (1962). *Am. J. Obstet. Gynecol.* **83,** 149.
MOGHISSI, K. S. & NEUHAUS, O. W. (1966). *Am. J. Obstet. Gynecol.* **96,** 91.
MOGHISSI, K. S., NEUHAUS, O. W. & STEVENSON, C. S. (1960). *J. Clin. Invest.* **39,** 1358.
NEUHAUS, O. W. & MOGHISSI, K. S. (1962). *Fertility Sterility,* **13,** 550.
NOYES, R. W. (1966). In *Ovulation*, p. 319. Ed. Greenblatt, R. B. Philadelphia : Lippincott.
NOYES, R. W., HERTIG, A. T. & ROCK, J. (1950). *Fertility Sterility,* **1,** 3.
NOVAK, E. R. & WOODRUFF, J. D. (1962). *Gynecologic and Obstetric Pathology*, 5th ed. Philadelphia : Saunders.
PAPANICOLAOU, G. N. (1946). *Am. J. Obstet. Gynecol.* **51,** 316.
PAPANICOLAOU, G. N. (1954). *Atlas of Exfoliative Cytology.* Cambridge : Harvard University Press.
PAPANICOLAOU, G. N. & TRAUT, H. F. (1943). *Diagnosis of Cancer of the Uterus by the use of Vaginal Smears.* New York : The Commonwealth Fund.
PAPANICOLAOU, G. N., TRAUT, H. F. & MARCHETTI, A. A. (1948). *The Epithelia of Women's Reproductive Organs.* New York : The Commonwealth Fund.
PARKES, A. S. (1965). In *Public Health and Population Change*, p. 417. Eds. Sheps, M. C. and Ridley, J. C. Pittsburgh : University of Pittsburgh Press.
DA PAZ, C. A. (1951). *Am. J. Obstet. Gynecol.* **61A,** 790.
RAKOFF, A. E. (1966). In *Ovulation*, p. 299. Ed. Greenblatt, R. B. Philadelphia : Lippincott.
REINL, C. (1887). *Klin. Med. Gynäk.* **3,** 1737.
REYNOLDS, S. R. M. (1947). *J. Am. Med. Assoc.* **135,** 552.
RILEY, G. M. (1959). *Gynecologic Endocrinology.* New York : Hoeber-Harper.

ROBINSON, M. F. & WATSON, P. E. (1965). *Brit. J. Nutr.* **19,** 225.
ROCK, J. & BARTLETT, M. K. (1937). *J. Am. Med. Assoc.* **107,** 2022.
RYDBERG, E. (1949). *Acta Obstet. Gynecol. Scand.* **28,** 172.
SCHUMACHER, G. F. B., STRAUSS, E. K. & WIED, G. L. (1965). *Am. J. Obstet. Gynecol.* **91,** 1035.
SIEGLER, S. L (1945). *Fertility in Women.* London : Heinemann.
SOUTHAM, A. L. & GONZAGA, F. P. (1965). *Am. J. Obstet. Gynecol.* **91,** 142.
SPECK, G. (1959). *Obstet. Gynecol. Survey,* **14,** 798.
TAGGART, N. (1962). *Brit. J. Nutr.* **16,** 223.
THORN, G. W., NELSON, K. R. & THORN, D. W. (1938). *Endocrinology,* **22,** 155.
TOMPKINS, P. (1944). *J. Am. Med. Assoc.* **124,** 698.
TOMPKINS, P. (1945). *J. Obstet. Gynaecol. Brit. Empire,* **52,** 241.
VAN DE VELDE, E. H. (1904). Quoted by Siegler, S. L. (1945). *Fertility in Women.* London : Heinemann.
VIERGIVER, E. & POMMERENKE, W. T. (1944). *Am. J. Obstet. Gynecol.* **48,** 321.
VINCZE, L. O., TAFT, P. D. & McARTHUR, J. W. (1959,. *J. Clin. Endocrinol. Metab.* **19,** 281.
VON FRICKE, E. (1838). *Z. Ges. Med.* **9,** 289.
WATSON, P. E. & ROBINSON, M. F. (1965). *Brit. J. Nutr.* **19,** 237.
ZAK, B., VOLINI, F., BRISKI, J. & WILLIAMS, L. A. (1960). *Am. J. Clin. Path.* **33,** 75.
ZILVA, J. F. & PATSTON, V. J. (1966). *Lancet,* **i,** 459.
ZONDEK, B. (1957). In *Progress in Gynecology,* vol. 3, p. 86. Eds. Meigs, J. V. and Sturgis, S. H. London : Heinemann.

CHAPTER VI

Hormone Levels in Abnormal Gynaecological Conditions

INTRODUCTION

AT the time of writing, the literature on endogenous hormone levels in the body fluids of patients with gynaecological disorders is very limited indeed. It has been customary to attempt to evaluate endocrine function in such diseases by histological examination of the endometrium and by vaginal cytology (see Chapter V). Both of these methods of assessment are indirect in nature and frequently fail to provide accurate information on the hormonal status of the individual. A much more reliable index of endocrine activity in patients with abnormal gynaecological conditions is provided by conducting assays of hormones and their metabolites in blood and urine, and in recent years such an approach has been greatly facilitated by the improvements which have been made in methods for the quantitative determination of these substances (see Chapter III). Such improvements have been especially marked in the case of urinary assays, and as a result it is now possible to study in detail interrelationships between the various endocrine glands, with special reference to the pituitary, ovaries and adrenals. It can be confidently predicted that with the passage of time information of this type will become progressively more important, not only in elucidating the pathogenesis of gynaecological disorders, but also in developing rational as opposed to empirical forms of treatment for these diseases.

The first topic to be discussed in this chapter will be hormonal interrelationships in ovulatory menstrual cycles in which abnormalities of urinary steroid excretion are encountered. Subsequently endocrine function in abnormal gynaecological conditions will be reviewed, consideration being given in turn to anovulatory cycles, dysmenorrhoea, oligomenorrhoea, amenorrhoea, galactorrhoea, the Stein-type syndrome, dysfunctional uterine haemorrhage, ovarian tumours, cervical carcinoma and endometrial carcinoma. Mention will not be made of excretion patterns in premenstrual tension, fibroid tumours, endometriosis, cervicitis, " senile " vaginitis and the menopausal syndrome, because, at present reliable information on hormonal interrelationships in these conditions is virtually non-existent.

Two major review articles in the literature form the basis of this chapter. The first of these is the paper by Brown *et al.* (1959) in which oestrogen assays alone were reported. The second is the publication of Loraine and Bell (1967) in which excretion patterns for oestrogens, pregnanediol and HPG were investigated.

OVULATORY CYCLES WITH ABNORMAL URINARY STEROID PATTERNS

Increasing experience with serial hormone assays in women during reproductive life has emphasised the variability in steroid excretion patterns during the ovulatory menstrual cycle (see Bell and Loraine, 1967 *a*; Loraine and Bell, 1968). The aim of this section is to illustrate this fact by presenting the results obtained in five cycles from three such individuals.

The subject shown in Figure 56 gave a history of irregular periods of variable length from the age of 18. Following her marriage she was infertile, and on the basis of evidence obtained from basal temperature records a diagnosis of anovular menstruation was made. In spite of this diagnosis it will be noted that the two cycles shown in Figure 56 were ovulatory in character as judged by assays of urinary pregnanediol and pregnanetriol. The first cycle was unduly long occupying 35 days, while the second was of normal length (28 days). In the first cycle the luteal phase rise in pregnanediol output was very pronounced, the mean level during this time being approximately four times higher than that for the follicular phase ; in the second cycle the increase in pregnanediol in the luteal phase was less marked while the pattern of pregnanetriol output in both cycles did not deviate from normality.

In the first cycle the curve of oestrogen excretion was completely atypical. It is probable that ovulation, judged on the basis of oestrone and oestriol output, occurred on the 19th

Mrs N McL. AGE 33 YEARS. PARA O+O.

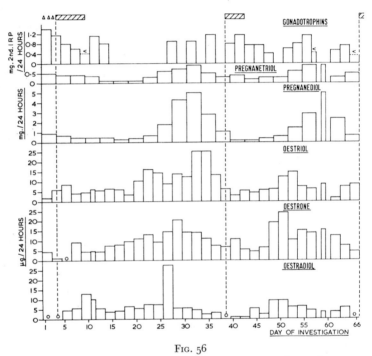

FIG. 56

Hormone excretion pattern during two consecutive cycles.

△ = spotting ; //// = menstrual bleeding.

(From Loraine and Bell 1968, *J. Obstet. Gynaecol. Brit. Commonwealth*).

or 20th day of the cycle ; this was followed by a luteal phase rise in oestriol excretion maximal on days 32 to 35 of the study. Oestradiol readings were grossly abnormal, showing high levels during menstruation and an isolated peak on days 26 and 27 ; in particular, ovulatory and luteal phase rises in oestradiol output did not occur.

In the second cycle the pattern of oestrogen excretion deviated less from normality, midcycle and luteal phase peaks for oestrone being reasonably well marked. Ovulation probably occurred on days 12 or 13 of the cycle, but following ovulation the luteal phase peaks of oestriol and oestradiol output were ill-defined. In both cycles HPG levels, measured by the mouse uterus test, were within the normal range for a woman during reproductive life ; no definite pattern of HPG excretion was observed.

The subject shown in Figure 57 had a previous history of regular 28 day menstrual cycles with bleeding lasting for four

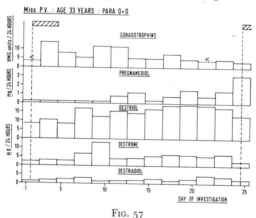

FIG. 57

Hormone excretion pattern during the menstrual cycle.

//// = menstrual bleeding.

From Loraine and Bell 1968, *J. Obstet. Gynaecol. Brit. Commonwealth*).

days. The cycle was probably ovulatory in type although the pattern of pregnanediol output was grossly abnormal. Levels of this steroid in the follicular phase were exceedingly low, and although values in the luteal phase were higher, readings still remained at the lower end of the normal range with the exception of one value of 3·12 mg. per 24 hours on days 25 and 26 of the study. The pattern of excretion of the three classical oestrogens was also atypical. Oestriol levels rose steadily until days 19 and 20 and gradually fell with the onset of menstruation. Oestrone output remained relatively constant apart from a well defined peak on days 9 and 10, while oestradiol levels remained below 5 µg. per 24 hours throughout and showed little or no fluctuation. The exact time of ovulation is difficult to estimate with accuracy, but in view of the fact that the increase in pregnanediol output commenced on days 10 and 11 of the cycle, it must be assumed that the event took place prior to this time presumably on days 8 or 9. As in

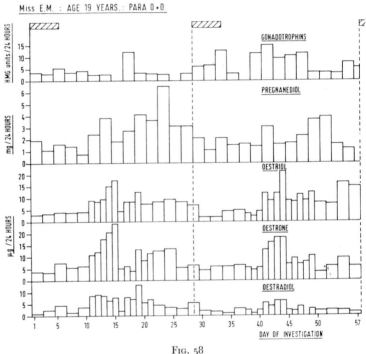

Fig. 58

Hormone excretion pattern during two consecutive menstrual cycles.

//// = menstrual bleeding.

(From Loraine and Bell 1968, *J. Obstet. Gynaecol. Brit. Commonwealth*).

Figure 56 HPG readings were within the normal range for a woman during reproductive life and failed to show any cyclic pattern.

Figure 58 presents two consecutive cycles collected from a 19 year old subject who had a previous history of regular 28 day menstrual cycles with bleeding lasting for five days. In both the pattern of oestrogen excretion was reasonably normal, midcycle and luteal phase peaks being well marked especially in the case of oestrone ; the sharp fall in oestrone and oestriol output immediately after the midcycle peak is noteworthy. Pregnanediol output was atypical in both cycles ; in each a luteal phase increase occurred, but, in addition, values for the follicular phase rose to levels in the same range as those encountered following ovulation. HPG readings tended to be higher in the second than in the first cycle, but a definite midcycle peak did not occur in either.

Comment

The data in Figures 56 to 58 indicate the great variations which can occur in steroid excretion patterns in women with ovulatory menstrual cycles. The results presented emphasise yet again the necessity for conducting serial assays, since if isolated determinations had been performed it is unlikely that these abnormalities would have been detected. Of especial interest is the finding of relatively high pregnanediol values in the follicular phase of the cycle in the third subject (see also Bell *et al.*, 1966). The cause of such high readings is not at present clear, but it is possible that they result from lack of specificity of the assay method in use as a consequence of which material other than pregnanediol is determined in the final extract. In this connection it will be of interest to apply to studies of this type the newer and more specific assay methods for pregnanediol having as their end point gas liquid chromatography rather than colorimetry (see Chapter III).

ANOVULATORY CYCLES

This term describes cyclic uterine bleeding occurring in the absence of ovulation and corpus luteum formation. The condition is more frequent at the beginning and towards the end of reproductive life, but may also be found at any time during the child-bearing age. It is probable that in anovular menstruation bleeding occurs from a proliferative rather than from a secretory endometrium. In clinical practice the diagnosis is generally made by endometrial biopsy although the finding of a monophasic temperature chart may be suggestive of the condition.

On the basis of urinary oestrogen excretion patients with anovulatory cycles can be classified into two groups. In the first of these oestrogen levels fluctuate markedly, while in the second they remain relatively constant.

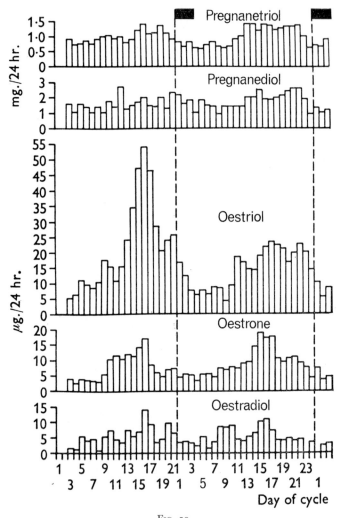

FIG. 59

Steroid excretion pattern during two consecutive anovulatory cycles.

■ = menstrual bleeding. (After Brown *et al.*, 1962).

146

1. Anovulatory Cycles with Fluctuating Oestrogen Levels

This type is well illustrated by Figure 59 which shows excretion values for pregnanediol and pregnanetriol in addition to oestrogens throughout two cycles. The subject had a history of regular 26 day menstrual cycles with bleeding lasting for five days. Severe dysmenorrhoea had been present for several

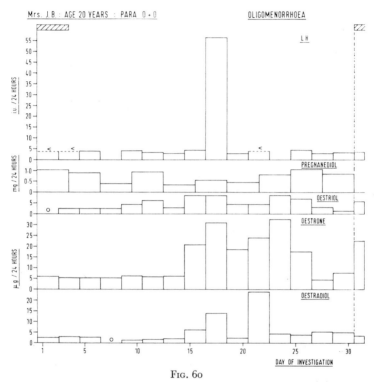

Fig. 60

Hormone excretion pattern in a patient with oligomenor-rhoea.

//// = menstrual bleeding.

years, and at the time of the investigation the patient was under considerable emotional stress. In the first cycle pregnanediol and pregnanetriol levels remained relatively constant, indicating the absence of ovulation. Oestrogen levels were low in the early part of the study ; they rose rapidly to a peak on day 16 and thereafter fell rapidly ; menstruation occurred on day 22 and lasted for four days. The second cycle was also anovulatory as judged by pregnanediol and pregnanetriol assays. Fluctuating oestrogen readings were again observed, but the sharp peak of excretion noted in the first cycle was absent. Maximum levels of oestrone were encountered from days 14 to 17 of the cycle, and values decreased prior to menstruation on day 25.

In the woman shown in Figure 60 the menarche had occurred at the age of 11. Subsequently there were regular cycles for two years followed by amenorrhoea for seven years. For the three years prior to the present investigation infrequent

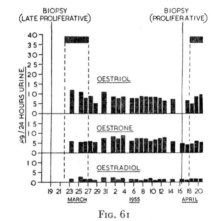

FIG. 61

Steroid excretion pattern during an anovulatory cycle.

■■■■ = menstrual bleeding.

(From Brown *et al.*, 1959, *J. Obstet. Gynaecol. Brit. Empire.*)

periods had occurred and a diagnosis of oligomenorrhoea was made. The patient was studied over a period of 31 days, during which time there was an anovulatory cycle. This was associated with fluctuating oestrogen levels, values for oestrone being at their maximum from days 15 to 26 of the study and falling prior to menstruation which commenced on day 31. Pregnanediol levels were generally below 1·1 mg. per 24 hours. Urinary LH assays were performed by the hypophysectomised rat prostate test ; readings were generally less than 5 i.u. per 24 hours, apart from a marked peak of excretion of 57 i.u. per 24 hours on days 17 and 18 of the investigation. The presence of a midcycle LH peak in a patient with an anovulatory cycle is of especial interest and has not to our knowledge been previously reported.

2. Anovulatory Cycles with Relatively Constant Oestrogen Levels

Such an excretion pattern is illustrated in Figure 61 which is taken from the paper of Brown *et al.* (1959). In this woman the menarche occurred at the age of 13 ; subsequently there were irregular menstrual periods of variable length. During

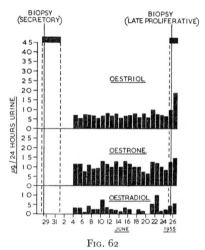

Fig. 62

Steroid excretion pattern during an anovulatory cycle.

▆▆▆▆ = menstrual bleeding.

(From Brown *et al.*, 1959, *J. Obstet. Gynaecol. Brit. Empire.*)

the period of study oestrogen levels were relatively constant, the value for " total oestrogens " remaining at or about 17 μg. per 24 hours. An endometrial biopsy taken on the 28th day of the investigation showed a proliferative pattern ; bleeding commenced on the 30th day and lasted for seven days.

A similar study in a patient with a history of regular menstrual cycles is shown in Figure 62. It will be noted that from the 9th day until bleeding commenced on the 30th day, the excretion of " total oestrogens " remained relatively constant at a figure of approximately 20 μg. per 24 hours. An endometrial biopsy performed on the 30th day of the investigation showed a proliferative pattern.

3. Comment

In patients with fluctuating oestrogen levels it must be assumed that the rising titre in body fluids stimulates endometrial growth, while in the presence of falling levels the endometrium is not maintained and bleeding occurs. The high excretion values in this group probably indicate that follicular development has occurred in the absence of corpus luteum formation. The reason for the failure of ovulation remains obscure but might conceivably result from inadequate LH production by the anterior pituitary. That such a hypothesis may well not be tenable is suggested by the findings in Figure 60 in which an LH peak occurred at or about the middle of an anovulatory cycle, and it is obvious that further work on this problem is necessary before any firm conclusions can be drawn.

In patients with anovulatory cycles in whom the pattern of oestrogen excretion remains relatively constant, the cause of the bleeding is also poorly understood. Brown *et al.* (1959) have suggested that oestrogen levels in such women are sufficiently high to cause growth of the endometrium, but as the latter increases in thickness under this form of stimulation it becomes unstable and disintegrates at intervals. This results in bleeding from an endometrium which is in the proliferative phase.

Brown *et al.* (1959) have emphasised that in patients with anovulatory cycles oestrogen levels are in general higher than in subjects with complete amenorrhoea and with an atrophic endometrium. In a series of 11 anovulatory cycles in six women reported by these investigators the mean "total oestrogen" excretion was $18 \cdot 2$ µg. per 24 hours and the range from $9 \cdot 0$ to 33 µg. per 24 hours. These figures must be compared with the lower values found in amenorrhoeic patients (see p. 173).

DYSMENORRHOEA

At the time of writing the role of the endocrine system in the aetiology of dysmenorrhoea is far from clear. An earlier hypothesis suggesting that the dysmenorrhoea was associated with excessive oestrogen secretion has not been substantiated, and the role of progesterone in the pathogenesis of the condition remains obscure. A comparison of hormone excretion patterns in normally menstruating women and in patients with dysmenorrhoea has recently been made by Bell and Loraine (1966 a) and part of the present section describes the results obtained. In addition, hormone excretion studies in a subject with dysmenorrhoea who was investigated on three occasions over a period of seven years are reported.

1. Comparison of Hormone Excretion Patterns in Normal and Dysmenorrhoeic Subjects

The study of Bell and Loraine (1966 a) was concerned only with patients suffering from so-called " incapacitating " dysmenorrhoea. This was defined as dysmenorrhoea of such severity that it necessitated absence from work or continuation at work only under analgesic therapy. Composite cycles for normal and dysmenorrhoeic subjects are shown in Figure 63. The composite cycle for the patients with dysmenorrhoea was derived from data obtained from six cycles in which oestrogens, pregnanediol and HPG were measured, and four in which pregnanetriol was also determined. The cycle was constructed in the same way as for the normally menstruating women, having the same four phases, i.e. menstruation, follicular phase, ovulatory phase and luteal phase (see p. 97). The average length of the cycles was $26 \cdot 8 \pm 1 \cdot 9$ days (S.D.). The composite data for the normal subjects were the same as that shown in Figure 29, being based on 18 menstrual cycles collected from 12 women.

The major difference to emerge between the two groups related to oestrogen excretion, the output of these hormones throughout the cycle tending to be lower in dysmenorrhoeic than in normal subjects. Significant differences in oestriol excretion were noted during the greater part of the follicular, ovulatory and luteal phases ; for oestrone and oestradiol such differences were mainly restricted to the latter two phases. Both midcycle and luteal phase peaks of oestrogen output tended to be poorly defined in the dysmenorrhoeic women.

Pregnanetriol levels in the ovulatory and luteal phases of the cycle were generally lower in dysmenorrhoeic than in normal women. However, on only four days of the composite cycle shown in Figure 63 were such differences significant. During the first three phases of the cycle mean excretion values for pregnanediol were virtually identical in the two categories ; however, following ovulation the luteal phase rise in this steroid occurred more rapidly in the dysmenorrhoeic group.

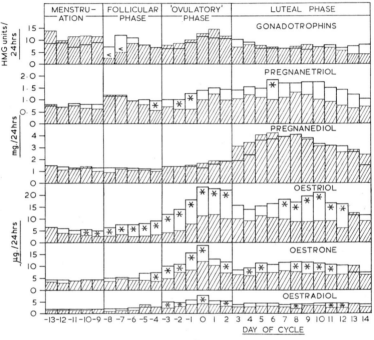

FIG. 63

Mean hormone excretion during the normal menstrual cycle (unhatched columns) and in patients with dysmenorrhoea (hatched columns).

Asterisks indicate days on which significant differences between the two groups of subjects were noted.

(From Bell and Loraine, 1966 a).

2. Hormone excretion patterns in a dysmenorrhoeic subject studied over a period of seven years

This woman had a history of regular 28 day menstrual cycles with bleeding generally lasting for six days and with the features of " incapacitating " dysmenorrhoea for many years.

Three investigations each involving one complete menstrual cycle were performed over a seven year period—the first in 1959, the second in 1962 and the third in 1966. In the first two studies dysmenorrhoea was present ; in the third this symptom was absent.

The cycle studied during 1959 (Figure 64) was of an ovulatory character, this being indicated by the pronounced luteal phase rise in pregnanediol output. The pattern of oestrone and oestradiol excretion was typical of a normal

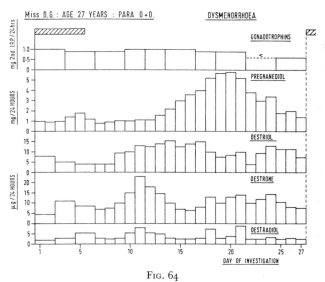

FIG. 64

Hormone excretion pattern in a patient with dysmenorrhoea.

//// = menstrual bleeding.

(After Brown *et al.*, 1962).

menstrual cycle, but the midcycle and luteal phase peaks of oestriol output were ill-defined. HPG excretion, measured by the mouse uterus test, remained within the normal range for a woman during reproductive life ; the absence of a midcycle peak will be noted.

Three years later the cycle (Figure 65) was also ovulatory in type, this being indicated by the luteal phase rise in preg-nanediol output. The midcycle peak of oestrogen excretion was ill-defined, but it is probable that ovulation took place on day 12 or 13 of the 28 day cycle ; the luteal phase rise in oestrogen output was more pronounced than the midcycle peak. HPG levels were relatively high towards the end of menstruation and on days 15 and 16 of the study ; readings in the luteal phase were lower than in the follicular, but all values were within the normal range.

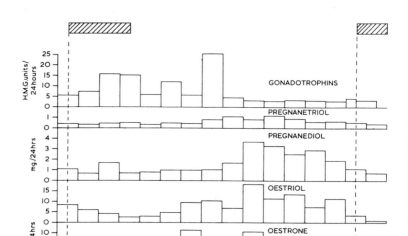

Mrs. D.G. AGE 30YEARS   PARA O+O   DYSMENORRHOEA

Fig. 65

Hormone excretion pattern in a patient with dysmenorrhoea.
//// = menstrual bleeding.
(After Bell and Loraine, 1965).

In the cycle collected during 1966 (Figure 66) ovulation as judged by oestrogen excretion again occurred, and from days 11 to 17 of the study levels of oestrone were considerably higher than those for oestriol. In contrast to the previous two cycles pregnanediol levels failed to show a marked rise in the luteal phase, readings being elevated only on days 21 to 23 of the investigation and immediately prior to menstruation which commenced on day 33.

3. Comment

Bell and Loraine (1966 *a*) have postulated that the low urinary levels of oestrogens and pregnanetriol found in dysmenorrhoeic women may result from an impairment of ovarian steroid biosynthesis, analagous to the hydroxylation defects believed to occur in the ovaries of patients with the Stein-Leventhal syndrome, and claimed to be of aetiological significance in relation to this disease (see Axelrod and Goldzieher, 1962). In dysmenorrhoea such a defect could affect the 17-hydroxylating mechanism and thus result in the formation

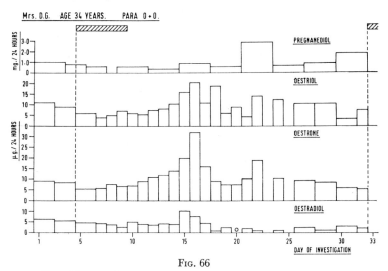

FIG. 66

Steroid excretion pattern in a patient with dysmenorrhoea.

//// = menstrual bleeding.

of inadequate amounts of the important biosynthetic precursors, 17α-hydroxyprogesterone and 17α-hydroxypregnenolone. Such a situation might in turn be reflected in low urinary excretion values for oestrogens and pregnanetriol. The hydroxylation defect could also cause progesterone to accumulate in the ovaries and might be expected to result in the appearance of increased quantities of pregnanediol in the urine especially during the luteal phase. The latter part of the hypothesis is difficult to reconcile with data indicating that the differences in pregnanediol output between normal and dysmenorrhoeic women are small and are probably within the limits of error of the assay method in use. On the other hand, support for this part of the hypothesis comes from the results shown in Figure 66, as in this cycle absence of dysmenorrhoea was associated with relatively low pregnanediol readings in association with high oestrogen values.

Figures 64 to 66 clearly indicate that the pattern of steroid excretion does not remain constant in the same individual over long periods of time. Thus in the cycles collected during 1959 and 1966 excretion values for " total oestrogens " were in general higher and the midcycle peak of oestrogen output was more clearly defined than in the cycle collected during 1962. Furthermore, in the first and second cycles the luteal phase rise in pregnanediol output was pronounced whereas in the third cycle it was ill-defined. In view of the fact that during the third cycle dysmenorrhoea was slight or absent, it appears reasonable to suggest that alterations in the secretion of progesterone, rather than of oestrogens, were associated with the occurrence of this symptom.

OLIGOMENORRHOEA

In the present chapter as in the review of Loraine and Bell (1967) a patient is considered to suffer from oligomenorrhoea in the presence of infrequent, irregular menstrual periods which are either ovulatory or anovulatory, the bleeding itself being scanty or normal in amount. In the four women reported herein (Figures 67 to 72) consecutive urine samples were collected over relatively long periods of time, making it possible to study hormone excretion patterns during different phases of the condition.

In the subject shown in Figures 67 and 68 the menarche occurred at the age of 15. Thereafter, she had scanty irregular periods which continued even after the birth of her two children ; for one year prior to the study the patient had been amenorrhoeic. During the first 22 days of the investigation oestrogen levels were similar to those normally encountered in the follicular phase of the menstrual cycle, while pregnanediol values were variable, ranging from 0·5 to 1·9 mg. per 24 hours. An ovulatory peak of oestrogen excretion probably occurred on

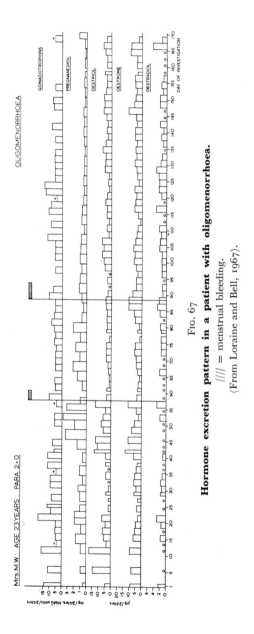

FIG. 67

Hormone excretion pattern in a patient with oligomenorrhoea.

//// = menstrual bleeding.

(From Loraine and Bell, 1967).

day 42 ; this was followed by a luteal phase rise in pregnanediol output and by menstruation which commenced on day 58. Oestrogen excretion in the luteal phase of this cycle was atypical, the peak being ill-defined.

During the cycle that occurred between days 58 and 89 the pattern of steroid output was unusual. Urinary oestrogens showed little fluctuation, but readings tended to be higher in the second than in the first half of the cycle, the highest oestrone level coinciding with bleeding on day 89. During the first 12 days of this cycle pregnanediol values gradually rose, reaching a maximum of 2·2 mg. per 24 hours on days 67 to 69 ; thereafter, levels fluctuated but tended to be low just prior to menstruation.

During the remaining 208 days of the study menstruation did not occur. From days 89 to 210 oestrogen levels showed only minor fluctuations and were generally within the post-menopausal range. Pregnanediol values gradually fell from day 89 onwards and, with the exception of one reading of 1·2 mg. per 24 hours on days 169 and 170, were at their lowest between days 145 and 210. From day 210 onwards oestrogen levels were somewhat higher than in the preceding phase of the study, being frequently within the range normally encountered in menstruating women ; the rise in oestrone output between days 217 and 237 was especially marked. Pregnanediol levels also tended to rise during this time and were generally above 1 mg. per 24 hours from day 235 onwards. Throughout the whole period of investigation HPG levels ranged from less than 5 to 19·2 HMG units per 24 hours, the majority of the readings being within the normal range for a subject of this age.

From her menarche until 10 months prior to the commencement of the investigation shown in Figures 69 and 70 the patient had a history of regular 28 day menstrual cycles with bleeding lasting for two or three days ; thereafter, her periods became irregular and of variable duration. The study occupied a total of 248 days during which time there were four periods of bleeding.

The first menstruation occurred from days 9 to 11 ; this probably represented ovulatory bleeding in view of the relatively high pregnanediol and oestriol figures immediately

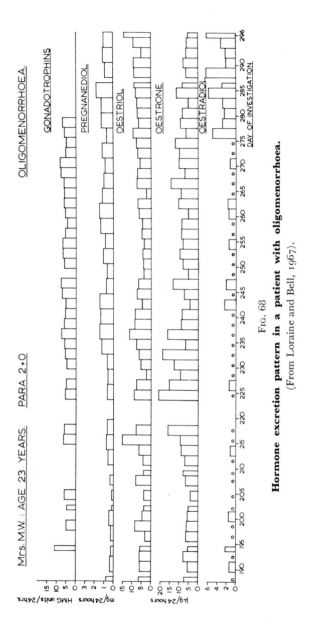

Fig. 68

Hormone excretion pattern in a patient with oligomenorrhoea.

(From Loraine and Bell, 1967).

prior to its onset. Between days 9 and 28 there was a further ovulatory cycle characterised by a marked luteal phase rise in pregnanediol output. In this latter cycle the pattern of

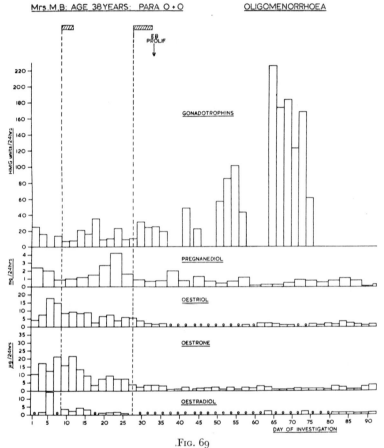

.FIG. 69

Hormone excretion pattern in a patient with oligomenorrhoea.

E.B. = endometrial biopsy ; //// = menstrual bleeding.
(From Loraine and Bell, 1967.)

oestrogen excretion was atypical, but it appears probable that ovulation, based on oestrone levels, occurred on day 11 or 12 ; menstruation commenced on day 28 and lasted for five days. For the first 27 days of the study urinary HPG levels showed no consistent pattern and were within the normal range for a woman during reproductive life.

From days 33 to 194 bleeding did not occur. Oestrogen readings were very low from days 28 to 129, levels of oestriol and oestradiol being frequently undetectable ; during this time pregnanediol values ranged from 0·2 to 2·0 mg. per 24 hours. From days 130 to 194 oestrogen levels were in general higher than in the preceding 100 days while pregnanediol readings were below 1·0 mg. per 24 hours. Between the 152nd and 195th day the pattern of oestrone excretion was cyclic, high levels being encountered from day 152 to 165 and 178 to 193. These high values were not associated with ovulation since pregnanediol readings failed to increase, and it must therefore be assumed that the bleeding which took place from days 195 to 198 was anovulatory in character. From day 28 onwards HPG levels started to rise reaching the abnormally high level of 225 HMG units per 24 hours on day 64 and 65 ; thereafter readings fell but until day 149 generally remained elevated for a subject in this age group. From day 159 until bleeding recommenced on day 195 HPG levels were lower being within the normal range for a woman during reproductive life.

From days 195 to 220 there was a further cycle ; during this time excretion values for oestradiol and oestriol showed no consistent pattern while oestrone output was cyclic in character. It is probable that ovulation did not take place during this cycle although a definite conclusion on this point cannot be reached because pregnanediol assays were not performed from days 215 to 220. Bleeding commenced on day 221 and lasted for eight days. During the last 28 days of the study ovulation again failed to occur, levels of oestrogens and pregnanediol remaining low and relatively constant. On the other hand, HPG output fluctuated considerably, the majority of the readings being abnormally high for a woman of this age.

In Figure 71 are presented the results in a patient who, following her menarche at 11, had regular periods until the age of 13. Subsequently her periods became irregular and variable in amount and for four and a half months prior to the inception of the study menstruation had not occurred. The data obtained during the first 21 days of the investigation

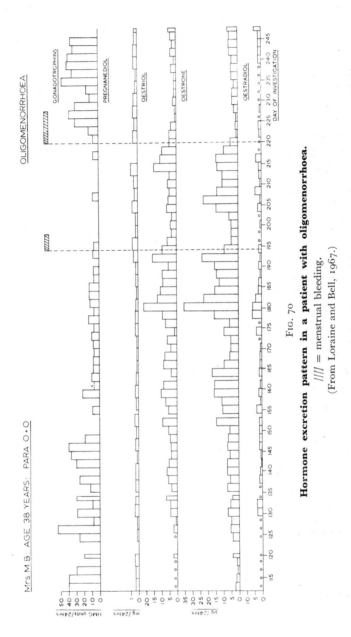

Hormone excretion pattern in a patient with oligomenorrhoea.

//// = menstrual bleeding.

(From Loraine and Bell, 1967.)

Fig. 70

therefore represented the findings obtained at the end of a period of amenorrhoea. Ovulation judged by oestriol excretion probably occurred on days 5 or 6. This was followed by a luteal phase rise in oestriol and pregnanediol output, readings of the latter steroid being maximal between days 13 and 18 ; during this cycle the luteal phase peaks of oestrone and oestradiol were ill-defined. Bleeding commenced on day 22 and lasted for three days. From days 22 to 29 oestrogen and pregnanediol levels were relatively low, being within the postmenopausal range. Bleeding recommenced on day 30 and lasted for four days ; during this time oestrogen levels started to rise and continued to do so until day 43 when bleeding again occurred. The cycle from day 43 until the recommencement of bleeding on day 68 was of an ovulatory character. An ovulatory peak of oestrogen output was present on the 10th or 11th day, and the luteal phase rise in pregnanediol was maximal on the 20th to 22nd day (days 61 to 63 of the investigation). It is noteworthy that oestradiol levels remained relatively constant throughout this cycle, failing to show the fluctuations present in the case of oestrone and oestriol.

A heavy menstruation commenced on day 68 and lasted for five days. Bleeding occurred 11 days after the completion of the study, and it must therefore be assumed that the period of investigation extending from day 68 onwards represented approximately half of a cycle during which ovulation did not take place. Throughout the whole investigation HPG readings remained within the normal range ; the absence of any cyclic pattern of gonadotrophin excretion is noteworthy.

Excretion values for oestrogens, pregnanediol and testo-sterone in a patient with a history of oligomenorrhoea in association with hirsutism and infertility have recently been reported by Ismail et al. (1967) ; the results are shown in Figure 72. During the first 38 days of the investigation pregnanediol readings remained reasonably constant ranging from $1 \cdot 4$ to $2 \cdot 0$ mg. per 24 hours. Bleeding which commenced on day 43 was associated with a fall in pregnanediol output. The pattern of oestrogen excretion was more typical of the anovulatory than of the ovulatory menstrual cycle. Oestriol levels remained relatively constant from day 3 to 29 ; there-after the output of this steroid decreased only to rise again from

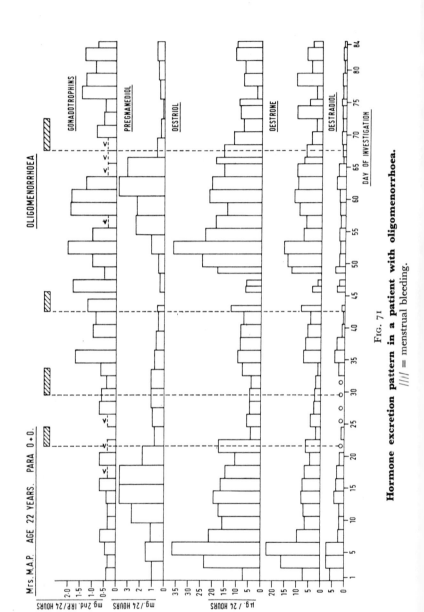

FIG. 71

Hormone excretion pattern in a patient with oligomenorrhoea.

//// = menstrual bleeding.

days 49 to 53 during the period of bleeding. Likewise readings of oestrone and oestradiol fluctuated in an irregular manner. Urinary testosterone levels were generally above the range for a woman during reproductive life, the highest reading of 23 μg. per 24 hours being encountered on days 26 and 27 of the study. The rise in urinary testosterone excretion from days 20 to 31 was associated with the increase in the output of oestrone.

Following the study shown in Figure 72 this patient was treated with Clomiphene and ovulated as a result of therapy. Ovulation was associated with a rise in testosterone as well as in pregnanediol output. In a subsequent ovulatory cycle produced by Clomiphene the subject became pregnant and eventually delivered a normal male child.

Comment

In the patient shown in Figures 67 and 68, HPG levels changed little throughout the period of observation suggesting the lack of any seasonal variation in pituitary gonadotrophic activity. On the other hand, spontaneous variations were noted in ovarian function as judged by oestrogen and pregnanediol assays. Thus between days 100 and 150 levels of pregnanediol, oestrone and oestriol were low and relatively constant, while oestradiol was detectable in the majority of the samples assayed ; the period between days 190 and 275 was characterised by a slow rise in pregnanediol output, by the virtual absence of oestradiol from the urine, and by relatively high excretion values for oestrone and oestriol. During the last 20 days of the investigation the presence of oestradiol could again be detected, and at this time levels of pregnanediol, oestrone and oestriol were reasonably high. It is noteworthy that during the whole period of observation only one ovulatory cycle occurred, this being indicated by the high luteal phase levels of pregnanediol from days 45 to 55.

The pattern of hormone excretion in the woman shown in Figures 69 and 70 bore little resemblance to that in the previous case. The major difference was the fact that in this subject considerable alterations in pituitary gonadotrophic function occurred. These were especially marked during the period of amenorrhoea which lasted from days 30 to 195, and during

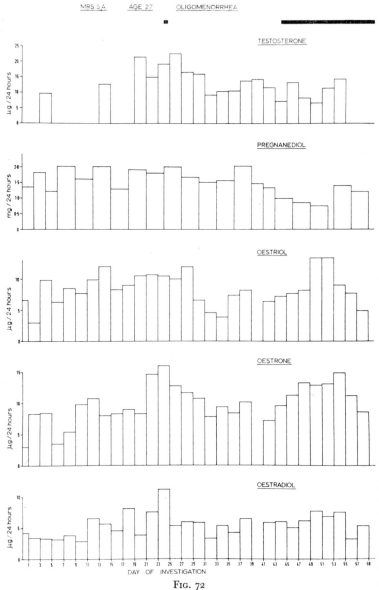

FIG. 72

Steroid excretion pattern in a patient with oligomenorrhoea.

━━ = menstrual bleeding.

which time many of the HPG readings were within and some were above the postmenopausal range. It is apparent that the high HPG levels from days 50 to 80 and from day 220 until the end of the investigation were associated with low figures for oestrogen excretion, while the much lower HPG readings from days 150 to 190 were accompanied by higher oestrogen values.

During the first half of the period of amenorrhoea from day 30 to 195 levels of the three classical oestrogens in urine were very low ; the ratio of oestrone to oestriol was approximately unity, this ratio being similar to that in Group 3 of the patients with secondary amenorrhoea (see page 173). In the second half of the amenorrhoeic phase oestrogen output was higher and levels were fluctuant ; relatively more oestrone than oestriol was excreted and the ratio oestrone/oestriol was similar to that in Group 2 of the patients with secondary amenorrhoea. Changes in pregnanediol output in this subject were less marked than in the woman shown in Figures 67 and 68, but with the exception of the ovulatory cycle which occurred from days 9 to 20, levels of this steroid tended to be low when oestrogen readings were relatively high.

In the third patient (Figure 71) the main point of interest was the occurrence of three separate periods of bleeding without evidence of ovulation between days 22 and 45 of the investigation. The cycles immediately prior to menstruation on day 21 and between days 42 and 67 were ovulatory in character. It should, however, be noted that, due to the prolonged period of amenorrhoea prior to the commencement of the investigation, the " follicular " phase of the first ovulatory cycle lasted for nearly five months, whereas in the second ovulatory cycle the corresponding duration of this phase was only 10 or 11 days.

In the fourth patient (Figure 72) the major abnormality was the finding of relatively high excretion values for urinary testosterone. This observation suggests the presence of a partial block in oestrogen biosynthesis resulting in the accumulation of androgenic precursors in the ovaries. Such an accumulation might well lead to raised androgen levels in body fluids which might in turn be responsible for the development of the hirsutism.

AMENORRHOEA

On clinical grounds it is customary to divide amenorrhoea into two main types—*primary* and *secondary*. In true *primary amenorrhoea* menstruation has failed to occur in patients well beyond the age of puberty ; the term *secondary amenorrhoea* is reserved for the condition in which menstrual function has ceased after having been completely established. Both primary and secondary amenorrhoea can be associated with either pituitary or ovarian failure. In *pituitary amenorrhoea* excretion values for both oestrogens and HPG are below the normal range for women during reproductive life, while in *ovarian amenorrhoea* an abnormally low oestrogen output is usually associated with increased excretion values for HPG. At the time of writing the literature on endocrine function in secondary amenorrhoea is much more extensive than is the case for primary amenorrhoea.

1. Primary Amenorrhoea

An early study of oestrogen and HPG excretion in patients with this condition was that of Pedersen-Bjergaard and Tønnesen (1951). They found normal oestrogen readings in some 20 per cent of their cases and abnormally low levels in 80 per cent ; increased excretion values were not observed. In 35 per cent of the women a low oestrogen output was associated with a normal or high HPG excretion, indicating that the amenorrhoea was of the ovarian type. In 46 per cent of the subjects excretion values for both HPG and oestrogens were below the normal range suggesting that the site of the lesion lay in the pituitary. The remaining cases (19 per cent) had oestrogen and HPG readings which were within the normal range. It must be emphasised that, although the overall conclusions drawn by Pedersen-Bjergaard and Tønnesen (1951) may well be valid, the assay methods used by these investigators were unreliable by modern standards, and accordingly the quantitative significance of the results quoted in individual cases is open to doubt.

Bjøro (1965) measured oestrogen excretion in 43 patients with primary amenorrhoea and in all cases found levels within the postmenopausal range. Bell and Loraine (1967 *b*) estimated HPG output by the mouse uterus test in 28 such subjects. In

16 (58 per cent) levels were within the normal range for women during reproductive life ; in 6 (21 per cent) they were abnormally high and in 6 they were low. Bjøro (1965) performed urinary HPG assays in 55 patients with primary amenorrhoea and reported normal values in the majority of cases.

In three subjects with primary amenorrhoea due to a congenital absence of the uterus Brown *et al.* (1959) observed a cyclic pattern of urinary oestrogen excretion with levels in the same range as those in the ovulatory menstrual cycle.

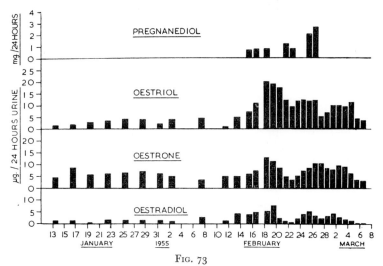

FIG. 73

Steroid excretion pattern in a patient with congenital absence of the uterus.

(From Brown *et al.*, 1959, *J. Obstet. Gynaecol. Brit. Empire.*)

This finding indicates that normal ovarian activity can occur in the absence of the target organ, the uterus. The results obtained in one such woman are shown in Figure 73. It will be noted that an ovulatory peak of oestrogen excretion was present on the 36th day of the investigation ; this followed a long period of time during which oestrogen levels were in the same range as those in the proliferative phase of the menstrual cycle. After ovulation a normal luteal phase peak of oestrogen excretion occurred in association with a rise in pregnanediol output.

2. Secondary Amenorrhoea

Pedersen-Bjergaard and Tønnesen (1951) conducted oestrogen assays by a biological method in a relatively large series of patients with this condition. They found normal levels in approximately one-third and low readings in some two-thirds of cases. In a limited number of their subjects serial assays were performed, and considerable variations in excretion patterns which were sometimes of a cyclic nature were found.

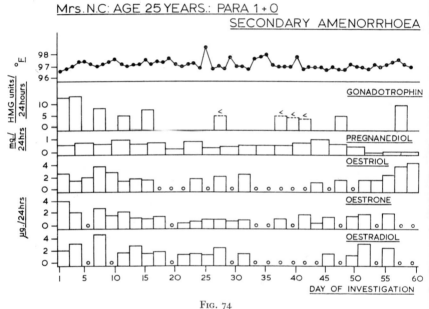

FIG. 74

Hormone excretion pattern in a patient with secondary amenorrhoea.

(From Loraine and Bell, 1967.)

Oestrogen assays by more reliable chemical methods have been performed in patients with secondary amenorrhoea by Brown *et al.* (1959), Bjøro (1965) and Loraine and Bell (1967). In Bjøro's series of 25 women values for " total oestrogens " were within or slightly above the postmenopausal range, readings being, in general, higher than in patients with primary amenorrhoea. In eight women studied by Brown *et al.* (1959) and classified as " menopause praecox " the mean excretion value for " total oestrogens " was 6·3 µg. per 24 hours and the range was from 1·8 to 10·0 µg. per 24 hours.

In a series of 109 patients with secondary amenorrhoea reported by Bjøro (1965) urinary HPG readings were within the normal range in 73 per cent ; levels were abnormally high in 14 and unduly low in 13 per cent. In 44 patients studied by Bell and Loraine (1967 b) HPG excretion was normal in 76 per cent, abnormally high in 4 and below the normal range in 20 per cent.

Serial hormone assay studies in six patients with secondary amenorrhoea have recently been published by Loraine and Bell (1967). The results obtained in three of their cases will be presented as illustrative examples of the hormonal patterns encountered.

In the woman shown in Figure 74 the menarche occurred at age 12 ; thereafter there were regular menstrual cycles varying in length from 21 to 35 days with bleeding generally lasting five days. For a period of 31 months prior to the initiation of the investigation the subject was amenorrhoeic. During the 60 days of the study urinary steroid levels remained within the postmenopausal range. Estimations of HPG could only be made in a proportion of the urine samples tested because some of the extracts proved toxic to the experimental animals. In the specimens in which assays were possible levels were either within or below the range normally encountered in women during reproductive life. Throughout the study basal temperature readings fluctuated in an irregular manner and failed to show a biphasic curve.

In the patient illustrated in Figure 75 menstruation first occurred at age 14 ; there had been a period of continuous amenorrhoea for 10 years prior to the commencement of the investigation, the latter continuing for a period of 85 days. In the majority of urine samples assayed the presence of oestriol could not be detected while oestrone was present in all but one ; throughout the study levels for " total oestrogens " were within the postmenopausal range. Pregnanediol output was generally low, apart from readings of 1·9 and 2·4 mg. per 24 hours on days 56 to 58 and 68 to 70 respectively ; these relatively high values were not associated with the occurrence of ovulation, and it is probable that the material estimated in the urine was

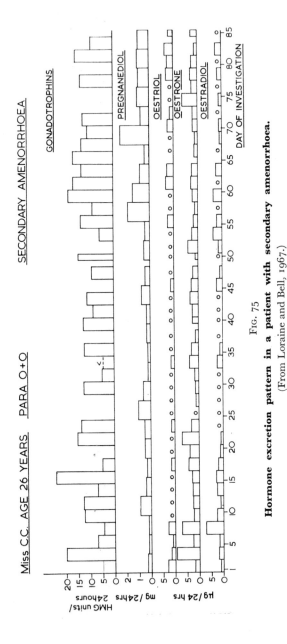

FIG. 75

Hormone excretion pattern in a patient with secondary amenorrhoea.

(From Loraine and Bell, 1967.)

derived from percursors secreted by the adrenal cortex rather than by the ovary. HPG levels were within the normal range for a woman during reproductive life.

Figure 76 shows the results obtained in a subject in whom the menarche had occurred at age 14. This was followed by a phase of oligomenorrhoea lasting for approximately nine years, and for 16 months prior to the investigation menstruation had not occurred. Throughout the study which occupied 32 days, values for pregnanediol and oestrogens remained low,

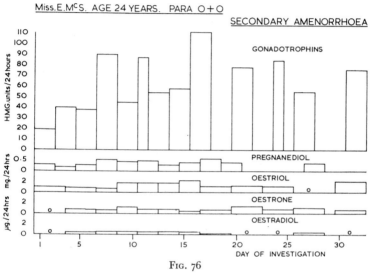

FIG. 76

Hormone excretion pattern in a patient with secondary amenorrhoea.

(From Loraine and Bell, 1967.)

being within the postmenopausal range. Urinary HPG readings were higher than in the previous two patients, ranging from 19 to 111 HMG units per 24 hours but being in general typical of the postmenopausal state.

Classification of patients with secondary amenorrhoea on the basis of hormone assays.—In Table 6 are shown mean values for oestradiol, oestrone, oestriol, pregnanediol and HPG in the six subjects with secondary amenorrhoea reported by Loraine and Bell (1967). It is evident that the cases can be divided into three groups depending on their HPG output. In Group 1, of

TABLE 6

MEAN HORMONE EXCRETION IN PATIENTS WITH SECONDARY AMENORRHOEA

(From Loraine and Bell, 1967)

Group	Oestradiol μg./24 hours	Oestrone μg./24 hours	Oestriol μg./24 hours	Pregnanediol mg./24 hours	HPG HMG units/24 hours
1	1·6	1·8	2·6	0·71	<5·8
2	2·6	3·2	1·5	1·15	<10·2
3	0·5	1·2	1·0	0·88	35·4

which Figure 74 is an example, HPG levels were at the lower end of or below the normal range for a woman during reproductive life. In Group 2 (see Figure 75) they were within, while in Group 3 (Figure 76) they were at the upper end of or above this range. In all three groups excretion values for oestrogens and pregnanediol were similar to those encountered in the postmenopausal state. However, in Group 2 levels for oestrone, oestradiol and pregnanediol were slightly higher than in Groups 1 and 3. It must be emphasised that all the oestrogen readings shown in the table were very low indeed, many of the figures being below the limits of reliability of the assay method used, and therefore being of doubtful quantitative significance.

3. Comment

It is now well recognised that in *primary amenorrhoea* hormone assays may be useful in providing information regarding the aetiology of the condition. Thus, in patients in whom the amenorrhoea is associated with a congenital absence of the uterus and vagina and in whom the ovaries are functioning normally, oestrogen levels show a cyclic pattern of excretion and are within the normal range for women during reproductive life. On the other hand, in subjects in whom the primary amenorrhoea is due to ovarian or pituitary failure, oestrogen levels remain relatively constant and are often so low that they cannot be accurately estimated by methods currently in use. A good example of the latter type of situation is provided by the condition of Turner's syndrome (ovarian agenesis).

Pituitary gonadotrophic function in patients with primary amenorrhoea has been little studied, and the work that has been reported has been concerned exclusively with the estimation in urine of " total gonadotrophic activity " rather than with the separate determination of FSH and LH. Evidence accumulated by Bell and Loraine (1967 *b*) indicates that a higher percentage of patients with primary than with secondary amenorrhoea show abnormally large quantities of HPG in their urine (21 as against 4 per cent in their series). On the other hand, the percentage of women with an abnormally low HPG output was virtually the same in the two groups. These observations suggest that the incidence of any ovarian lesion is higher in patients with primary than with secondary amenorrhoea.

In amenorrhoeic patients knowledge of endogenous excretion values for HPG and oestrogens is likely to be of considerable value in relation to the management of the condition. Thus Bell and Loraine (1966 *b*) and Townsend *et al.* (1966) have shown that oestrogen output can be useful in predicting the response to the ovarian stimulant Clomiphene (see also Chapter VII). Both groups of investigators found that the patients most likely to ovulate as a result of Clomiphene administration are those showing definite evidence of ovarian activity as judged by urinary oestrogen assays. On the other hand, patients with a low oestrogen output characteristic of the menopause or post-menopause, are more likely to respond satisfactorily to gonadotrophins than to Clomiphene.

The classification of patients with *secondary amenorrhoea* into three groups on the basis of their HPG excretion is also likely to be useful in relation to therapy. Thus patients in Groups 1 and 2 of Table 6 in whom HPG levels are within or below the normal range are more likely to respond to treatment by Clomiphene or by gonadotrophic hormones than those in Group 3 in whom HPG readings are within the postmenopausal range and the site of the lesion is in the ovaries rather than in the pituitary.

GALACTORRHOEA

Two main clinical syndromes involving galactorrhoea have been described. The first is the *Chiari-Frommel syndrome* characterised by lactation, amenorrhoea and sterility following childbirth. The second has been termed the *Forbes* or *del-Castillo syndrome* ; in this condition the symptomatology is similar to that of the Chiari-Frommel syndrome, but lactation can occur without a preceding pregnancy. The aetiology of both conditions remains obscure, and none of the hypotheses put forward to explain them is completely satisfactory.

Hormone assay studies in patients with the Chiari-Frommel syndrome have previously been described by Loraine *et al.* (1966), and Figure 77 is illustrative of the results obtained. In this subject the menarche occurred at age 13 ; thereafter menstruation was regular for some 16 years. Following the delivery of a normal male child she developed amenorrhoea and sterility in association with lactation, the latter still being present at the time at which the hormone assays were conducted. The study shown in Figure 77 was performed over a period of 43 days during which time menstruation did not occur. Excretion values for 17-hydroxycroticosteroids (17-OHCS) were normal but the output of total 17-oxosteroids, dehydroepiandrosterone (DHA) and pregnanediol was low. Oestrogen levels were generally within the postmenopausal range, oestradiol being detectable in only a relatively small proportion of the samples assayed. A small peak of oestrone excretion occurred on days 32 and 33 of the study, but this was not followed by a luteal phase rise in either oestrogen or pregnanediol output or by menstruation. Throughout the period of investigation HPG levels were at the lower end of or below the normal range for a woman during reproductive life.

Even less is known regarding hormone excretion patterns in the Forbes than in the Chiari-Frommel syndrome. In a patient with the former condition investigated by Charles *et al.* (1967) endogenous excretion values for FSH and LH were abnormally low (see p. 215).

Comment

In the woman shown in Figure 77 both HPG and oestrogen readings were low, and the hormone excretion pattern was therefore similar to that in Group 1 of the patients with secondary amenorrhoea (see Table 6). In another subject with the same syndrome reported by Loraine *et al.* (1966) levels of both groups of hormones were within the normal range ; such a subject would therefore resemble those in Group 2 of Table 6.

The patient shown in Figure 77 was lactating during the period of investigation, and it is of interest to note that lactation did not appear to produce any marked alteration in either pituitary or ovarian function. Assays of the lactogenic hormone, prolactin, might have been especially informative in this particular case, but at the time of writing, methods for the quantitative determination of this hormone are not yet suitable for application to clinical problems (see Loraine and Bell, 1966).

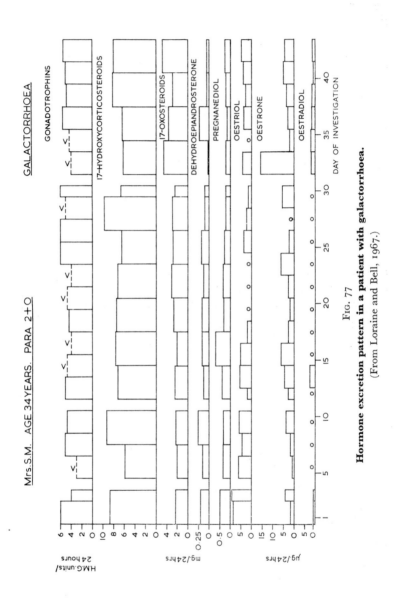

FIG. 77

Hormone excretion pattern in a patient with galactorrhoea.

(From Loraine and Bell, 1967.)

THE STEIN-LEVENTHAL SYNDROME

The symptomatology of the Stein-Leventhal syndrome has been reviewed in numerous publications, among the more recent of which are those by Goldzieher and Green (1962), Stein (1966) and Roberts (1966). The main clinical features are menstrual abnormalities, usually amenorrhoea or oligo-menorrhoea, in association with hirsutism and bilateral ovarian enlargement. In addition, infertility is a relatively frequent complaint in married women with the disease. The precise aetiology of the Stein-Leventhal syndrome is poorly understood, but the disease is thought to be associated with a defect in one or more of the enzyme systems responsible for ovarian steroid biosynthesis (see Shearman and Cox, 1966 ; Jenkins, 1966). The traditional treatment of the condition has been by wedge resection of the ovaries, but the mechanism by which this operation produces its beneficial effect is far from clear (see Zander et al., 1962). In recent years it has been demonstrated that patients with the Stein-Leventhal syndrome can be treated satisfactorily either by Clomiphene or by gonado-trophic hormones. (See Chapters VII and VIII for references.)

A serial study of hormone levels in the Stein-Leventhal syndrome has been undertaken by Loraine and Bell (1967). On the basis of urinary steroid assays these workers classified their patients into two main groups, designated respectively *anovulatory* and *ovulatory*. Representative diagrams of hormone excretion patterns in the two categories of subject are illustrated in Figures 78 and 79.

The patient in Figure 78 had a previous history of oligo-menorrhoea, and when subjected to laparotomy her ovaries were found to contain cystic follicles. The period of study extended over 29 days during which time oestrogen output remained low, being within the postmenopausal range. Pregnanediol values fluctuated in an irregular manner, figures ranging from 1·1 to 3·1 mg. per 24 hours. In the presence of low urinary oestrogen readings it must be assumed that the pregnanediol present in the urine was derived from progesterone which was of adrenal rather than ovarian origin. Levels of 17-OHCS and total 17-oxosteroids were at the upper end of the normal range ; pregnanetriol readings were typical of the follicular phase of the normal menstrual cycle, and were in the same range as those reported by Lanthier and Sandor (1964) who investigated a series of 33 women with the Stein-Leventhal syndrome.

In Figure 79 are shown the results obtained in a patient who ovulated during the period of observation. The subject had

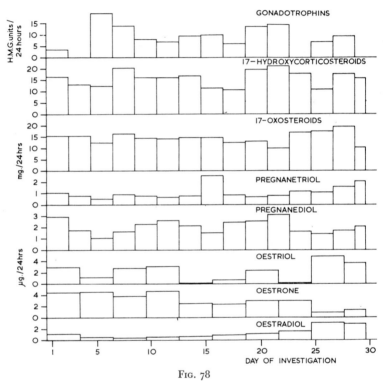

FIG. 78

Hormone excretion pattern in a patient with the Stein-type syndrome.

(From Loraine and Bell, 1967.)

suffered from oligomenorrhoea since her menarche at the age of 16 ; in addition, she exhibited moderate hirsutism together with bilateral ovarian enlargement. At laparotomy her ovaries showed fibrous cortical sclerosis with numerous follicular cysts. From days 7 to 41 of the investigation there was an ovulatory menstrual cycle as judged by pregnanediol assays. However, the pattern of oestrogen excretion was atypical. Ovulation occurred relatively late on the 20th or 21st day of the cycle and was followed by a luteal phase rise in oestrone and oestriol output ; levels fell immediately prior to menstruation on day 42. High HPG readings were noted from days 13

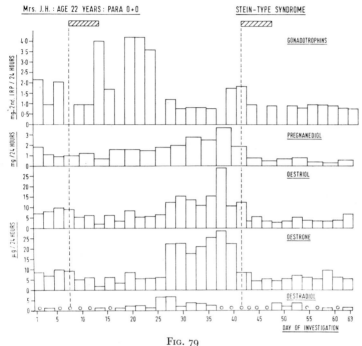

Fig. 79

Hormone excretion pattern in a patient with the Stein-type syndrome.

//// = menstrual bleeding.

to 24 of the study during the follicular phase ; values subsequently fell in the luteal phase and rose slightly prior to the commencement of menstruation on day 42. For the last 24 days of the study levels of oestrogens, pregnanediol and HPG were low and remained relatively constant.

The studies of Loraine and Bell (1967) concentrated mainly on estimations of oestrogens, pregnanediol and HPG in the Stein-Leventhal syndrome. Assays of total and fractionated 17-oxosteroids in patients with this condition have been reported by Jailer and Vande Wiele (1954), Dorfman and Shipley (1956), Gallagher et al. (1958), Lanthier (1960), Goldzieher and Axelrod (1962) and others. In general, such estimations have proved to be of limited diagnostic value, and in a series of 29 patients collected from the literature by Dorfman and Shipley (1956) the total 17-oxosteroid excretion was abnormally high in only five instances. A more recent study involving 27 patients is that of Lanthier (1960). He found that the mean value for total 17-oxosteroid excretion was significantly higher in the Stein-Leventhal series than in control subjects, although there was a considerable overlap between the two categories. He also noted that the higher mean figure in the patients with the Stein-Leventhal syndrome was due to an increase in the fraction containing androsterone and aetiocholanolone.

Mahesh and Greenblatt (1964) and Goldzieher and Axelrod (1962) have shown that in most cases of the Stein-Leventhal syndrome the output of 11-deoxy-17-oxosteroids does not fall significantly after adrenal suppression with dexamethasone. This observation presumably indicates that these compounds are being produced by the ovaries rather than by the adrenals. On the other hand, a few patients do show a marked fall in 11-deoxy-17-oxosteroids after this form of treatment and in these cases it must be presumed that the steroids originate from the adrenals. Plasma testosterone levels in patients with the Stein-type syndrome have been estimated by Korenman et al. (1965) and by Lloyd et al. (1966). Both groups of workers reported abnormally high levels and, on the basis of studies involving the parenteral administration of HCG, concluded that the ovaries were secreting increased amounts of this hormone.

Comment

One of the major problems in relation to the Stein-Leventhal syndrome is that of diagnosis, there still being considerable controversy in the literature regarding which patients should be included in this category. It is now established that endogenous hormone levels in patients with the Stein-Leventhal syndrome vary greatly from one subject to another and when assays are conducted on a serial basis considerable variations in the same individual are encountered. This is especially so in the case of the oestrogens, and the investigations of Loraine and Bell (1967) have emphasised that such variations can occur both in the ovulatory and anovulatory groups. In addition, in patients in the ovulatory group, the pattern of oestrogen excretion is frequently different from that found in normally menstruating women. Studies of testosterone excretion in patients with the Stein-Leventhal syndrome are at present very limited indeed, and it is to be hoped that in the future serial assays of this hormone and of other C-19 steroids such as androstenedione will be conducted in an attempt to clarify the role of the androgens in the pathogenesis of the condition.

In the four patients with the Stein-Leventhal syndrome reported by Loraine and Bell (1967) levels of " total gonadotrophic activity " were generally within the normal range for a woman during reproductive life. This observation suggests that the disease is not associated with any major disturbance of pituitary gonadotrophic function. However, it might be of interest in this connection to perform separate determinations of urinary FSH and LH, particularly in view of the claim of McArthur *et al.* (1958) that levels of the latter hormone tend to be abnormally high in patients with the Stein-Leventhal syndrome.

DYSFUNCTIONAL UTERINE HAEMORRHAGE

This is an imprecise term used to cover all forms of abnormal bleeding for which an organic cause cannot be found. Although the classification of dysfunctional uterine haemorrhage is difficult most investigators recognise two types, designated respectively ovulatory and anovulatory ; within the latter group is included the condition of metropathia haemorrhagica. Up till now hormone assay studies in patients with dysfunctional uterine haemorrhage have been performed on a very limited scale. Serial assays of oestrogens have been reported by Brown *et al.* (1959) while Loraine and Bell (1967) have performed estimations of pregnanediol and HPG in addition to oestrogens. Typical hormone excretion patterns in patients with dysfunctional uterine haemorrhage are shown in Figures 80 and 81.

In Figure 80 from the paper by Brown *et al.* (1959) is shown the pattern of oestrogen excretion in a 27 year old patient who had a history of prolonged phases of amenorrhoea interspersed with irregular periods of bleeding. A diagnosis of cystic glandular hyperplasia was made on the basis of an endometrial biopsy. During the period of study " total oestrogen " excretion was reasonably constant, remaining in the range 20 to 40 μg. per 24 hours, with a mean level of approximately 30 μg. per 24 hours. It should be noted that

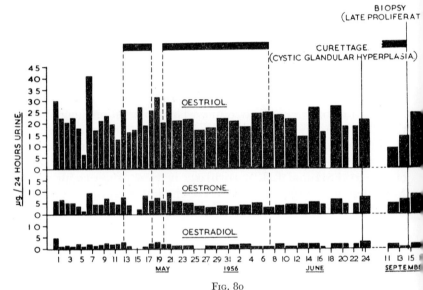

Fig. 80

Steroid excretion pattern in a patient with cystic glandular hyperplasia.

■■■ = menstrual bleeding.

(From Brown *et al.*, 1959, *J. Obstet. Gynaecol. Brit. Empire.*)

menstrual bleeding occurred in spite of these relatively high levels. The pattern of oestrogen output was similar to that observed in anovulatory menstrual cycles with constant levels (see p. 149) except that in the present condition oestrogen readings tended to be somewhat higher.

In the patient shown in Figure 81 a diagnosis of cystic glandular hyperplasia was made following a dilatation and curettage performed six months before the commencement of the study, the subject having had a two year history of heavy irregular bleeding. In the first 12 days of the investigation during a period of bleeding oestrogen levels fluctuated markedly, oestriol values ranging from 6·5 to 44 µg. per 24 hours. Thereafter, levels tended to fall, and from days 29 to 46 were within the range normally encountered in postmenopausal subjects. On day 47 oestrogen readings started to rise reaching a maximum on days 63 and 64 at which time the oestriol figure was 40·2 µg. per 24 hours. Subsequently, levels fell and remained relatively constant from days 75 to 86. In the next 28 day period oestrogen values rose to an ovulatory peak on days 91 and 92, and this was followed by a luteal phase rise from days 101 to 104 ; low values were found during the remaining eight days of the investigation. Pregnanediol readings were very low throughout the study up to day 97 ; subsequently higher values were noted, probably representing a luteal phase rise following the ovulatory peak of oestrogen excretion on day 91 or 92. It will be seen that bleeding occurred almost continuously for the first 61 days of the investigation and that the rise in oestrogen excretion commencing on day 47 was associated with cessation of bleeding on day 62. No further bleeding occurred during the next eight days during which time oestrogen levels remained high. Thereafter " spotting " was present, this being associated with a precipitous fall in oestrogen output. From days 85 to 93 there was again heavy bleeding with the ovulatory peak of oestrogen excretion mentioned above occurring during the bleeding on days 90 and 91.

HPG readings throughout the study were within the normal range for a woman during reproductive life, ranging from less than 4 to 25 HMG units per 24 hours. Relatively high levels were encountered from days 50 to 67, coinciding with the end of a protracted period of bleeding and with a rise in oestrogen output. No correlation could be demonstrated between the HPG readings on the one hand and the duration and severity of bleeding on the other.

Comment

Patients with dysfunctional uterine haemorrhage resemble those with the Stein-Leventhal syndrome in that their hormone

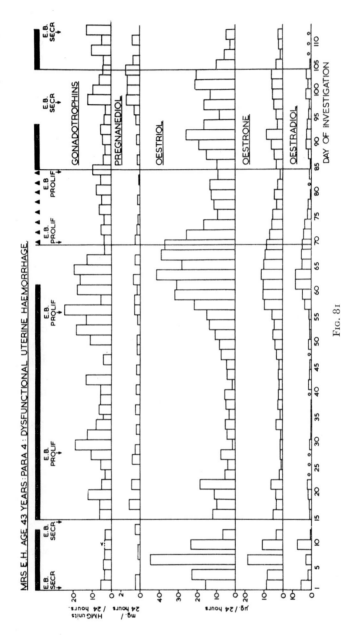

FIG. 81

Hormone excretion pattern in a patient with dysfunctional uterine haemorrhage.

E.B. = endometrial biopsy; ▲ = spotting; ■ = menstrual bleeding.

(From Loraine and Bell, 1966.)

excretion patterns vary not only between subjects but in the same subject at different times. The variability in oestrogen output between individuals was noted by Brown *et al.* (1959) who reported some women with reasonably constant levels over relatively long periods of time and others in whom readings fluctuated markedly from day to day. Variations in oestrogen output in the same subject are well illustrated by the results presented in Figure 81 in which a long period of anovulation was associated with fluctuating oestrogen levels, this being followed by a shortened ovulatory cycle with a peak of oestrogen excretion occurring during menstruation itself.

Another characteristic feature of oestrogen excretion patterns in dysfunctional uterine haemorrhage is the fact that at certain stages of the disease levels may be very high indeed and may approximate those found in early pregnancy. This observation was originally made by Brown *et al.* (1959) and has been commented upon by others ; its precise significance is not at present clear. The exact relationship between oestrogen excretion on the one hand and periods of bleeding on the other in patients with dysfunctional uterine haemorrhage remains to be established. Brown *et al.* (1959) concluded that no such correlation existed ; however, it will be noted that in the patient shown in Figure 81 cessation of bleeding was associated with rising oestrogen levels while recommencement of bleeding occurred in the presence of a decreasing output of these hormones. Pituitary gonadotrophic function in patients with dysfunctional uterine haemorrhage has not yet been satisfactorily investigated, and a study of alterations in the FSH/LH ratio of body fluids at different stages of the disease might well yield useful information in relation to pathogenesis.

OVARIAN TUMOURS

The classification of ovarian tumours on a pathological basis is outside the scope of this book and for recent reviews on this subject the reader is referred to articles by Jeffcoate (1962) and Scully (1963). In the present chapter the classification adopted by Jeffcoate (1962) will be followed. This involves dividing such tumours into three categories designated *feminising*, *virilising* and *neuter* (*non-functioning*). It must be emphasised that the literature on hormone excretion patterns in patients with ovarian tumours remains very meagre (see Scott *et al.*, 1967), and the ensuing discussion will be limited to those types of neoplasm in which reasonably complete endocrine investigations have been performed. Among the tumours considered herein will be granulosa and thecal cell types, arrhenoblastoma and dysgerminoma.

1. Feminising Tumours

The most important members of this group are granulosa and thecal cell tumours ; these can occur either in pure or in mixed form. Oestrogen assays by biological methods in patients with *granulosa cell tumours* have been reported by Glass and McKennon (1937) and Stohr (1942) amongst others. Pre-operatively abnormally high oestrogen levels are generally found both in blood and urine ; removal of the tumour causes a sharp fall in oestrogen output, while recurrence of the lesion in the contralateral ovary is associated with an increase in oestrogen excretion. Brown *et al.* (1959) and Brown and Matthew (1962) reported isolated oestrogen assays in three patients with combined granulosa and thecal cell tumours of the ovary. Two of the women were within the child-bearing age and showed normal excretion values ; the third who was postmenopausal had abnormally high levels which fell rapidly following operation.

The pre-operative pattern of hormone excretion in a subject with a granulosa cell tumour studied by the Edinburgh group is shown in Figure 82. It will be noted that oestrogen output was not abnormally high, readings being within the postmenopausal range. Values for HPG, pregnanediol, pregnanetriol and 17-OHCS did not deviate from normality, while the excretion of total 17-oxosteroids was at the lower end of or just below the normal range.

2. Virilising Tumours

In patients with *arrhenoblastoma* the output of total 17-oxosteroids may be normal even in the presence of marked signs of virilisation (Cohen *et al.*, 1958 ; Wiest *et al.*, 1959 ; Savard *et al.*, 1961). Such subjects generally show an increase in excretion values for some of the individual 17-oxosteroids, especially androsterone and to a lesser extent aetiocholanolone. Pesonen and Mikkonen (1958) found that in patients with arrhenoblastoma the output of DHA was not abnormal.

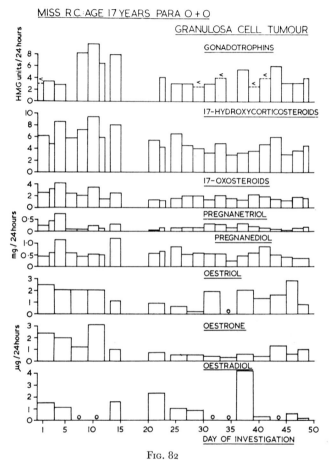

FIG. 82

Hormone excretion pattern in a patient with a granulosa cell tumour.

Plasma testosterone levels in a woman with an arrhenoblastoma have been reported by Coppage and Cooner (1965) ; readings were abnormally high pre-operatively and fell rapidly after surgical intervention.

3. Neuter (non-functioning) Tumours

The most important member of this group is the *dysgerminoma*. Reliable information on steroid excretion patterns in patients with this type of neoplasm is virtually non-existent, but recently Hobson and Baird (1966) have measured urinary HPG levels in a 16 year old girl with this disease. Assays were performed by the test depending on ovulation in the female toad, *Xenopus laevis*, and the results were expressed in terms of the international standard for HCG. Estimations were made both before and following operative treatment by total hysterectomy and bilateral oöphorectomy. Before surgical intervention the mean output was 1,624 i.u. per 24 hours. Following operation a marked fall in HPG excretion occurred, and seven days post-operatively biological activity could no longer be detected in the urine. On the basis of the available evidence the authors concluded that the type of gonadotrophin being excreted was luteinising rather than follicle-stimulating in nature. They were unable to draw any definite conclusion regarding the site of elaboration of the hormone and suggested that either the anterior pituitary or the tumour itself might be responsible.

CARCINOMA OF THE CERVIX

Information regarding hormone excretion patterns in patients with this disease is extremely scanty. In the experience of Brown *et al.* (1959), who measured urinary oestrogen levels in five such patients, readings were within the range normally encountered in postmenopausal women. Further work in this field should obviously be undertaken.

ENDOMETRIAL CARCINOMA

It has long been believed that oestrogens may be of aetiological importance in the pathogenesis of endometrial carcinoma (see Becker, 1904 ; Taylor, 1932 ; Jeffcoate, 1962 for reviews). However, there are few reports in the literature of endogenous hormone levels in patients with this disease, and, in particular, the relationship of oestrogen levels in body fluids to the course and prognosis of the condition has, until recently, been little studied. That abnormalities of endocrine function may have some part to play in the development of endometrial carcinoma is suggested by the fact that in a proportion of subjects a previous history of hormonal disturbances can be elicited. Such a history may include such complaints as infertility, menstrual abnormalities, an unduly late menopause, obesity and diabetes mellitus.

Charles *et al.* (1965) estimated endogenous hormone levels in a series of nine patients with endometrial carcinoma before and following operative treatment, usually by hysterectomy and by salpingo-oöphorectomy. Weighted mean levels for oestrogens, 17-OHCS, total 17-oxosteroids and HPG in the pre-operative period are shown in Table 7 from which it will be noted that all the readings were within the postmenopausal range. Results obtained in two subjects are presented in Figures 83 and 84.

TABLE 7

WEIGHTED MEAN HORMONE EXCRETION IN PATIENTS WITH ENDOMETRIAL CARCINOMA PRIOR TO OPERATION

(From Loraine and Bell, 1967)

Hormone	Excretion value	No. of patients	No. of observations
Oestradiol (μg./24 hours)...	0·6	9	29
Oestrone (μg./24 hours) ...	1·0	9	31
Oestriol (μg./24 hours) ...	2·5	9	31
17-OHCS (mg./24 hours)	10·0	4	17
Total 17-oxosteroids (mg./24 hours)	4·3	4	17
HPG (HMG units/24 hours)...	48·5	9	40

The patient shown in Figure 83 had a previous history of postmenopausal bleeding lasting for three months. During the pre-operative period excretion values for 17-OHCS, total 17-oxosteroids and oestrogens were within the normal range for a postmenopausal subject ; on the other hand, HPG levels were abnormally low. Following operation a marked rise in hormone output was observed. In the case of HPG the highest level was found on the 11th day of the study, while increased values for 17-OHCS, total 17-oxosteroids and oestrogens were noted in the immediate post-operative period only. It is apparent that the rise in oestriol output postdated that of 17-OHCS and 17-oxosteroids. By the 16th day of the investigation readings had fallen and were similar to those encountered pre-operatively.

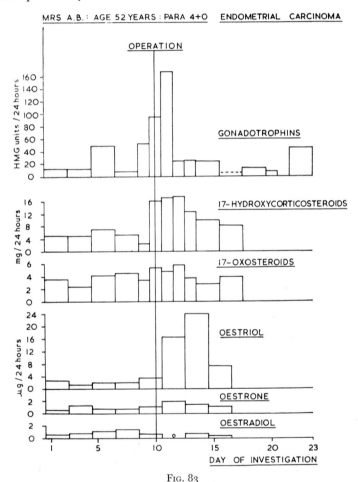

FIG. 83

Hormone excretion pattern in a patient with endometrial carcinoma.

(From Charles *et al.*, 1965.)

In Figure 84 are shown hormone assay data in a patient with a two-month history of postmenopausal bleeding. Prior to the operation excretion values for HPG and oestrogens did not deviate from normality. Following surgical treatment a slight increase in HPG excretion occurred on day 12 of the study ; there was, however, no effect on oestrogen output.

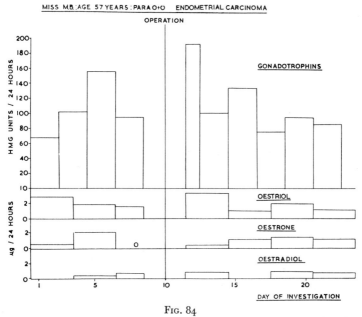

FIG. 84

Hormone excretion pattern in a patient with endometrial carcinoma.

(From Charles *et al.*, 1965.)

Comment

In all the nine patients investigated by Charles *et al.* (1965) urinary oestrogen levels in the pre-operative period were within the normal range for postmenopausal subjects. Following surgical treatment a rise in oestrogen, total 17-oxosteroid and 17-OHCS output was noted, and it is reasonable to conclude that this increase resulted from adrenocortical stimulation. In six of the nine women HPG excretion in the pre-operative period was within the normal range for hospitalised post-menopausal subjects (see Apostolakis and Loraine, 1960), while in the remainder abnormally low values were encountered. Operation produced an increase in HPG output in only three subjects, there being no effect in the remainder. The reason for the variation in HPG output following operative stress is not at present clear and clearly this subject merits further investigation. It is of interest to note that Sherman and Woolf (1959), using the ventral prostatic weight test in hypophysectomised rats, have noted abnormally high levels of urinary LH in 31 patients with endometrial carcinoma. Unfortunately, these investigators did not express their results in terms of a reference preparation, and for this reason the data they reported are of little or no quantitative significance.

There have been suggestions on the basis of cytological evidence that patients with endometrial carcinoma might be expected to show abnormally high oestrogen levels in body fluids. Thus Ayre and Bauld (1946), Berg and Durfee (1958), and Wachtel (1956) have reported that the cornification index in patients with this disease is generally higher than that in normal postmenopausal subjects. In the study of Charles et al. (1965) cytological features consistent with significant oestrogenic activity were noted in eight out of the nine patients studied, the remaining subject showing an atrophic vaginal smear. If hormone assays had not been performed it might have been postulated that the women in question showed definite evidence of abnormally high oestrogenic activity in their body fluids. Such a conclusion would obviously not have been justified since, in fact, urinary oestrogen levels in these cases were low, suggesting that ovarian activity was slight or absent. Accordingly it appears reasonable to conclude that in patients with endometrial carcinoma cytological evidence *per se* provides an unreliable estimate of the oestrogenicity of body fluids and that such evidence should not be used to assess oestrogen production in this disease.

SUMMARY AND CONCLUSIONS

Abnormalities in urinary steroid excretion are relatively frequent during the ovulatory menstrual cycle. These may affect the midcycle oestrogen peak and the luteal phase rise in oestrogen and pregnanediol output.

Anovular menstruation is associated either with fluctuating or with relatively constant values for oestrogen excretion. The precise relationship between oestrogen levels in body fluids and the occurrence and duration of bleeding remains to be elucidated.

In dysmenorrhoeic women cycles are generally of an ovulatory character. However, oestrogen levels tend to be lower than in normally menstruating women and, in particular, the midcycle and luteal phase peaks of oestrogen output are ill-defined. During the ovulatory and luteal phases of the cycle urinary pregnanetriol readings are lower in dysmenorrhoeic than in normal subjects.

When serial assays are conducted over relatively long periods of time in patients with oligomenorrhoea marked alterations in pituitary gonadotrophic and ovarian function occur.

In subjects with primary amenorrhoea in whom the condition is due to ovarian or pituitary failure, urinary oestrogen levels remain low and relatively constant. When the amenorrhoea is associated with a congenital absence of the uterus or vagina, a cyclic pattern of oestrogen excretion is encountered.

Patients with secondary amenorrhoea can be classified into three categories on the basis of their HPG output. In the first group levels are low, in the second normal and in the third abnormally high. Such a classification may be of value in relation to the therapy of the condition.

In patients with galactorrhoea and amenorrhoea the pattern of steroid and gonadotrophin output is similar to that encountered in secondary amenorrhoea. The presence of lactation itself does not appear to affect excretion values for oestrogens, pregnanediol and HPG.

The main characteristic of hormone excretion patterns in the Stein-Leventhal syndrome is their variability. Patients with this diagnosis can be classified on the basis of hormone assays into ovulatory and anovulatory groups.

In dysfunctional uterine haemorrhage very variable patterns of hormone excretion are encountered, such variations being especially marked in the case of the oestrogens. In a proportion of such subjects urinary oestrogen levels are greatly increased, being within the range normally encountered in early pregnancy.

Little information is at present available on hormone excretion patterns in patients with ovarian tumours.

In postmenopausal women with endometrial carcinoma excretion values for oestrogens and HPG are within the normal range. The fact that in such subjects low oestrogen levels are frequently associated with high cornification indices suggests that the latter parameter does not provide a reliable guide to the oestrogenic activity present in the body fluids of patients with this disease.

REFERENCES

APOSTOLAKIS, M. & LORAINE, J. A. (1960). *J. Clin. Endocrinol. Metab.* **20**, 1437.
AXELROD, L. R. & GOLDZIEHER, J. W. (1962). *J. Clin. Endocrinol. Metab.* **22**, 431.
AYRE, J. E. & BAULD, W. A. G. (1946). *Science*, **103**, 441.
BACKER, J. (1904). *Zentr. Gynakol.* **28**, 735.
BELL, E. T. & LORAINE, J. A. (1965). *Lancet*, **i**, 403.
BELL, E. T. & LORAINE, J. A. (1966 *a*). *Lancet*, **ii**, 519.
BELL, E. T. & LORAINE, J. A. (1966 *b*). *Lancet*, **i**, 626.
BELL, E. T. & LORAINE, J. A. (1967 *a*). *Acta Endocrinol.* Suppl. 119, 182.
BELL, E. T. & LORAINE, J. A. (1967 *b*). Unpublished observations.
BELL, E. T., MUKERJI, S., LORAINE, J. A. & LUNN, S. F. (1966). *Acta Endocrinol.* **51**, 578.
BERG, J. W. & DURFEE, G. R. (1958). *Cancer*, **11**, 158.
BJØRO, K. (1965). *Acta Obstet. Gynec. Scand.* **44**, Suppl. 4.
BROWN, J. B. & MATTHEW, G. D. (1962). *Recent Prog. Hormone Res.* **18**, 337.
BROWN, J. B., FOTHERBY, K. & LORAINE, J. A. (1962). *J. Endocrinol.* **25**, 331.
BROWN, J. B., KELLAR, R. J. & MATTHEW, G. D. (1959). *J. Obstet. Gynaecol. Brit. Empire*, **66**, 177.
CHARLES, D., BELL, E. T., LORAINE, J. A. & HARKNESS, R. A. (1965). *Am. J. Obstet. Gynecol.* **91**, 1050.
CHARLES, D., LORAINE, J. A., BELL, E. T. & HARKNESS, R. A. (1967). *Proceedings of Fifth World Congress on Fertility and Sterility*. Stockholm, 1966. Excerpta. Med. Inter. Cong. Series. No. 133 p. 92.
COHEN, M., MALTBY, E. J. & LAIDLAW, J. C. (1958). *J. Clin. Endocrinol. Metab.* **18**, 794.
COPPAGE, W. S., Jr. & COONER, A. E. (1965). *New Engl. J. Med.* **273**, 902.
DORFMAN, R. I. & SHIPLEY, R. A. (1956). *The Androgens*. New York : Wiley.
GALLAGHER, T. F., KAPPAS, A., HELLMAN, L., LIPSETT, M. B., PEARSON, O. H. & WEST, C. D. (1958). *J. Clin. Invest.* **37**, 794.
GLASS, S. J. & MCKENNON, B. J. (1937). *West J. Surg.* **45**, 467.
GOLDZIEHER, J. W. & AXELROD, L. R. (1962). *J. Clin. Endocrinol. Metab.* **22**, 425.
GOLDZIEHER, J. W. & GREEN, J. A. (1962). *J. Clin. Endocrinol. Metab.* **22**, 325.
HOBSON, B. M. & BAIRD, D. T. (1966). *J. Obstet. Gynaecol. Brit. Commonwealth*, **73**, 131.
ISMAIL, A. A. A., HARKNESS, R. A. & LORAINE, J. A. (1967). *Acta Endocrinol*, Suppl. 119, 50.
JAILER, J. W. & VANDE WIELE, R. L. (1954). *Gynaecologia*, **138**, 276.
JEFFCOATE, T. N. A. (1962). *Principles of Gynaecology*. London : Butterworths.
JENKINS, J. S. (1966). *Hospital Medicine*, **1**, 37.

KORENMAN, S. G., KIRSCHNER, M. A. & LIPSETT, M. B. (1965). *J. Clin. Endocrinol. Metab.* **25,** 798.
LANTHIER, A. (1960). *J. Clin. Endocrinol. Metab.* **20,** 1587.
LANTHIER, A. & SANDOR, T. (1964). *Acta Endocrinol* **46,** 245.
LLOYD, C. W., LOBOTSKY, J., SEGRE, E. J., KOBAYASHI, T., TAYMOR, M. L. & BATT, R. E. (1966). *J. Clin. Endocrinol. Metab.* **26,** 314.
LORAINE, J. A. & BELL, E. T. (1966). *Hormone Assays and their Clinical Application,* 2nd Ed. Edinburgh : Livingstone.
LORAINE, J. A. & BELL, E. T. (1967). *Obstet. Gynec. Surv.* **22,** 463.
LORAINE, J. A. & BELL, E. T. (1968). *J. Obstet Gynaecol. Brit. Commonwealth. In press.*
LORAINE, J. A., BELL, E. T., HARKNESS, R. A. & HARRISON, M. T. (1966). *Acta Endocrinol.* **52,** 527.
MCARTHUR, J. W., INGERSOLL, F. M. & WORCESTER, J. (1958). *J. Clin. Endocrinol. Metab.* **18,** 1202.
MAHESH, V. B. & GREENBLATT, R. B. (1964). *Recent Prog. Hormone Res.* **20,** 341.
PEDERSEN-BJERGAARD, K. & TØNNESEN, M. (1951). *Acta Endocrinol.* **7,** 270.
PESONEN, S. & MIKKONEN, R. (1958). *Acta Endocrinol.* **27,** 170.
ROBERTS, D. (1966). *Hospital Medicine,* **1,** 35.
SAVARD, K., GUT, M., DORFMAN, R. I., GABRILOVE, J. L. & SOFFER, L. J. (1961). *J. Clin. Endocrinol. Metab.* **21,** 165.
SCOTT, J. S., LUMSDEN, C. E. & LEVELL, M. J. (1967). *Am. J. Obstet. Gynecol.* **97,** 161.
SCULLY, R. E. (1963). In *Progress in Gynaecology,* vol. 4, p. 335. Eds. Meigs, J. V. and Sturgis, S. H. London : Heinemann.
SHEARMAN, R. P. & COX, R. I. (1966). *Obstet. Gynec. Surv.* **21,** 1.
SHERMAN, A. E. & WOOLF, R. B. (1959). *Am. J. Obstet. Gynecol.* **77,** 233.
STEIN, I. F. (1966). In *Ovulation,* p. 150. Ed. Greenblatt, R. B. Philadelphia : Lippincott.
STOHR, C. (1942). *Am. J. Obstet. Gynecol.* **43,** 586.
TAYLOR, H. C., Jr. (1932). *Am. J. Obstet. Gynecol.* **23,** 309.
TOWNSEND, S. L., BROWN, J. B., JOHNSTONE, J. W., ADEY, F. T., EVANS, J. H. & TAFT, H. P. (1966). *J. Obstet. Gynaecol. Brit. Commonwealth,* **73,** 529.
WACHTEL, E. (1956). *J. Obstet. Gynaecol. Brit. Empire,* **63,** 176.
WIEST, W. G., ZANDER, J. & HOLMSTROM, E. G. (1959). *J. Clin. Endocrinol. Metab.* **19,** 297.
ZANDER, J., WIEST, W. G. & OBER, K. G. (1962). *Arch. Gynäkol.* **196,** 481.

CHAPTER VII

Induction of Ovulation by Clomiphene

INTRODUCTION

CLOMIPHENE (Clomid, MRL-41) bears a close structural relationship to the potent synthetic oestrogen chlorotri-anisene (TACE). It is also related to the compound MER-25 (1-p-2-diethylaminoethoxyphenyl)-1-phenyl-2-p-methoxyphenylethanol), a substance which was shown by Tyler *et al.* (1960) and by Kistner and Smith (1961) to be capable of stimulating ovulation in human subjects, but which proved to be too toxic for clinical use. The structural formulae of Clomiphene, TACE and MER-25 are shown in Figure 85.

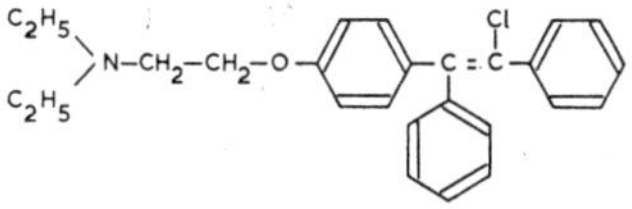

CLOMIPHENE

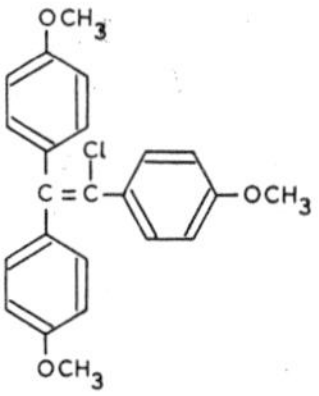

TACE

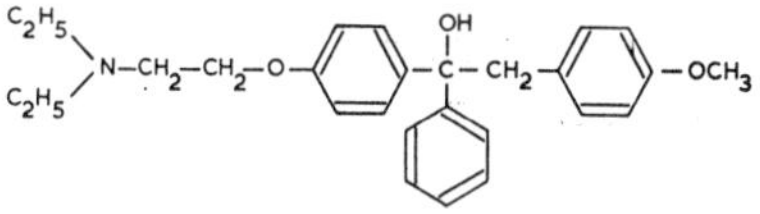

MER 25

FIG. 85
Structural formulae of Clomiphene, TACE and MER 25.

The effects of Clomiphene in animals were first investigated by Holtkamp *et al.* (1961) and have been recently summarised (see Holtkamp, 1966). In adult female rats the compound, given in dosages ranging from 0·1 to 0·3 mg. per kg. body weight per day, showed marked antifertility properties, being capable of preventing conception and subsequent pregnancy; following withdrawal of Clomiphene normal fertility was restored. Barnes and Meyer (1962) showed that the compound was a potent inhibitor of endogenous pituitary gonadotrophic activity in rats as judged by its effect on ovarian weight. The experiments of Segal and Nelson (1961) in adult male rats demonstrated that Clomiphene, given at dose levels ranging from 1·0 to 5·0 mg. per kg. body weight, reduced the sperm count and decreased fertility; as in the case of female animals these effects were reversed when treatment was withdrawn. In immature female mice Clomiphene had two apparently opposite actions, the first to increase uterine weight, and the second to prevent the effect of oestradiol in causing uterine enlargement (Holtkamp, 1966).

Early studies by Greenblatt and his associates, summarised in a review by Greenblatt and Mahesh (1965), indicated that the effects of Clomiphene in human subjects were very different from those in rodents. These workers noted that the compound lacked contraceptive activity in women and observed that, when it was administered to patients with unduly short menstrual cycles, the latter reverted to a normal length. Greenblatt and his colleagues (Greenblatt, 1961; Greenblatt et al., 1961) subsequently showed that, far from having an antifertility effect, Clomiphene actually stimulated ovulation in a proportion of women in whom this event failed to occur. Recently Boutselis et al. (1967) have given Clomiphene to normally menstruating women in an attempt to control the time of ovulation and cycle length and thereby to increase the efficiency of the rhythm method of contraception (see p. 131). This interesting approach requires further investigation.

SELECTION OF PATIENTS FOR CLOMIPHENE THERAPY

Clomiphene is generally administered by the oral route in the form of the citrate. It has been given to patients with a large number of disorders characterised by infertility including primary and secondary amenorrhoea, oligomenorrhoea, the Stein-Leventhal syndrome, the Chiari-Frommel syndrome, dysfunctional uterine haemorrhage, the adrenogenital syndrome and various types of pituitary and ovarian failure. In earlier studies the selection of patients for Clomiphene therapy depended entirely on clinical assessment. Recently Bell and

Loraine (1966) and Townsend *et al.* (1966) have demonstrated the value of hormone assay studies in predicting the response of infertile patients to treatment with the compound.

According to Kistner (1965 *a*), who used mainly clinical parameters, the type of patient most likely to derive benefit from Clomiphene therapy is one in whom ovulation does not occur, but who, nevertheless, shows evidence of adequate endogenous oestrogen production as judged by vaginal cytology endometrial biobsy, and by the fact that that a withdrawal bleeding takes place following progesterone administration. This worker has emphasised that, prior to the initiation of Clomiphene therapy, careful pelvic examination is necessary, special attention being paid to the size of the ovaries. If a definite ovarian cyst is present the administration of the compound is contra-indicated; however, it can be given with safety in the presence of the moderate ovarian enlargement encountered in patients with the Stein-Leventhal syndrome.

Bell and Loraine (1966) were the first to investigate the value of serial hormone assays in urine in predicting the therapeutic response to Clomiphene. They studied a series of 14 women suffering from various forms of infertility; clinical details of their patients are shown in Table 8. The estimations performed were those for oestrogens, pregnanediol and HPG, and the response to therapy was assessed on the basis of the steroid excretion pattern. Three types of response were recognised (i) *ovulation*; (ii) *oestrogen increase without ovulation*, presumably indicating follicular development in the absence of corpus luteum formation and (iii) *no effect*.

Assay results prior to therapy are shown in Table 9 from which it will be noted that in patients who ovulated in response to Clomiphene the mean urinary oestrogen excretion before treatment was higher than in the other two groups. The lowest oestrogen readings were encountered in the women who failed to respond, while in the patients showing an increase in oestrogen output in the absence of ovulation, the mean figure occupied a position intermediate between the other two groups. Pregnanediol assays were not found to be of assistance in predicting the response to Clomiphene therapy. HPG readings were highest in women in whom Clomiphene did not affect steroid output, lowest in the group in which ovulation

TABLE 8

CLINICAL DETAILS OF PATIENTS

(After Bell and Loraine, 1966)

Patient	Age years	Parity	Diagnosis	Response
1	26	0	Secondary amenorrhoea	Ovulation
2	24	0	Secondary amenorrhoea	
3	29	0	Stein-Leventhal syndrome	
4	32	1 + 0	Post partum galactorrhoea	
5	34	1 + 0	Post partum galactorrhoea	
6	33	0	Secondary amenorrhoea	Oestrogen rise in the absence of ovulation
7	31	0	Secondary amenorrhoea	
8	20	0	Stein-Leventhal syndrome	
9	19	0	Stein-Leventhal syndrome	
10	30	2 + 0	Secondary amenorrhoea	No effect
11	31	1 + 0	Secondary amenorrhoea	
12	22	0	Secondary amenorrhoea	
13	32	0	Secondary amenorrhoea and galactorrhoea	
14	23	0	Secondary amenorrhoea and galactorrhoea	

occurred and intermediate in the subjects showing an oestrogen rise in the absence of ovulation.

The observations of Bell and Loraine (1966) suggest that the patients most likely to ovulate as a result of Clomiphene therapy are those already showing definite evidence of ovarian activity as judged by urinary oestrogen assays, and in whom HPG excretion is either low or undetectable. On the other hand, patients with the very low oestrogen output characteristic of the menopause or postmenopause and with relatively high HPG levels are much less likely to show a favourable response. Similar results to those of Bell and Loraine (1966) have been reported by Townsend et al. (1966) who stated that ovulation as a result of Clomiphene therapy could be anticipated in patients in whom the excretion of " total oestrogens " (see p. 30) prior to treatment exceeded 10 μg. per 24 hours.

DOSAGE OF CLOMIPHENE TO INDUCE OVULATION

As emphasised by Greenblatt and Mahesh (1965) and by others, individual patients differ greatly in their response to the same dosage of Clomiphene. For this reason it is difficult to recommend a dosage schedule which is universally applicable. In earlier studies in this field dosages of the compound ranging from 25 to 150 mg. per day were administered continuously for weeks or even months. On such a regime ovulatory menstrual cycles frequently occurred, but pregnancies were few and the incidence of cystic enlargement of the ovaries was high. In later work the compound has been given for shorter periods of time, and the regime now recommended by Kistner (1965 a) consists of the administration of 50 or 100 mg. of Clomiphene per day for five days. Charles et al. (1963) originally recommended that the compound be given at a dose level of from 25 to 100 mg. per day for 14 to 21 days. In the light of subsequent experience the same group of investigators (Charles et al., 1967) concluded that the most satisfactory clinical response was produced with a dosage of 100 mg. per day for 5 to 14 days.

It is generally recognised that patients with the Stein-Leventhal syndrome are especially sensitive to Clomiphene administration, showing a relatively high incidence of cystic

TABLE 9

STEROID AND GONADOTROPHIN EXCRETION BEFORE CLOMIPHENE THERAPY IN PATIENTS WITH PROBLEMS OF INFERTILITY

(After Bell and Loraine, 1966)

Group	"Total oestrogens"			Pregnanediol			HPG		
	Number of patients	Number of assays	Mean excretion —μg. per 24 hours	Number of patients	Number of assays	Mean excretion —mg. per 24 hours	Number of patients	Number of assays	Mean excretion —HMG units per 24 hours
Ovulation ...	5	54	14·0	5	37	0·7	5	50	<6·5
Oestrogen rise in the absence of ovulation ...	4	41	6·5	4	31	0·8	4	37	<7·9
No effect ...	3	65	3·6	4	47	1·1	2	48	<13·5

204

enlargement of the ovaries. Accordingly, in such women smaller rather than larger doses of the compound should be given, and, in addition, the duration of administration should probably be relatively short. In the opinion of Greenblatt and Mahesh (1965) infertile women showing ovarian insensitivity and failing to ovulate following a short course of Clomiphene, should be treated with a larger dose for a longer period. In patients of this type these investigators have given courses of 100 mg. per day for as long as 20 days. It is now established that, after withdrawal of cyclic Clomiphene therapy, ovulatory cycles may continue for relatively long periods of time, and that, following a Clomiphene induced pregnancy, ovulatory cycles generally recommence.

INCIDENCE OF OVULATION AS A RESULT OF CLOMIPHENE THERAPY

This has been determined by a large number of investigators including Greenblatt et al. (1961), Southam and Janovski (1962), Smith et al. (1963), Roy et al. (1963), Charles et al. (1963, 1966, 1967), Kaiser (1963), Whitelaw (1963, 1966), Payne and Karow (1963), Naville et al. (1964), Puebla and Greenblatt (1964), Riley and Evans (1964), Vorys et al. (1964), Whitelaw et al. (1964), Wall et al. (1964), Thompson and Mellinger (1965), Kistner (1965 b), Bishop (1965), Jones and Moraes-Ruehsen (1965), Pildes (1965), Beck et al. (1966), Cudmore and Tupper (1966), Cohen (1966) and Johnson et al. (1966). In such studies ovulation was assessed by numerous criteria including basal body temperature records, endometrial biopsies, urinary pregnanediol assays, the demonstration of fresh corpora lutea at laparotomy and the occurrence of pregnancy. The most extensive individual clinical experience in this field remains that of Kistner (1965 a) and of Greenblatt and Mahesh (1965).

The results obtained in the 2,616 patients reported by Johnson et al. (1966) are shown in Table 10. The high total incidence of ovulation in the series (69 per cent) should be noted, together with the fact that ovulatory cycles were especially frequent in patients with secondary amenorrhoea and with the Stein-Leventhal syndrome. Ovulation occurred after the first course of Clomiphene in 2,014 women (76 per cent). Kistner (1965 *a*) found that patients with panhypopituitarism generally did not ovulate as a result of Clomiphene therapy in spite of the fact that they were receiving adequate replacement therapy. Likewise, women with ovarian agenesis and with a premature menopause failed to show a satisfactory response. Kistner (1965 *a*) has also emphasised that in some

TABLE 10

INCIDENCE OF OVULATION FOLLOWING CLOMIPHENE ADMINISTRATION

(After Johnson *et al.*, 1966)

Diagnosis	Number of patients	Occurrence of ovulation	
		Number of patients	%
Secondary amenorrhoea, oligomenorrhoea and anovulatory cycles... ...	1,718	1,238	72
Polycystic ovary syndrome ...	569	433	76
Chiari-Frommel syndrome ...	83	48	58
Adrenal hyperplasia	40	29	72
Pituitary failure	17	8	47
Pituitary tumour	12	5	42
Pituitary amenorrhoea ...	77	27	35
Ovarian failure	100	17	17
Total	2,616	1,805	69

patients ovulation occurs following each course of the compound, while in others a response is noted to some but not to all courses of treatment.

The clinical experience of Greenblatt and Mahesh (1965) with Clomiphene is shown in Table 11. The high incidence of ovulatory cycles in patients with so-called " functional " and secondary amenorrhoea, the Stein-Leventhal syndrome and dysfunctional uterine haemorrhage is noteworthy.

TABLE 11

INCIDENCE OF OVULATION FOLLOWING CLOMIPHENE ADMINISTRATION

(After Greenblatt and Mahesh, 1965)

Diagnosis	Number of patients	Incidence of ovulation		Number of treatment cycles	Incidence of ovulation	
		Number of patients	%		Number of treatment cycles	%
"Functional" amenorrhoea ...	87	74	85	418	343	82
Secondary amenorrhoea ...	75	54	72	465	299	64
Primary amenorrhoea ...	18	5	28	109	26	24
Stein-Leventhal syndrome ...	42	36	86	165	149	90
Dysfunctional uterine haemorrhage	35	31	89	174	147	85
Total	257	200	77	1,331	962	73

PREGNANCY FOLLOWING THERAPY BY CLOMIPHENE

It is clear that the number of patients in whom ovulation occurs as a result of Clomiphene therapy bears little or no relationship to the pregnancy rate produced by the administration of the compound. This arises because many of the patients who have received such treatment were either unmarried or were not desirous of bearing children. Furthermore, in a proportion of the cases reported in the literature conception may have been prevented because the husband was infertile. In the series of 1,809 women who ovulated following Clomiphene administration, 704 (27 per cent) subsequently became pregnant (Johnson et al., 1966). In the patients studied by Roy et al. (1963) 28 out of 179 (16 per cent) conceived as a result of treatment, while in the subjects studied by Charles et al. (1967) 16 out of 71 (22·5 per cent) became pregnant. In a proportion of patients receiving Clomiphene multiple pregnancies occur. Thus, in 25 out of 300 conceptions reported by Kistner (1965 a) there were 22 twins, two sets of triplets and one set of quadruplets; in Kistner's series neonatal deaths occurred in three sets of twins and one set of quadruplets. However, it must be emphasised that at the time of writing, there is no evidence to suggest that the administration of Clomiphene increases the incidence of congenital malformations in the foetus.

THE EFFECT OF CLOMIPHENE ON HORMONE EXCRETION PATTERNS

Serial hormone assays in patients receiving Clomiphene have been reported by Smith et al. (1963), Roy et al. (1963), Dickey et al. (1965), Townsend et al. (1966), Shearman (1966) and by the Edinburgh group (Charles et al., 1963, 1966, 1967; Loraine et al., 1966 a; Bell et al., 1966 a). Isolated assays have been performed by several investigators, but the results obtained are of very limited importance and will not be considered herein. The present section concentrates mainly on the work of the Edinburgh group and provides examples of the effect of Clomiphene on endocrine function in patients with secondary amenorrhoea, galactorrhoea and the Stein-Leventhal syndrome. A comparison of the effects of Clomiphene and of gonadotrophins on hormone excretion in infertile patients will be found on p. 253.

1. Secondary Amenorrhoea

Investigations in three patients with this disease are shown in Figures 86 to 88. In the first (Figure 86) both TACE and Clomiphene were administered, ovulation occurring following

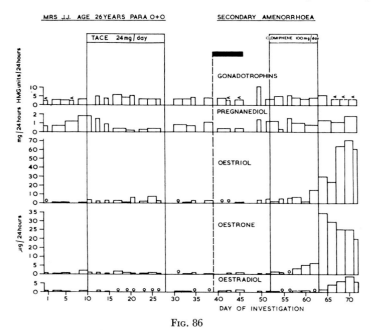

FIG. 86

Hormone excretion pattern in a patient with secondary amenorrhoea treated with TACE and Clomiphene.

■ = menstrual bleeding.

(From Charles *et al.*, 1966.)

therapy with the latter but not with the former compound. In the second subject Clomiphene produced a rise in oestrogen output in the absence of ovulation, while in the third Clomiphene therapy was followed by ovulation and conception.

The patient in Figure 86 had a history of irregular and infrequent periods from her menarche at the age of 16; prior to the investigation she had been amenorrhoeic for approximately three years. Her endometrium showed an inactive proliferative pattern; her ovaries were slightly enlarged but, on histological examination, were not typical of the Stein-Leventhal syndrome. After an initial control period of 10 days TACE was administered orally at a dose-level of 24 mg. per day for 18 days. Twenty-four days later Clomiphene was given daily for 11 days at a dose-level of 50 mg. b.i.d.

During the control period excretion values for HPG and oestrogens were abnormally low for a woman during reproductive life. Pregnanediol values were within the normal range for the follicular phase of the menstrual cycle. Treatment with TACE produced no effect on HPG, oestrone or oestradiol excretion. Pregnanediol levels tended to fall slightly during therapy and rose again after cessation of treatment. Levels of oestriol showed a slight increase during drug administration, but the sum of excretion values for oestrone, oestriol and oestradiol remained within the postmenopausal range. It should be emphasised that an ovulatory cycle as judged by the pattern of steroid excretion did not result from the administration of TACE. Bleeding occurred on day 40 and lasted for seven days.

Therapy with Clomiphene was initiated 13 days after the start of bleeding. During the treatment period there was no effect on HPG, pregnanediol and oestradiol excretion, but levels of oestrone and oestriol tended to rise. Immediately after cessation of therapy there was a slight rise in pregnanediol output. On days 64 and 65 a sharp increase in oestrone excretion occurred, this being associated with a smaller rise in oestriol output. From day 66 until the end of the study, a marked rise in oestriol and oestradiol levels took place in association with falling oestrone values. On day 70 a dilatation and curettage was performed and the endometrium obtained showed a secretory pattern consistent with the 22nd or 23rd day of the normal menstrual cycle. Accordingly, it may be concluded on the basis both of the clinical and the endocrinological findings that in this subject Clomiphene therapy produced an ovulatory cycle.

In Figure 87 are shown hormone assay results in a 33 year old patient who had been amenorrhoeic for 14 years prior to the investigation, the amenorrhoea being probably of psychological origin. The control period lasted for 57 days during which time levels of oestrogens and pregnanediol were low and were within the postmenopausal range. The excretion of " total gonadotrophic activity " as measured by the mouse uterus test was also low, being generally less than 5 HMG units per 24 hours; however, a high value of 23·9 HMG units per 24 hours was encountered on days 51 and 52.

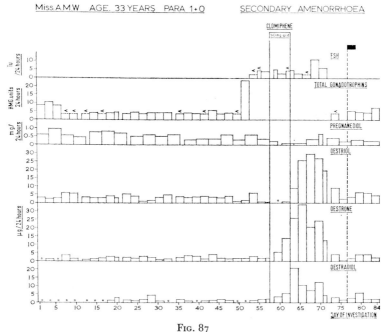

FIG. 87

Hormone excretion pattern in a patient with secondary amenorrhoea treated with Clomiphene.

▨ = menstrual bleeding.

(From Bell *et al.*, 1966 *a*, *J. Obstet. Gynaecol. Brit. Commonwealth.*)

Clomiphene was administered at a dose-level of 50 mg. q.i.d. from days 58 to 62 inclusive. It caused a marked increase in oestrone and oestradiol output but had no effect on oestriol or pregnanediol excretion. After withdrawal of medication, oestrogen levels continued to rise being at their maximum from days 63 to 70. Thereafter readings fell prior to menstruation, which occurred on day 77 and lasted for two days. It should be noted that the high oestrogen levels were not followed by an increase in pregnanediol output, indicating that the patient failed to ovulate as a result of treatment. During Clomiphene therapy there was no change in FSH excretion as measured by the mouse ovarian augmentation test; however, following cessation of medication a slight rise in the output of this hormone occurred. The excretion of " total gonadotrophic activity " during the last 12 days of the study was in the same range as in the control period.

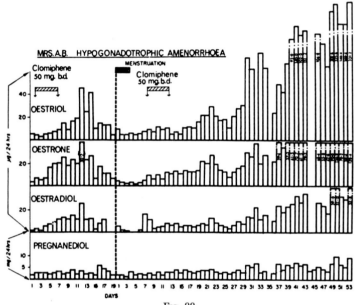

FIG. 88

**Steroid excretion pattern in a patient with secondary amenor-
rhoea treated with Clomiphene.**

(From Shearman, 1966.)

It is noteworthy that in the two patients with secondary amenorrhoea shown in Figures 86 and 87 and in one woman reported by Smith *et al.* (1963) the rise in oestrone output produced by Clomiphene occurred earlier than the increase in oestriol excretion. This finding has also been commented on by Bell *et al.* (1966 *a*) who observed that in Clomiphene induced ovulatory cycles the ratio of oestrone to oestriol tended to be different from that found in the normal cycle, proportionately more of the former steroid being excreted.

Information on the differential excretion of FSH and LH in patients with secondary amenorrhoea treated by Clomiphene is very limited indeed. In one such subject investigated by Dickey *et al.* (1965) the compound caused a transient rise in FSH output without any marked effect on LH excretion.

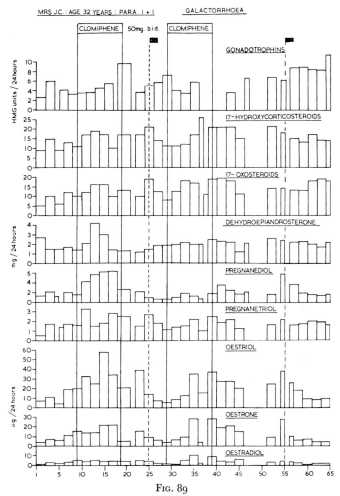

FIG. 89

Hormone excretion pattern in a patient with galactorrhoea treated with Clomiphene.

■ = menstrual bleeding.

(From Loraine *et al.*, 1966 *a*.)

213

In Figure 88 is shown the steroid excretion pattern in a woman with secondary amenorrhoea of 15 months duration who was investigated by Shearman (1966) and who became pregnant as a result of Clomiphene therapy. In the first cycle a rise in oestrogen output occurred at approximately midcycle, but the increase in pregnanediol excretion in the luteal phase was small and transitory. In the second cycle Clomiphene produced ovulation and this was followed by conception. The very high oestrogen levels in the latter part of the study are noteworthy and are within the range normally encountered soon after fertilisation of the ovum. The pregnancy itself was uneventful and resulted in the birth of a single normal male child.

2. Galactorrhoea

Hormone excretion patterns in patients with galactorrhoea treated by Clomiphene have been reported by Loraine et al. (1966 a) and by Charles et al. (1967). Two examples of the results obtained are included and are shown in Figures 89 and 90. In the first subject an ovulatory cycle was produced while in the second the compound caused a rise in oestrogen output in the absence of ovulation.

The patient shown in Figure 89 had a history of amenorrhoea and galactorrhoea following the birth of a normal male infant three years prior to the investigation. When Clomiphene was given at the dose level shown the galactorrhoea promptly ceased. The subject became pregnant one year after the last course of Clomiphene and gave birth to a normal female infant. Following a short period of breast feeding lactation ceased in a normal manner and the patient subsequently had regular menstrual cycles.

During the control period which lasted for nine days the urinary excretion values for HPG, 17-hydroxycorticosteroids (17-OHCS) and 17-oxosteroids were within the normal range for a woman during reproductive life. The output of dehydro-epiandrosterone (DHA) and pregnanetriol was somewhat high as was that of oestrogens and pregnanediol. However, in view of the fact that amenorrhoea had been present for several months prior to the commencement of the study, it was considered unlikely that the high values of these steroids were associated with the occurrence of a recent ovulation. The first course of Clomiphene was administered from days 10 to 19 inclusive, the dose-level being 50 mg. twice daily. During this time a rise in 17-OHCS, 17-oxosteroids, pregnanetriol and DHA occurred, the increase in the last mentioned steroid being especially pronounced. Ovulation as judged by oestrogen

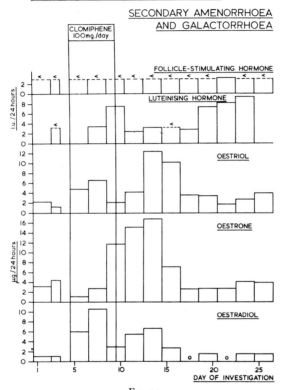

FIG. 90

Hormone excretion pattern in a patient with secondary amenorrhoea and galactorrhoea treated with Clomiphene.
(From Charles *et al.*, 1967.)

excretion probably occurred on days 11 or 12 and was followed by a luteal phase rise in pregnanediol which was maximal on days 17 and 18; pregnanediol levels fell prior to menstruation which occurred on days 26 and 27. Towards the end of the course of Clomiphene HPG readings rose, reaching a maximum of 9·8 HMG units per 24 hours from days 19 to 21.

The second course of Clomiphene was administered from days 30 to 39 inclusive at the same dose level. Again there was an increase in excretion values for 17-OHCS and 17-oxosteroids over control levels. Little or no effect was noted on the output of HPG or pregnanediol, but a small increase in levels of DHA and pregnanetriol was observed. Oestrogen excretion rose, reaching its maximum on days 35 and 36. This was probably an ovulatory peak and was followed by a small luteal phase rise in pregnanediol output which occurred immediately following withdrawal of medication. Menstruation commenced on day 56 and lasted for three days; it was immediately preceded by high levels of pregnanediol, pregnanetriol and oestrogens. Following menstruation, readings of HPG, 17-OHCS and 17-oxosteroids were higher than in the initial pre-treatment period. On the other hand, excretion values for DHA, pregnanediol, pregnanetriol and oestrogens were in the same range as in the control period.

The patient shown in Figure 90 was nulliparous and gave a history of secondary amenorrhoea in association with galactorrhoea for $3\frac{1}{2}$ years. The investigation was conducted over a period of 26 days, during which time assays of FSH by the mouse ovarian augmentation test, LH by the OAAD method and oestrogens were performed. Clomiphene was administered orally from day 5 to 9 at a dose-level of 100 mg. per day. FSH levels remained low throughout, being detectable in only one of the 13 samples assayed. Values for urinary LH were in the same range as those previously described by Bell et al. (1966 b) in normally menstruating women; Clomiphene produced no definite effect on the excretion of this hormone. Oestrogen levels before treatment were within the postmenopausal range; Clomiphene caused a rise in oestrogen excretion, the increase in oestradiol being maximal during therapy and that of oestriol and oestrone following withdrawal of medication. The treatment did not produce an ovulatory cycle and menstruation failed to occur.

3. Stein-Leventhal Syndrome

Serial hormone assays in patients with the Stein-Leventhal syndrome treated by Clomiphene have been reported by Roy et al. (1963), Charles et al. (1963), Dickey et al. (1965) and

Bell *et al.* (1966 *a*). A typical example of the results obtained by the Edinburgh group is shown in Figure 91. The patient had a history of oligomenorrhoea in association with hirsutism for 11 years. On culdoscopy her ovaries were found to be enlarged and to be characteristic of the Stein-Leventhal syndrome. Assays of FSH, " total gonadotrophic activity ", oestrogens and pregnanediol were performed.

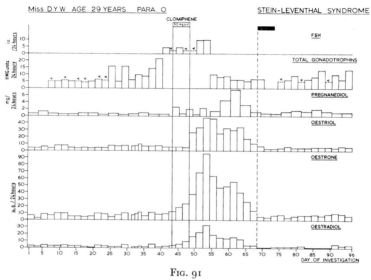

FIG. 91

Hormone excretion pattern in a patient with the Stein-Leventhal syndrome treated with Clomiphene.

▬ = menstrual bleeding.

(From Bell *et al.*, 1966 *a*, *J. Obstet. Gynaecol. Brit. Commonwealth.*)

During the control period, which lasted for 43 days, the urinary excretion of oestrogens and pregnanediol remained low, being at the lower end of the range normally encountered in the follicular phase of the menstrual cycle. Values for " total gonadotrophic activity " were variable, ranging from less than 4 to 22·9 HMG units per 24 hours and were therefore within the range characteristic of women during reproductive life. Clomiphene was administered at a dose-level of 50 mg. q.i.d. from days 44 to 48 inclusive of the investigation. During this time an increase in oestrone and oestradiol excretion occurred, with little or no effect on the output of oestriol or pregnanediol. Following cessation of therapy, oestrogen levels continued to rise reaching an ovulatory peak on days 53 and 54. This was followed by a luteal phase rise in pregnanediol output, maximal on days 61 to 63 of the study, and by menstruation which commenced on day 69 and lasted for four days.

Clomiphene therapy produced no effect on urinary FSH excretion, but following withdrawal of medication a slight rise

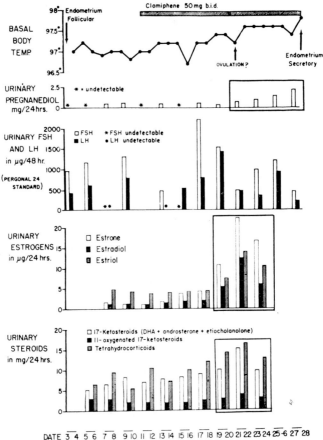

FIG. 92

Hormone excretion pattern and basal body temperature readings in a patient with the Stein-Leventhal syndrome treated with Clomiphene.

(From Roy *et al.*, 1963.)

in the output of this hormone occurred. Estimates of " total gonadotrophic activity " conducted from day 55 until the end of the study, were in the same range as in the control period. During the last 27 days of the investigation urinary steroid levels were also similar to those in the control period and, in particular, an ovulatory cycle did not occur.

The effect of Clomiphene on hormone excretion, basal temperature records and endometrial histology in a patient with the Stein-Leventhal syndrome studied by Roy *et al.* (1963) is shown in Figure 92. The compound was administered at a dose level of 50 mg. b.i.d. from day 9 of the investigation for 18 days. During the control period oestrogen and pregnanediol levels were within the postmenopausal range while FSH and LH readings were either low or undetectable; the endometrium was proliferative in character, and the basal body temperature record was of an anovulatory type. The administration of Clomiphene produced an ovulatory cycle as indicated by the pattern of pregnanediol and oestrogen output, and the fact that ovulation had occurred was confirmed by the finding of a secretory endometrium on day 26 of the investigation. Clomiphene produced a slight rise in the output of both FSH and LH, and following ovulation there was an increase in excretion values for tetrahydro derivatives of corticosteroids, total 17-oxosteroids and 11-oxygenated-17-oxosteroids.

OTHER EFFECTS OF CLOMIPHENE

1. Effects on the Endometrium

A number of investigators, including Charles (1962), Charles *et al.* (1964), Wall *et al.* (1964) and Kistner (1965 *b*) have studied the effects of Clomiphene on endometrial histology in patients with diseases associated with infertility. Endometrial patterns before and after the administration of the compound in a woman with secondary amenorrhoea, who had previously been subjected to wedge resection, are shown in Figures 93 and 94. Prior to treatment the endometrium showed atypical hyperplasia with a cribriform pattern; following therapy a secretory pattern was present. Endometrial histology before and after Clomiphene therapy in a patient with the Stein-Leventhal syndrome studied by Charles *et al.* (1963) is shown

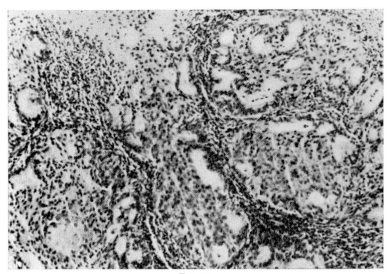

Fig. 93

**Endometrial biopsy in a patient with secondary amenor-
rhoea prior to Clomiphene therapy.**

(From Charles, 1962.)

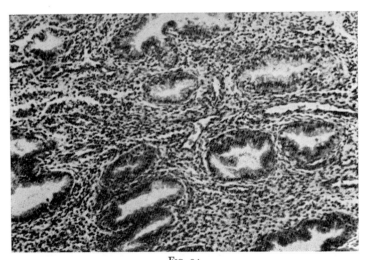

Fig. 94

**Endometrial biopsy in a patient with secondary amenor-
rhoea following Clomiphene therapy.**

(From Charles, 1962.)

in Figures 95 and 96. It will be noted that before treatment the pattern was proliferative in type while the post-treatment endometrium was typical of the early secretory phase.

Wall *et al.* (1964) found that following Clomiphene therapy reversal of both benign and malignant endometrial changes occurred. Kistner (1965 *b*) treated a series of patients with endometria classified either as hyperplastic or as anaplastic and found that in the majority of cases the post-treatment endometria showed a normal secretory pattern. Kistner *et al.* (1966) also studied the effect of continuous Clomiphene therapy on the endometria of women suffering from cystic adenomatous hyperplasia, anaplasia and carcinoma *in situ*; in many cases such therapy continued for weeks or months. For the first six to eight weeks of medication the endometrium was secretory in type; thereafter, it became atrophic and remained so for as long as the administration of the drug was continued. In a proportion of the women studied cessation of therapy was associated with reversion of the endometrium to a hyperplastic pattern, indicating that oestrogenic stimulation was now occurring, and suggesting that the effect produced during drug administration was a result of the well recognised anti-oestrogenic action of Clomiphene.

2. Effects on Vaginal Cytology

These have been reported by Thompson and Mellinger (1965) and by others. In a patient with Turner's syndrome Thompson and Mellinger (1965) found that Clomiphene produced anti-oestrogenic effects, diminishing the number of cornified superficial cells resulting from the administration of stilboestrol, and increasing the number of intermediate uncornified cells. These workers also noted that, despite its anti-oestrogenic effects on vaginal cytology, Clomiphene produced a biphasic temperature pattern and caused changes characteristic of the luteal phase of the cycle *e.g.* the absence of ferning of cervical mucus.

3. Effects on Lactation

Treatment of patients with galactorrhoea by Clomiphene has been reported by various investigators including Kaiser (1963), Thompson and Mellinger (1965), Greenblatt and Mahesh (1965), Loraine *et al.* (1966 *a*), Greenblatt *et al.* (1966)

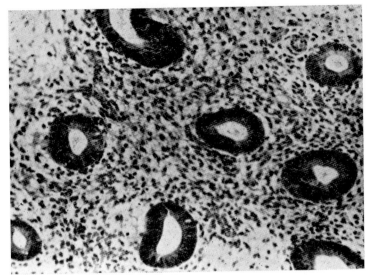

FIG. 95
**Endometrial biopsy in a patient with the Stein-Leventhal
syndrome prior to Clomiphene therapy.**
(From Charles *et al.*, 1963.)

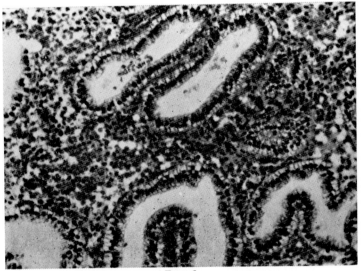

FIG. 96
**Endometrial biopsy in a patient with the Stein-Leventhal
syndrome following Clomiphene therapy.**
(From Charles *et al.*, 1963.)

and Charles *et al.* (1967). In a woman with amenorrhoea and galactorrhoea resulting from chlorpromazine therapy Thompson and Mellinger (1965) found that the compound did not affect the galactorrhoea although it produced an ovulatory cycle. In two patients with the Chiari-Frommel syndrome studied by Loraine *et al.* (1966 *a*) prompt cessation of galactorrhoea occurred as a result of Clomiphene therapy. In the five subjects reported by Greenblatt *et al.* (1966) the compound produced variable effects on lactation.

4. Side Effects

The two most important side effects resulting from Clomiphene administration are hot flushes and the occurrence of ovarian enlargement with or without cyst formation. The results obtained in a series of 179 patients quoted by Roy *et al.* (1963) are presented in Table 12 from which it will be noted that the incidence of hot flushes was 9·5 per cent and of ovarian enlargement with or without cyst formation 19·5 per cent. Emphasis must be given to the fact that the table includes subjects receiving a great variety of treatment schedules in some of which the compound was administered for relatively long periods of time. It is virtually certain that with the shorter courses of treatment now being used the incidence of side effects and especially of ovarian enlargement will be considerably reduced. Side effects other than hot flushes and ovarian enlargement, have been noted in a small proportion of patients. These include visual disturbances, frequency of micturition, nausea and vomiting, undue fatigue, increased appetite, giddiness and headache. Such complaints have rarely proved troublesome and have seldom caused treatment to be withdrawn. Side effects associated with Clomiphene therapy in a series of 2,616 patients reviewed by Johnson *et al.* (1966) are shown in Table 13.

SITE AND MODE OF ACTION OF CLOMIPHENE

At the time of writing neither the site nor the mode of action of Clomiphene is known with certainty. Some investigators have suggested that the compound acts directly on the ovaries, while others believe that the effects are produced via

TABLE 12

INCIDENCE OF OVULATION AND SIDE EFFECTS FOLLOWING CLOMIPHENE ADMINISTRATION

(After Roy et al., 1963)

Diagnosis	Number of patients	Incidence of ovulation		Incidence of ovarian enlargement		Incidence of hot flushes	
		Number of patients	%	Number of patients	%	Number of patients	%
" Functional " amenorrhoea	56	49	88	8	14	5	9
Secondary amenorrhoea ...	48	31	65	8	17	5	10
Primary amenorrhoea ...	11	3	27	5	45	2	18
Stein-Leventhal syndrome ...	35	32	91	10	29	4	11
Dysfunctional uterine haemorrhage	26	23	88	4	15	1	4
Total	179	138	77	35	20	17	9

the anterior pituitary and/or hypothalamus. A discussion of the subject has been published by Smith (1965). In the present section an attempt will be made to assess the site and mode of action of the compound by describing its effect on gonado-trophin and steroid excretion and on steroid biosyntheses.

TABLE 13

SIDE EFFECTS ASSOCIATED WITH CLOMIPHENE THERAPY IN A SERIES OF 2,616 PATIENTS

(After Johnson *et al.*, 1966)

Side effect	% occurrence
Vasomotor symptoms especially hot flushes ...	14
Ovarian enlargement	14
Abdominal discomfort	6
Nausea and/or vomiting	2
Visual complaints	2
Breast tenderness	1·8
Nervousness and insomnia	1·5
Headache	1·4
Giddiness	1·4
Increased frequency of micturition	1·4
Depression and/or fatigue	1·0
Menorrhagia	1·0
Dermatitis or rashes	0·8
Weight gain	0·6
Increased appetite	0·5
Hair loss	0·3
Miscellaneous	3

1. Effects on HPG Excretion

The effect of Clomiphene on the excretion of " total gonadotrophic activity ", as measured by the mouse uterus test, has been studied by numerous investigators including Smith *et al.* (1963), Charles *et al.* (1963, 1966), Riley and Evans (1964), Heinrichs and Zander (1964), Pildes (1965), Loraine *et al.* (1966 *a*) and Bell *et al.* (1966 *a*). Variable results have been reported, some workers claiming that such treatment caused a rise in HPG output, and others noting no change in levels. The experience of the Edinburgh group is illustrated in

Q   225

Figures 86 and 89 from which it will be noted that Clomiphene did not markedly affect the output of " total gonadotrophic activity ".

Preliminary studies on the differential excretion of FSH and LH in patients receiving Clomiphene have been published by Dickey *et al.* (1965), Roy *et al.* (1965), Thompson and Mellinger (1965), Mishell (1967) and Charles *et al.* (1967). Again, the results obtained have been conflicting, and it is not possible to draw any definite conclusions from the available data. In this connection one of the major points to establish in the future will be whether the pattern of excretion of FSH and LH in the patients who ovulate as a result of Clomiphene therapy differs from that in women who fail to ovulate following treatment.

2. Effects on Oestrogen Excretion

It is generally agreed that in patients in whom ovulation is produced by Clomiphene the output of urinary oestrogens is increased. In the majority of such women proportionately more oestrone than oestriol is excreted, suggesting that the compound affects oestrogen metabolism by retarding the conversion of oestrone and oestradiol to oestriol. Bell *et al.* (1966 *a*) have also called attention to the fact that in a proportion of subjects who do not ovulate as a result of therapy, a rise in oestrogen output occurs. These investigators have suggested that in such cases the treatment has caused follicular development in the absence of corpus luteum formation.

3. Effects on Excretion of Other Steroids

Following Clomiphene induced ovulation an increase in urinary pregnanediol excretion occurs (Roy *et al.*, 1963; Charles *et al.*, 1963, 1966, 1967; Kistner, 1965 *a*; Loraine *et al.*, 1966 *a*; Bell *et al.*, 1966 *a*). Clomiphene produces variable effects on the output of pregnanetriol, total 17-OHCS, total 17-oxosteroids and DHA, but the general tendency is for the excretion of these steroids to rise during and immediately following drug administration (Roy *et al.*, 1963; Loraine *et al.*, 1966 *a*; Bell *et al.*, 1966 *a*). Relevant information regarding the site of action of Clomiphene in male subjects has been obtained by Harkness *et al.* (1964) who measured these steroids in normal individuals and by Loraine *et al.* (1966 *b*) and Harkness *et al.* (1968) who performed similar studies in patients with Addison's disease and following castration. The data obtained from these investigations support the view that Clomiphene is capable of stimulating both testicular and adrenocortical function.

4. Effects on Steroid Biosynthesis

These have been extensively studied by Smith (1965) who was especially concerned with the effect of Clomiphene on the oestrogenic hormones. This investigator showed that the compound could increase the rate of incorporation of labelled acetate into oestradiol in the human ovary maintained under *in vitro* conditions. She also demonstrated that Clomiphene, when added to an *in vitro* placental aromatising system, increased the rate of conversion of testosterone and androstenedione to oestrone. At the same time it increased the availability of reduced pyridine nucleotides.

5. Comment

Definite conclusions regarding the mode and site of action of Clomiphene in the human female cannot be drawn at present and it is obvious that much further work in this important field requires to be done. In view of the fact that so little reliable information is available on the mechanisms responsible for ovulation in normally menstruating women (see Chapter II), it is hardly surprising that the processes involved in Clomiphene induced ovulation are so poorly understood.

SUMMARY AND CONCLUSIONS

The compound Clomiphene (MRL-41) was initially shown on the basis of experiments in rodents to have antifertility properties. However, when administered to the human female it was found to be capable of stimulating ovarian function and causing ovulation.

The patients most suitable for Clomiphene therapy are those suffering from primary and secondary amenorrhoea of pituitary rather than ovarian origin, the Stein-Leventhal syndrome and the Chiari-Frommel syndrome. Subjects most likely to ovulate as a result of Clomiphene administration are those who already show definite evidence of ovarian activity as judged by urinary oestrogen assays and in whom urinary HPG readings are either low or undetectable.

It is now generally agreed that short courses of Clomiphene, e.g. 50 to 100 mg. per day for five to seven days, are more satisfactory than continuous therapy with larger doses for relatively long periods of time.

In a series of 2,616 patients reviewed by Johnson *et al.* (1966) ovulation due to Clomiphene therapy occurred in 76 per cent of cases. The pregnancy rate following Clomiphene administration in the same series was 26 per cent.

Effects of Clomiphene on hormone excretion are variable, one of the more constant findings being a rise in oestrogen output affecting especially oestrone. The rise in oestrogen excretion may or may not be associated with ovulation as judged by pregnanediol assays. Levels of FSH, LH and " total gonadotrophic activity " show no consistent pattern following Clomiphene administration, but stimulation of adrenocortical as well as ovarian function may occur.

The two most important side effects resulting from medication by Clomiphene are hot flushes and the presence of ovarian enlargement with or without cyst formation.

Further work is necessary in order to elucidate the site and mode of action of Clomiphene in human subjects.

REFERENCES

BARNES, L. E. & MEYER, R. K. (1962). *Fertility Sterility,* **13,** 472.
BECK, P., GRAYZEL, E. F., YOUNG, I. S. & KUPPERMAN, H. S. (1966). *Obstet. Gynecol.* **27,** 54.
BELL, E. T. & LORAINE, J. A. (1966). *Lancet,* **i,** 626.
BELL, E. T., LORAINE, J. A., HARKNESS, R. A. & FOSS, G. L. (1966 a). *J. Obstet. Gynaecol. Brit. Commonwealth,* **73,** 766.
BELL, E. T., MUKERJI, S., LORAINE, J. A. & LUNN, S. F. (1966 b). *Acta Endocrinol.* **51,** 578.
BISHOP, P. M. F. (1965). *Proc. Roy. Soc. Med.* **58,** 905.
BOUTSELIS, J. G., VORYS, N. & ULLERY, J. C. (1967). *Am. J. Obstet. Gynecol.* **97,** 949.
CHARLES, D. (1962). *Lancet,* **ii,** 278.
CHARLES, D., BARR, W., BELL, E. T., BROWN, J. B., FOTHERBY, K. & LORAINE, J. A. (1963). *Am. J. Obstet. Gynecol.* **86,** 913.
CHARLES, D., BARR, W. & McEWAN, H. P. (1964). *J. Obstet. Gynaecol. Brit. Commonwealth,* **71,** 66.
CHARLES, D., LORAINE, J. A., BELL, E. T. & HARKNESS, R. A. (1966). *Fertility Sterility,* **17,** 351.
CHARLES, D., LORAINE, J. A., BELL, E. T. & HARKNESS, R. A. (1967). *Proceedings of Fifth World Congress on Fertility and Sterility.* Stockholm 1966. Excerpta Med. Inter. Cong. Series No. 133, p. 92.

COHEN, M. R. (1966). *Fertility Sterility*, **17**, 765.
CUDMORE, D. W. & TUPPER, W. R. C. (1966). *Fertility Sterility*, **17**, 363.
DICKEY, R. P., VORYS, N., STEVENS, V. C., BESCH, P. K., HAMWI, G. J. & ULLERY, J. C. (1965). *Fertility Sterility*, **16**, 485.
GREENBLATT, R. B. (1961). *Fertility Sterility*, **12**, 402.
GREENBLATT, R. B. & MAHESH, V. B. (1965). *Year Book of Endocrinology*, p. 248. Ed. Schwartz, T. B. Year Book Medical Publishers: Chicago.
GREENBLATT, R. B., BARFIELD, W. E., JUNGCK, E. C. & RAY, A. W. (1961). *J. Am. Med. Ass.* **178**, 101.
GREENBLATT, R. B., FAUCHER, G., MAHESH, V. B., LUNENFLED, B., RABAU, E., DAVID, A. & INSLER, V. (1966). *Fertility Sterility*, **17**, 742.
HARKNESS, R. A., BELL, E. T., ISMAIL, A. A. A., LORAINE, J. A. & MORSE, W. I. (1968). *Acta Endocrinol. In press.*
HARKNESS, R. A., BELL, E. T., LORAINE, J. A. & MORSE, W. I. (1964). *J. Endocrinol.* **31**, 53.
HEINRICHS, H. D. & ZANDER, J. (1964). *Klin. Wochschr.* **42**, 15.
HOLTKAMP, D. E. (1966). *Excerpta Medica International Congress Series* No. 111, p. 206. Excerpta Medica Foundation: Amsterdam.
HOLTKAMP, D. E., DAVIS, R. H. & RHOADS, J. E. (1961). *Federation Proc.* **20**, 419.
JOHNSON, J. E. Jr., BUNDE, C. A. & HOEKENGA, M. T. (1966). *Pacific Med. Surg.* **74**, 153.
JONES, G. S. & MORAES-REUHSEN, M. DE (1965). *Fertility Sterility*, **16**, 461.
KAISER, I. H. (1963). *Am. J. Obstet. Gynecol.* **87**, 149.
KISTNER, R. W. (1965 a). *Obstet. Gynecol. Surv.* **20**, 873.
KISTNER, R. W. (1965 b). *Am. J. Obstet. Gynecol.* **92**, 380.
KISTNER, R. W. & SMITH, O. W. (1961). *Fertility Sterility*, **12**, 121.
KISTNER, R. W., LEWIS, J. L. & STEINER, G. J. (1966). *Cancer*, **19**, 115.
LORAINE, J. A., BELL, E. T., HARKNESS, R. A. & HARRISON, M. T. (1966 a). *Acta Endocrinol.* **52**, 527.
LORAINE, J. A., HARKNESS, R. A., BELL, E. T. & ISMAIL, A. A. A. (1966 b). *Excerpta Medica Foundation Congress Series* No. 111, p. 207. Excerpta Medica Foundation: Amsterdam.
MISHELL, D. R. (1967). *Fertility Sterility*, **18**, 102.
NAVILLE, A. H., KISTNER, R. W., WHEATLEY, R. E. & ROCK J. (1964). *Fertility Sterility*, **15**, 290.
PAYNE, S. & KAROW, W. G. (1963). *Western J. Surg. Obstet. Gynecol.* **71**, 262.
PILDES, R. B. (1965). *Am. J. Obstet. Gynecol.* **91**, 466.
PUEBLA, R. A. & GREENBLATT, R. B. (1964). *J. Clin. Endocrinol. Metab.* **24**, 863.
RILEY, G. M. & EVANS, T. N. (1964). *Am. J. Obstet. Gynecol.* **89**, 97.
ROY, S., GREENBLATT, R. B., MAHESH, V. B. & JUNGCK, E. C. (1963). *Fertility Sterility*, **14**, 575.
SEGAL, S. J. & NELSON, W. O. (1961). *Anat. Record*, **139**, 273.
SHEARMAN, R. P. (1966). *Australasian Ann. Med.* **15**, 266.
SMITH, O. W. (1965). *Am. J. Obstet. Gynecol.* **94**, 440.
SMITH, O. W., SMITH, G. V. & KISTNER, R. W. (1963). *J. Am. Med. Ass.* **184**, 878.
SOUTHAM, A. L. & JANOVSKI, N. A. (1962). *J. Am. Med. Ass.* **181** 443.
THOMPSON, R. J. & MELLINGER, R. C. (1965). *Am. J. Obstet. Gynecol.* **92**, 412.
TOWNSEND, S. L., BROWN, J. B., JOHNSTONE, J. W., ADEY, F. D., EVANS, J. H. & TAFT, H. P. (1966). *J. Obstet. Gynaecol. Brit. Commonwealth*, **73**, 529.
TYLER, E. T., OLSON, H. J. & GOTLIB, M. H. (1960). *Intern. J. Fertility*, **5**, 429.
VORYS, N., GANTT, C. L., HAMWI, G. J., COPELAND, W. E. & ULLERY, J. C. (1964). *Am. J. Obstet. Gynecol.* **88**, 425.
WALL, J. A., FRANKLIN, R. R. & KAUFMAN, R. H. (1964). *Am. J. Obstet. Gynecol.* **88**, 1072.
WHITELAW, M. J. (1963). *Fertility Sterility*, **14**, 540.
WHITELAW, M. J. (1966). *Fertility Sterility*, **17**, 584.
WHITELAW, M. J., GRAMS, L. R. & STAMM, W. J. (1964). *Am. J. Obstet. Gynecol.* **90**, 355.

CHAPTER VIII

Induction of Ovulation by Gonadotrophic Hormones

INTRODUCTION

A NUMBER of gonadotrophic hormones have been used to stimulate ovarian function in women suffering from problems of sterility and infertility. These substances have included pregnant mare's serum gonadotrophin (PMSG), human chorionic gonadotrophin (HCG) and human gonadotrophins derived from anterior pituitary tissue and from menopausal and postmenopausal urine. Until the late 1950's the only preparations which had been employed on any scale clinically were PMSG and HCG, given either alone or in combination. As pointed out by Kotz and Herrmann (1961) and by others, the results obtained by the use of such treatment were generally unsatisfactory, being associated with a marked inconsistency of response and with the formation of antibodies to PMSG (see also Loraine and Schmidt-Elmendorff, 1963; Østergaard, 1964). Since the introduction of therapy by human gonadotrophins by Gemzell et al. (1958) treatment by PMSG has been virtually abandoned.

The present chapter is concerned only with therapy by gonadotrophins of human origin. Results obtained with pituitary gonadotrophins are first considered, and subsequently similar data obtained with gonadotrophins of urinary origin are discussed. For detailed accounts of some of the topics reviewed in this chapter articles by Gemzell and his associates (Gemzell, 1964, 1965 a; Gemzell et al., 1966) and by Lunenfeld (1967) should be consulted.

SELECTION OF PATIENTS FOR GONADOTROPHIN THERAPY

As in the case of Clomiphene (see Chapter VII) gonadotrophins have been administered to patients with a large number of clinical conditions in which infertility is a major symptom. These have included primary and secondary amenorrhoea, oligomenorrhoea, the Stein-Leventhal syndrome, the Chiari-Frommel syndrome and various types of pituitary and ovarian failure.

The selection of patients for gonadotrophin therapy has been discussed by Lunenfeld (1965), Crooke (1964), Gemzell (1965 a b), Vande Wiele and Turksoy (1965) and Townsend *et al.* (1966). Gemzell (1965 *a*) considers that an ideal subject for treatment is one suffering from primary amenorrhoea or from secondary amenorrhoea of long duration in whom the ovaries and uterus are normally developed and in whom, prior to therapy, gonadotrophic activity cannot be detected in the urine. In the opinion of Lunenfeld (1965) suitable cases should show low or undetectable urinary HPG levels, low oestrogen readings typical of the postmenopausal state and pregnanediol values of less than 1 mg. per 24 hours; furthermore, they should have an atrophic endometrium and should fail to show a withdrawal bleeding following the administration of HCG or progesterone. The criteria used by Crooke (1964) are similar to those described by Lunenfeld (1965) but the former investigator has emphasised that the patient should, in addition, have atrophic ovaries. According to Townsend *et al.* (1966) endogenous oestrogen excretion prior to therapy is of importance in the selection of patients. These workers state that, if in an otherwise suitable subject, the " total oestrogen " excretion is less than 10 µg. per 24 hours a satisfactory response to gonadotrophin therapy can be anticipated. If, on the other hand, the mean ocstrogen output before treatment is above 10 µg. per 24 hours the treatment of choice is Clomiphene rather than gonadotrophic hormones.

EFFECTS OF HUMAN PITUITARY GONADOTROPHINS

1. Preparation of Administered Material

The hormones have generally been derived from human pituitaries obtained at autopsy, the material being freeze-dried, fresh frozen or dried in acetone. The aim of all the extraction procedures has been to obtain a preparation rich in FSH activity and capable of initiating follicular growth in the ovaries. In the original procedure used by Gemzell *et al.* (1958) the freeze-dried glands were extracted with a calcium hydroxide solution, and the material containing the FSH was fractionated by means of ammonium sulphate. In later studies Gemzell and his associates employed the technique of Roos and Gemzell (1964, 1965) which involves extraction with phosphate buffer, fractionation with ammonium sulphate and on DEAE cellulose columns and gel filtration on Sephadex columns.

The method used by Butt et al., (1961, 1964) to extract gonadotrophins from anterior pituitary tissue involved initial extraction with ammonium acetate, separation of FSH from TSH and LH by chromatography on carboxy methyl cellulose, and subsequent purification of the FSH containing fraction using DEAE cellulose and calcium phosphate. By this means Butt and his collaborators obtained materials designated CP_1 and CP_2 which were extensively used in clinical studies by Crooke and his associates in Birmingham. Yields of FSH activity from human pituitary glands and the degree of LH contamination of the extracts have varied in the hands of different investigators (see Gemzell et al., 1966 for references).

2. Dosage of Administered Material

The literature on this subject is confused, mainly because a variety of standard preparations have been employed to assess the potency of the administered material. Reference preparations used have included the First and Second IRP's for HMG (see p. 57) and NIH-FSH-S1 and S2. It is to be hoped that, in the future, estimates of potency will be expressed only in terms of the Second IRP-HMG as international units (i.u.).

The total dosage of FSH administered to individual patients has varied greatly in the hands of different investigators. This has been mainly due to the fact that women differ to a considerable extent in their sensitivity to gonadotrophic hormones. Thus, Gemzell (1966) administered the equivalent of 4 to 6 mg. NIH-FSH-S1 (108 to 162 i.u.) daily i.m. for 10 days, and followed this course by three daily intramuscular dosages of HCG each of 3,000 i.u. Crooke and his associates (Crooke et al., 1963 a b, 1964 a b, 1966 a b) have employed a number of dosage regimes in the most recent of which a single injection of FSH mixed with HCG is given and is followed eight to 10 days later by a second injection of HCG. This form of treatment is repeated at approximately three weekly intervals, using increasing dosages of FSH, until a positive response is obtained, the latter being assessed by the increase in urinary oestriol and pregnanediol excretion. The rise in steroid levels following gonadotrophin therapy has been made the basis of a sensitivity test, details of which are given in a recent paper by Crooke et al. (1966 a). The dosage of FSH given to individual patients by these investigators has varied from 570 to 4,290 i.u.; the first injection of HCG contained 12,000 and the second 24,000 i.u.

3. Incidence of Ovulation and Pregnancy Following Treatment

The fact that ovulation can occur following gonadotrophin therapy has been documented by several authors including Buxton and Herrmann (1961), Apostolakis et al. (1962), Gemzell (1962, 1964, 1965 a b, 1966), Crooke et al. (1963 a b, 1964 a b, 1966 a b), Bettendorf (1964), Diczfalusy et al. (1964), Crooke (1964) and Gemzell and Roos (1966). The criteria of ovulation have varied greatly from one publication to another, and have included alterations in basal body temperature, elevation of urinary pregnanediol levels, the presence of a secretory endometrium and the occurrence of pregnancy. The most extensive clinical experience in this field is probably that of Gemzell and his associates on some of whose results the following account is based.

Gemzell (1966) has recently described the treatment of 35 infertile women with combinations of FSH and HCG in the manner described on p. 233. Sixty-six courses of therapy were administered and ovulation occurred on 47 occasions (71 per cent). As a result of treatment, 16 of the 35 women (46 per cent) became pregnant, and in two of the subjects pregnancy occurred twice. Of the 18 pregnancies obtained, 11 were single and seven multiple. The multiple pregnancies consisted of five sets of twins, in two of which an abortion occurred; there were two sets of quadruplets in one of which the pregnancy terminated in an abortion. In a series of 18 women reported by Crooke et al. (1966 a) 16 (89 per cent) became pregnant as a result of treatment.

4. Effect of Human Pituitary Gonadotrophins on Steroid Excretion

This subject has been studied by numerous investigators including Gemzell and his associates (Gemzell, 1966; Gemzell et al., 1958; Gemzell and Roos, 1966), Crooke and his collaborators (Crooke, 1964; Crooke et al., 1963 a, 1966 a b),

Apostolakis *et al.* (1962), Diczfalusy *et al.* (1964), J. B. Brown (1965) and Townsend *et al.* (1966). Assays of oestrogens, pregnanediol, pregnanetriol, 17-oxosteroids and 17-hydroxy-corticosteroids (17-OHCS) have been performed. Representative hormone excretion patterns during and immediately

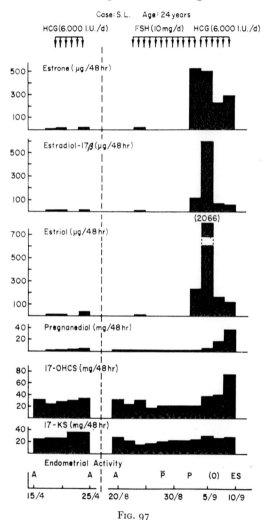

FIG. 97

Steroid excretion pattern in a patient with secondary amenorrhoea treated with HCG and FSH.

(From Gemzell, 1964.)

following treatment, together with results obtained following gonadotrophin induced pregnancy, are presented in the ensuing discussion.

In Figure 97, which is taken from a paper by Gemzell (1964), the effect of HCG alone and of FSH followed by HCG on the output of the three " classical " oestrogens, pregnanediol, total 17-oxosteroids (ketosteroids) and 17-OHCS is shown. HCG alone produced little or no effect on steroid output, whereas a combination of FSH and HCG caused a marked rise

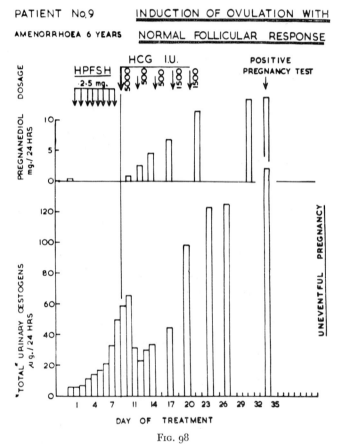

FIG. 98

Steroid excretion pattern in a patient with secondary amenorrhoea treated with human pituitary FSH and HCG.

(From Townsend *et al.*, 1966, *J. Obstet. Gynaecol. Brit. Commonwealth.*)

in oestrogen and pregnanediol excretion, indicating that ovulation had occurred. It should be emphasised that the rise in steroid output was very large indeed, being much greater than that normally encountered in the menstrual cycle; this observation suggests that considerable hyperstimulation of the ovaries had been produced. Following therapy with FSH and HCG the endometrial pattern changed from a proliferative to an early secretory pattern.

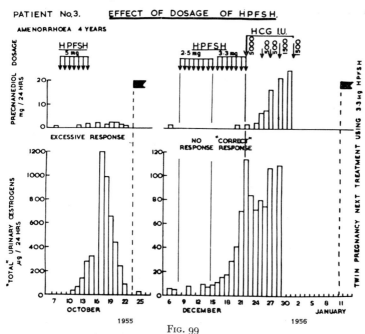

FIG. 99

Steroid excretion pattern in a patient with secondary amenorrhoea treated with human pituitary FSH and HCG.
//// = menstrual bleeding.
(From Townsend *et al.*, 1966, *J. Obstret. Gynaecol. Brit. Commonwealth*).

Townsend *et al.* (1966) have studied the effect of various dosages of FSH and HCG on steroid output in amenorrhoeic women. The results obtained in two of their subjects are shown in Figures 98 and 99. The woman in Figure 98 was treated with 2·5 mg. FSH per day for eight days followed by HCG. The rise in oestrogen excretion produced was similar to that observed during the normal menstrual cycle and was followed by an increase in pregnanediol output indicating that ovulation had taken place. As a result of this treatment a pregnancy occurred.

In Figure 99 are shown the results obtained when FSH at varying dose levels was administered to a patient with a four year history of amenorrhoea; FSH was given both alone and followed by HCG. It will be noted that a dosage of 5 mg. FSH per day for seven days produced oestrogen levels more than ten times greater than those normally found during the

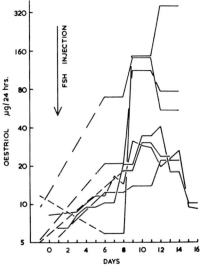

FIG. 100

Oestriol excretion in seven patients treated with FSH and HCG.

(From Crooke *et al.*, 1966 *a*.)

menstrual cycle (see Loraine and Bell, 1963), but that these high levels were not associated with the occurrence of ovulation as judged by pregnanediol assays. When the dosage was reduced to 2·5 mg. per day there was little or no effect on oestrogen output, while an intermediate dose of 3·3 mg. per day again produced marked over-stimulation of ovarian activity on the basis of oestrogen estimations. The administration of HCG immediately following the third course of FSH resulted in ovulation, this being indicated by the high levels of urinary oestrogens and pregnanediol. During a subsequent course of treatment with FSH at a dosage of 3·3 mg. per day the patient became pregnant and eventually delivered twins.

The effect of a single injection of FSH and HCG on oestriol excretion in seven women studied by Crooke *et al.* (1966 *a*) is

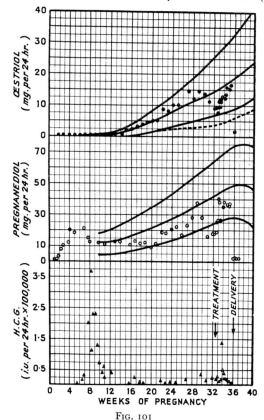

FIG. 101

Steroid and HCG excretion following gonadotrophin induced pregnancy.

(From Crooke *et al.*, 1964 *a*.)

shown in Figure 100. It will be noted that in all subjects an increase in oestriol output occurred, but that the effect of the hormone on the excretion of the steroid varied greatly. The dosage of FSH required to affect oestriol excretion ranged from 570 to 1,570 i.u., again emphasising that marked differences in ovarian sensitivity to gonadotrophins exist from one woman to another.

Patterns of excretion of steroids and HCG during pregnancies following the administration of FSH and HCG have been reported by Crooke *et al.* (1964 *a*); one of their cases is shown in Figure 101. In this patient oestriol and pregnanediol levels remained within the normal range until the 30th week of pregnancy. Thereafter they failed to show the expected rise, but increased again following the administration of various

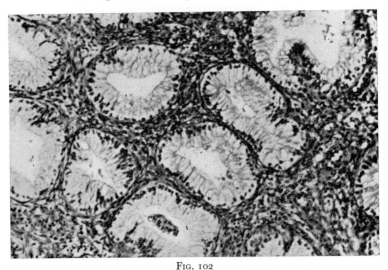

FIG. 102

Endometrial biopsy in a patient with primary amenorrhoea following treatment with FSH and HCG.

(From Buxton and Herrmann. 1961.)

steroids. Caesarean section was performed at the 36th week, at which time a healthy female child was delivered. The HCG assays shown in Figure 101 were performed by an immunological technique depending on haemagglutination-inhibition; the figures quoted are much higher than those generally obtained using bio-assays and are probably of doubtful quantitative significance (see Loraine and Bell, 1966).

5. Other Effects of Human Pituitary Gonadotrophins

(*a*) EFFECTS ON THE ENDOMETRIUM.—Many investigators have used endometrial biopsies as a method of determining

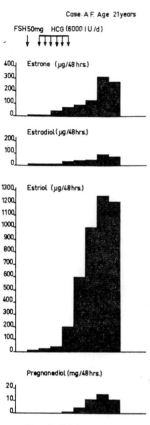

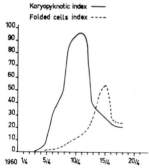

FIG. 103

Steroid excretion pattern and cytological data in a patient with primary amenorrhoea treated with FSH and HCG.

(From Johannisson *et al.*, 1961.)

whether ovulation has occurred as a result of gonadotrophin therapy. In Figure 102 which is taken from a paper by Buxton and Herrmann (1961) is shown the endometrium following the administration of FSH and HCG to a patient with primary amenorrhoea; the presence of a secretory pattern will be noted indicating that ovulation had taken place.

(b) EFFECT ON VAGINAL CYTOLOGY.—Johannisson et al. (1961) have reported detailed studies of vaginal cytology after a single injection of FSH followed by several injections of HCG. Measurements were made of the karyopyknotic and " folded cell " indices, the latter being regarded as a criterion of regression of the epithelium. A typical investigation is illustrated in Figure 103, which shows the findings in a patient who ovulated following gonadotrophin therapy. It will be noted that the treatment caused a marked increase in the karyopyknotic index; subsequently the index decreased, this being associated with a rise in urinary oestrogen and pregnanediol output. The increase in steroid excretion occurred at the same time as the rise in the folded cell index.

(c) INCIDENCE OF MULTIPLE PREGNANCY.—It is now agreed that the incidence of multiple pregnancy after gonadotrophin treatment is relatively high. The most extensive series so far reported in the literature is that of Gemzell and Roos (1966) who found that of 43 patients delivered following a gonadotrophin induced pregnancy, 14 (33 per cent) had twins and nine (20 per cent) had triplets or more. In two out of the 23 patients who delivered two or more foetuses an abortion occurred. Liggins and Ibbertson (1966) have reported a quintuplet pregnancy following FSH and HCG administration, while Gemzell and Roos (1966) described a pregnancy with seven foetuses which ended in an abortion. It must be presumed that these multiple pregnancies arise because of gross ovarian hyperstimulation resulting in the rupture of several follicles with subsequent fertilisation of the ova.

According to Gemzell and Roos (1966) urinary steroid assays conducted on the day following cessation of HCG therapy are of little or no value in differentiating patients who will have a single pregnancy from those in whom a multiple pregnancy will occur. The results of these investigators are shown in Table 14. The only positive finding was that the

TABLE 14

URINARY STEROID EXCRETION IN PATIENTS WITH SINGLE OR MULTIPLE PREGNANCY

(Mean ± S.E.)

(After Gemzell and Roos, 1966)

Type of pregnancy	Number of women	Oestrone µg./24 hours	Oestradiol µg./24 hours	Oestriol µg./24 hours	Pregnanediol mg./24 hours
Single	20	100 ± 28	39 ± 11	119 ± 37	7·3 ± 1·4
Twin	14	93 ± 15	36 ± 4	203 ± 33	7·6 ± 1·1
Triplet or more ...	9	166 ± 44	42 ± 7	152 ± 43	16·9 ± 5·3

mean pregnanediol level in women conceiving three or more foetuses was higher than that in subjects conceiving a single foetus or twin foetuses.

(*d*) Side Effects.—Apart from multiple pregnancy the main complication resulting from gonadotrophin therapy is the so-called " hyperstimulation syndrome " (see p. 252). This comprises rapid ovarian enlargement associated with intra-peritoneal effusions and/or haemorrhage. The syndrome has been encountered by Gemzell (1963) in approximately two

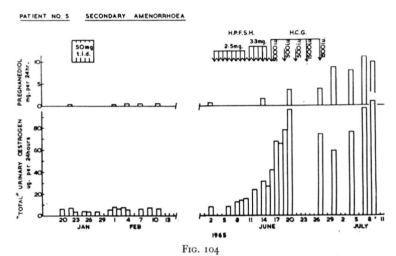

Fig. 104

Steroid excretion pattern in a patient with secondary amenorrhoea treated with Clomiphene (50 mg. t.i.d.) and with human pituitary FSH and HCG.

(From Townsend *et al.*, 1966, *J. Obstret. Gyneacol. Brit. Commonwealth*).

per cent of his courses of treatment. Thrombo-embolic phenomena rarely occur when FSH is administered and foetal abnormalities are uncommon.

(*e*) Comparison of the Effects of Clomiphene and Human Pituitary Gonadotrophins.—Such a comparison in relation to hormone excretion has recently been made by Townsend *et al.* (1966), and the results obtained in one of the subjects investigated are shown in Figure 104. This was a patient with secondary amenorrhoea in whom serial oestrogen assays were performed and who was first treated by Clomiphene at a dose level of 50 mg. t.i.d. for five days. She was subsequently given two different dosages of FSH followed by HCG, the latter being administered in varying amounts. It is apparent that neither Clomiphene nor the low dose of FSH produced any effect on steroid excretion. However, the higher dosage of FSH (3·3 mg. per day) caused an increase in urinary oestrogen output, and when this was followed by the administration of HCG, ovulation occurred. The results of this study are compatible with the view that, when endogenous oestrogen levels prior to therapy are low, a satisfactory response in terms of ovulation is more likely to be produced by gonadotrophin therapy than by Clomiphene (see also p. 201).

EFFECTS OF HUMAN URINARY GONADOTROPHINS

1. Preparation of Administered Material

Most investigators have employed the substance known as " Pergonal " (Serono, Rome) which is derived from postmenopausal urine. The method of preparation of this material has been described in detail in publications by Donini *et al.* (1964) and by Lunenfeld (1965). The main steps are as follows:

(*a*) Kaolin adsorption of gonadotrophins.

(*b*) Ammonium hydroxide elution.

(*c*) Acetone precipitation.

(*d*) Purification of the crude kaolin extract using ammonium acetate-ethanol and DEAE cellulose.

(*e*) Further purification by column chromatography on permutit.

For clinical administration Pergonal is available in ampoules each containing 75 i.u. FSH and 75 i.u. LH. When administered to human subjects the material has no effect on liver function tests, plasma protein levels and haematological indices. Minor increases in body temperature following treatment by Pergonal have been reported.

2. Dosage of Administered Material

At the time of writing it is a matter of considerable difficulty to recommend a standard dosage of Pergonal for use in clinical studies. This arises from the fact that, as in the case of the pituitary gonadotrophins, the sensitivity of individual patients to the material varies enormously. The dosage of Pergonal most frequently employed has been 75 to 150 i.u. FSH per day. Three different dosage schedules have been used and these will be briefly described.

(*a*) TREATMENT OF THE PATIENT WITH A SPECIFIC DOSAGE OF PERGONAL FOR A PREDETERMINED TIME.—This schedule has been employed with success by Pasetto and Montanino (1964) who treated their patients with various total dosages of Pergonal for periods of time ranging from 10 to 14 days. The Pergonal was followed by the administration of HCG at a dose level ranging from 1,500 to 5,000 i.u.

(*b*) TREATMENT OF THE PATIENT WITH A SPECIFIC DOSAGE OF PERGONAL FOR A VARIABLE PERIOD OF TIME.—This design has been recommended by Vande Wiele and Turksoy (1965) who assessed the response to treatment by examination of vaginal smears and cervical mucus, and by pelvic examination. The dosage of HCG employed by these investigators was 4,000 to 5,000 i.u. per day for four days, this being combined with the last four days of Pergonal administration. A treatment schedule somewhat similar to that of Vande Wiele and Turksoy (1965) has been employed by Taymor (1967).

(*c*) TREATMENT OF THE PATIENT WITH VARIABLE DOSAGES OF PERGONAL FOR VARIABLE LENGTHS OF TIME.—This is the schedule favoured by Lunenfeld and his associates (Lunenfeld, 1967; Lunenfeld *et al.*, 1962 *a b*, 1963) who assessed the response by ferning of cervical mucus, basal body temperature records, vaginal cytology and urinary oestrogen assays. If after four days of treatment the patient failed to show a response, the dosage of Pergonal was increased. Therapy with HCG was generally commenced on the 10th day of the investigation, the dosage being 5,000 to 10,000 i.u. per day for three or four days.

3. Incidence of Ovulation and Pregnancy Following Treatment

The most extensive experience in this field has been that of the Tel Aviv group (Lunenfeld *et al.*, 1962 *a b*, 1963; Lunenfeld, 1965; Rabau *et al.*, 1967). A Searle memorandum (1966) has quoted the results of these investigators in 87 patients who received a total of 157 courses of Pergonal. Ovulation was produced in 142 instances (91 per cent); eighty-five of the patients were married and of these 43 (51 per cent) became pregnant. In three subjects abortion occurred following gonadotrophin therapy. Twin pregnancy was noted in 13 per cent of cases, while triplets and quadruplets were not produced as a result of treatment.

In a series of 21 patients who received 44 courses of treatment Pasetto achieved a pregnancy rate of 72 per cent (see Searle memorandum, 1966). Of 20 patients with various forms of infertility studied by Vande Wiele and Turksoy (1965) 14 conceived following Pergonal therapy and six of the subjects became pregnant on two occasions. In eight women an abortion occurred; three patients gave birth to a single child while two subjects produced twins and one quadruplets.

4. Effects of Urinary Gonadotrophins on Steroid Excretion

Such effects have been studied by various investigators including Rosemberg *et al.* (1963, 1964), Lunenfeld *et al.* (1962 *a b*), Pasetto and Montanino (1964), Diczfalusy *et al.* (1964), Shearman (1965, 1966) and Taymor *et al.* (1967). Illustrative examples of the results obtained are presented in Figures 105 to 108.

Figure 105, which is taken from a paper by Shearman (1966), shows the effect of FSH and HCG in a patient with secondary amenorrhoea. It will be noted that the therapy produced a marked rise in oestrogen output with an ovulatory peak of excretion occurring probably on the 12th day of the study. This peak was followed by a marked rise in urinary pregnanediol levels, and during this cycle the patient became pregnant.

Unsuccessful therapy with gonadotrophins in a patient suffering from obesity, galactorrhoea and secondary amenorrhoea (the Forbes-Albright syndrome) is shown in Figure 106. This subject received three courses of therapy with FSH in association with HCG, the dosage of both hormones being increased in successive treatment periods. With all three courses a rise in oestrogen output occurred; however, this was not associated with an increase in pregnanediol excretion, thus indicating that ovulation had not been produced.

The effects of HCG, two gonadotrophic preparations of urinary origin (HMG-O and HMG-S) and one preparation of pituitary origin (HHG) on steroid output and vaginal cytology are shown in Figure 107 which is taken from Diczfalusy *et al.* (1964). It will be noted that HCG and the first course of HMG-O had no effect on endocrine function. On the other

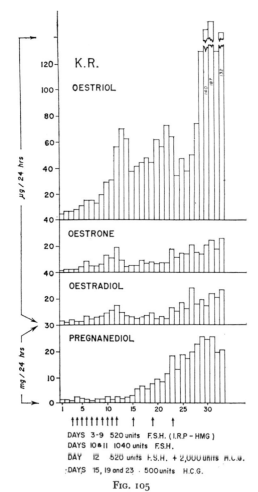

Fig. 105

Steroid excretion pattern in a patient with secondary amenorrhoea treated with FSH and HCG.

(From Shearman, 1966.)

248

hand, treatment with the pituitary material produced an ovulatory response which was associated with a marked rise in the output of 17-OHCS and a lesser rise in the excretion of total 17-oxosteroids. The second course of treatment with a higher dosage of HMG-O followed by HCG had no effect on steroid output, while treatment with HMG-S produced ovulation as judged both by urinary assays and by vaginal

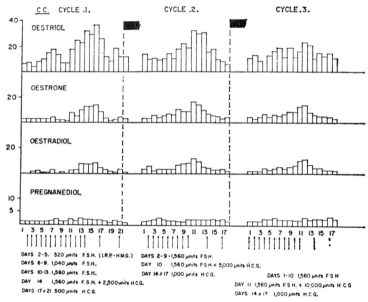

Fig. 106

Steroid excretion pattern in a patient with the Forbes-Albright syndrome treated with FSH and HCG.

■■■ = menstrual bleeding.

(From Shearman, 1966.)

cytology. Diczfalusy *et al.* (1964), using assay methods specific for FSH and LH, demonstrated that the HMG-O material contained a relatively greater proportion of LH than of FSH while in the HMG-S the ratio was reversed. On the basis of their results they concluded that, with gonadotrophins of urinary origin, a satisfactory response to treatment is more likely to be obtained in the presence of a relatively high content of FSH in the administered material.

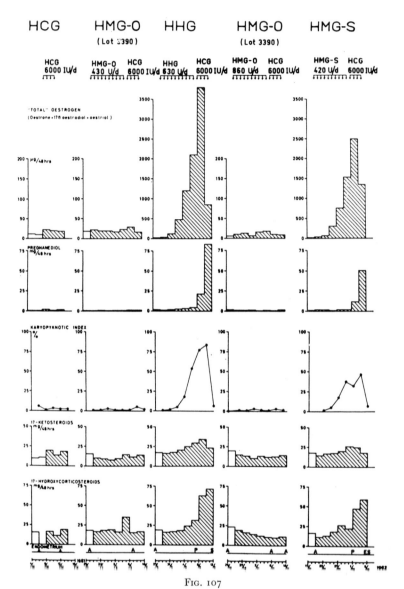

FIG. 107

Steroid excretion pattern and cytological data in a patient with secondary amenorrhoea treated with HCG and with gonadotrophins of pituitary and urinary origin.

(From Diczfalusy *et al.*, 1964.)

In Figure 108 taken from Lunenfeld *et al.* (1962 *b*) hormone excretion patterns in a subject during and following treatment by Pergonal and HCG are shown; the patient became pregnant as a result of the treatment and assays were conducted for the

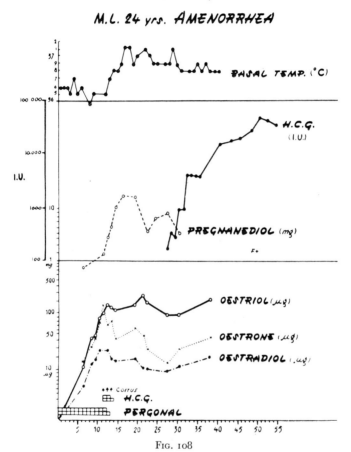

FIG. 108

Hormone excretion pattern and basal body temperature in a patient with amenorrhoea treated with Pergonal and HCG.

(From Lunenfeld *et al.*, 1962 *b*.)

first 40 days of the gestation period. The marked rise in HCG output characteristic of the first trimester of pregnancy should be noted together with the increased levels of urinary oestrogens. It is, however, noteworthy that the pattern of excretion of pregnanediol was atypical, levels rising immediately following treatment and subsequently falling during the first few days after the occurrence of conception. Recently Abrams *et al.* (1967) have reported the results obtained when a 15 year old girl with panhypopituitarism and infantilism was treated with Pergonal and HCG. This form of therapy induced ovulation as judged by oestriol and pregnanediol assays ; menstruation occurred approximately two weeks following cessation of HCG treatment. Further investigations in patients of this type will be awaited with interest.

5. Other Effects of Urinary Gonadotrophins

(*a*) VAGINAL CYTOLOGY.—Effects of FSH on vaginal cytology have been studied by various workers including Diczfalusy *et al.* (1964) and Lunenfeld *et al.* (1962 *a*), (see also Searle memorandum, 1965). Results obtained by Diczfalusy *et al.* (1964) are shown in Figure 107 from which it will be noted that both a pituitary (HHG) and a urinary material (HMG-S) caused an increase in the karyopyknotic index in association with ovulation; the other gonadotrophins studied, HCG and HMG-O, did not affect vaginal cytology. Lunenfeld *et al.* (1962 *a*), using Pergonal, have reported results very similar to those of Diczfalusy *et al.* (1964).

(*b*) SIDE EFFECTS.—These have been described by Vande Wiele and Turksoy (1965), Mozes *et al.* (1965) and Lunenfeld (1967), and have been collectively termed the " hyperstimulation syndrome ". In the mild form of this syndrome the main symptoms are abdominal pain and distension associated with varying degrees of ovarian enlargement. In the severe form of the condition ascites with or without pleural effusions, abdominal tenderness and peripheral circulatory failure may be present. The syndrome, which is a relatively rare complication, generally occurs four to eight days after HCG administration. In the mild cases no specific treatment is indicated; severe cases should be admitted to hospital where appropriate symptomatic therapy should be instituted. According to Lunenfeld (1967) patients developing the severe form of the hyperstimulation syndrome tend to show abnormally high levels of urinary pregnanetriol. This worker showed that the high pregnanetriol levels were not reduced by therapy with dexamethasone and concluded that the site of production of the steroid was the ovary rather than the adrenal.

6. Comparison of the Effects of Clomiphene and Urinary Gonadotrophins

Such a comparison involving hormone assays has recently been conducted by Bell *et al.* (1968) in a patient with a previous history of secondary amenorrhoea of five years duration. The

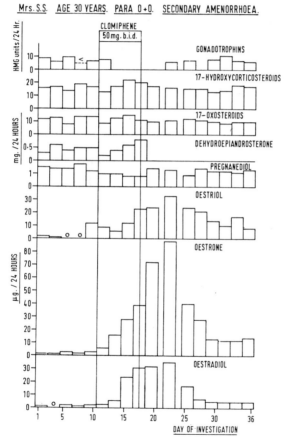

FIG. 109

Hormone excretion pattern in a patient with secondary amenorrhoea treated with Clomiphene.

(From Bell *et al.*, 1968, *J. Obstet. Gynaecol. Brit. Commonwealth.*)

results are shown in Figures 109 and 110. Following a control period of 10 days the subject was treated with Clomiphene at a dose level of 50 mg. b.i.d. for seven days (Figure 109). During

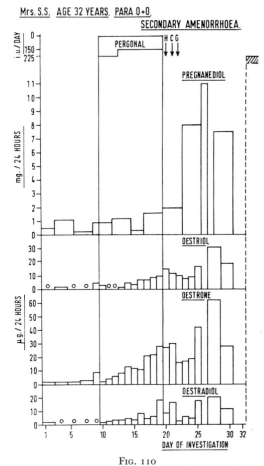

FIG. 110

Steroid excretion pattern in a patient with secondary amenorrhoea treated with Pergonal and HCG.

//// = menstrual bleeding.

(From Bell *et al.*, 1968, *J. Obstet. Gynaecol. Brit. Commonwealth.*)

the control period levels of HPG, 17-OHCS, 17-oxosteroids and dehydroepiandrosterone were within the normal range for a woman during reproductive life; treatment by Clomiphene had no effect on excretion values for these substances. Oestrogen excretion prior to therapy was very low, being within the postmenopausal range. Clomiphene produced a marked rise in urinary oestrogen output, this being particularly evident in the case of oestrone, levels of which were maximal on the 22nd and 23rd days of the study. The compound had no effect on pregnanediol output which remained within the range normally encountered in the follicular phase of the menstrual cycle. Ovulation was not produced as a result of Clomiphene therapy.

Approximately 16 months later the same patient was treated with Pergonal, the results being shown in Figure 110. Following a control period of nine days Pergonal was administered at a dose level of 225 i.u. FSH per day for three days; subsequently the dosage was decreased to 150 i.u. per day for seven days and this was followed by the administration of 3,000 i.u. HCG per day for three days. The treatment caused an increase in urinary oestrogen and pregnanediol output, indicating that ovulation had been produced. It is probable that conception also occurred as a result of therapy, this being indicated by the rising steroid levels between days 23 and 28 of the study. However, vaginal bleeding commenced on day 33 and continued for six days. This was preceded by abdominal pain, backache and nausea for two days, and it is virtually certain that the bleeding was associated with an early abortion.

Kistner (1966) has compared treatment by combinations of gonadotrophins and Clomiphene with therapy by Clomiphene alone in a series of 19 women suffering from secondary amenorrhoea and in one patient with primary amenorrhoea. Prior to treatment all these subjects showed very low endogenous levels of urinary oestrogens and HPG in association with small ovaries and uteri. In none of the patients did Clomiphene alone or HCG alone cause ovulation. However, it was found that HMG (Pergonal) plus Clomiphene produced ovulation in nine per cent of the treatment cycles while the corresponding figure with Clomiphene plus HCG was as high as 68 per cent. On the basis of his observations Kistner (1966) has concluded that Clomiphene is more effective as a follicle-stimulating than as a luteinising agent.

COMMENT

The data presented in this chapter indicate that gonadotrophins of both pituitary and urinary origin when administered in association with HCG are capable of producing ovulation in suitably selected patients. It would also appear that the two types of material are equally efficient in this respect. One of the major limitations of both forms of treatment is the widely varying sensitivity of individual patients to the same dosage of administered FSH. Because of this, there is always the possibility that side effects or multiple pregnancy may occur due to excessive stimulation of ovarian function as a result of treatment. At the time of writing a definite dosage schedule of either pituitary or urinary FSH which would be suitable for use in all patients cannot be recommended. However, it is of the utmost importance that when this type of therapy is being administered the patient's hormonal status be investigated as thoroughly as possible. Only in this way will the incidence of side effects and especially of the hyperstimulation syndrome be reduced.

SUMMARY AND CONCLUSIONS

Ovulation can be produced in a proportion of infertile women by the administration of human gonadotrophins of pituitary or urinary origin given in association with HCG. Individual patients vary greatly in their sensitivity to gonadotrophin therapy.

The main clinical conditions in which treatment by gonadotrophins has been successful are primary and secondary amenorrhoea, the Stein-Leventhal syndrome and the Chiari-Frommel syndrome. Results are most satisfactory in patients in whom endogenous HPG levels prior to therapy are low or undetectable and in whom the excretion of " total oestrogens " is less than 10 μg. per 24 hours.

The schedule of gonadotrophin administration has varied greatly in the hands of different investigators. The most favoured regime has been one in which FSH has been given for seven to 10 days, HCG generally being administered for three days towards the end of, or immediately following, the course of FSH. Crooke et al. (1966 a b) have recently suggested that a single injection of FSH followed by HCG is a more satisfactory therapeutic regime.

The conception rate following gonadotrophin therapy in suitably selected patients is relatively high, more than 50 per cent of women becoming pregnant as a result of treatment.

Gonadotrophin administration produces variable effects on urinary steroid output. Overdosage of the hormones causes ovarian hyperstimulation which is associated with grossly elevated excretion values for oestrogens and pregnanediol.

The major complications of gonadotrophin therapy are the occurrence of multiple pregnancy and the development of the " hyperstimulation syndrome ".

REFERENCES

ABRAMS, C. A. L., GRUMBOCH, M. M., DYRENFURTH, I. & VANDE WIELE, R. L. (1967). *J. Clin. Endocrinol. Metab.* **27**, 467.

APOSTOLAKIS, M., BETTENDORF G. & VOIGT, K. D. (1962). *Acta Endocrinol.* **41**, 14.

BELL, E. T., LORAINE, J. A. & STRONG, J. A. (1968). *J. Obstet. Gynaecol. Brit. Commonwealth. In press.*

BETTENDORF, G. (1964). *Intern. J. Fertil.* **9**, 351.

BROWN, J. B. (1965). In *Recent Advances in Ovarian and Synthetic Steroids*, p. 61. Ed. Shearman, R. P. Sydney: Globe Commercial Ltd.

BUTT, W. R., CROOKE, A. C. & CUNNINGHAM, F. J. (1961). *Biochem. J.* **81**, 596.

BUTT, W. R., CUNNINGHAM, F. J. & STOCKELL-HARTREE, A. (1964). *Proc. Roy. Soc. Med.* **57**, 107.

BUXTON, C. L. & HERRMANN, W. (1961). *Am. J. Obstet. Gynecol.* **81**, 584.

CROOKE, A. C. (1964). *Proc. Roy. Soc. Med.* **57**, 111.

CROOKE, A. C., BUTT, W. R. & BERTRAND, P. V. (1966 a). *Acta Endocrinol Suppl.* 111.

CROOKE, A. C., BUTT, W. R. & BERTRAND, P. V. (1966 b). *Lancet*, **ii**, 514.

CROOKE, A. C., BUTT, W. R., CARRINGTON, S. P., MORRIS, R., PALMER, R. F. & EDWARDS, R. L. (1964 a). *Lancet*, **i**, 184.

CROOKE, A. C., BUTT, W. R., PALMER, R. F., BERTRAND, P. V., CARRINGTON, S. P., EDWARDS, R. L. & ANSON, C. J. (1964 b). *J. Obstet Gynaecol. Brit. Commonwealth*, **71**, 571.

CROOKE, A. C., BUTT, W. R., PALMER, R. F., MORRIS, R., EDWARDS, R. L. & ANSON, C. J. (1963 a). *J. Obstet. Gynaecol. Brit. Commonwealth*, **70**, 604.

CROOKE, A. C., BUTT, W. R,. PALMER, R. F., MORRIS, R., EDWARDS, R. L., TAYLOR, C. W. & SHORT, R. V. (1963 b). *Brit. Med. J.* **1**, 1119.

DICZFALUSY, E., JOHANNISSON, E., TILLINGER, K-G. & BETTENDORF, G. (1964). *Acta Endocrinol. Suppl.* **90**, 35.

DONINI, P., PUZZUOLI, D. & MONTEZEMOLO, R. (1964). *Acta Endocrinol.* **45**, 321.

GEMZELL, C. A. (1962). *Fertility Sterility*, **13**, 153.

GEMZELL, C. A. (1963). In *Modern Trends in Gynaecology*, **3**, 133. Ed. Kellar, R. J. London: Butterworths.

GEMZELL, C. A. (1964). *Vitamins Hormones*, **22**, 129.

GEMZELL, C. A. (1965 a). *Recent Prog. Hormone Res.* **21**, 179.

GEMZELL, C. A. (1965 b). *Proc. Second Int. Cong. Endocrinology*, p. 805. Ed. Taylor, S. Amsterdam: Excerpta Medica Foundation.

GEMZELL, C. A. (1966). *Fertility Sterility*, **17**, 149.

GEMZELL, C. A. & ROOS, P. (1966). *Am. J. Obstet. Gynecol.* **94**, 490.

GEMZELL, C. A., DICZFALUSY, E. & TILLINGER, K-G. (1958). *J. Clin. Endocrinol. Metab.* **18**, 1333.

GEMZELL, C. A., ROOS, P. & LOEFFLER, F. E. (1966). *J. Reprod. Fertil.* **12**, 49.
JOHANNISSON, E., GEMZELL, C. A. & DICZFALUSY, E. (1961). *J. Clin. Endocrinol. Metab.* **21**, 1068.
KISTNER, R. W. (1966). *Fertility Sterility,* **17**, 569.
KOTZ, H. L. & HERRMANN, W. (1961). *Fertility Sterility,* **12**, 375.
LIGGINS, G. C. & IBBERTSON, H. K. (1966). *Lancet,* **i**, 114.
LORAINE, J A. & BELL, E. T. (1963). *Lancet,* **i**, 1340.
LORAINE, J. A. & BELL, E. T. (1966). *Hormone Assays and their Clinical Application.* Second ed. Edinburgh: Livingstone.
LORAINE, J. A. & SCHMIDT-ELMENDORFF, H. W. (1963). In *Modern Trends in Human Reproductive Physiology,* p. 18. Ed. Carey, H. M. London: Butterworths.
LUNENFELD, B. (1965). *Proc. Second Int. Cong. Endocrinology,* p. 814. Ed. Taylor, S. Amsterdam: Excerpta Medica Foundation.
LUNENFELD, B. (1967). In *Recent Research on Gonadotrophic Hormones,* p. 257. Eds. Bell, E. T. and Loraine, J. A. Edinburgh: Livingstone.
LUNENFELD, B., ESHKOL, A., DONINI, P., PUZZUOLI, D. & SHELESNYAK, M. C. (1963). *Harokeach Haivri.* **9**, 766.
LUNENFELD, B., SULIMOVICI, S. & RABAU, E. (1962 a). *Compt. Rend. Soc. Francaise Gynecol.* **32**, 292.
LUNENFELD, B., SULIMOVICI, S., RABAU, E. & ESHKOL, A. (1962 b). *Compt. Rend. Soc. Francaise Gynecol.* **32**, 346.
MOZES, M., BOGOKOWSKY, H., ANTEBI, E., LUNENFELD, B., RABAU, E., SERR, D. M., DAVID, A. & SALOMY, M. (1965). *Lancet,* **ii**, 1213.
ØSTERGAARD, E. (1964). *Acta Endocrinol. Suppl.* **90**, 235.
PASETTO, N. & MONTANINO, G. (1964). *Acta Endocrinol.* **47**, 1.
RABAU, E., DAVID, A., SERR, D. M., MASHIACH, S. & LUNENFELD, B. (1967). *Am. J. Obstet. Gynecol.* **98**, 92.
ROOS, P. & GEMZELL, C. A. (1964). *Biochim. Biophys. Acta,* **82**, 218.
ROOS, P. & GEMZELL, C. A. (1965). *Ciba Found. Study Group,* No. 22, 11.
ROSEMBERG, E., COLEMAN, J., DEMANY, M. & GARCIA, C-R. (1963). *J. Clin. Endocrinol. Metab.* **23**, 181.
ROSEMBERG, E., MAHER, R. E., STERN, A. & DEMANY, M. (1964). *J. Clin. Endocrinol. Metab.* **24**, 105.
SEARLE, G. D. & Co. Ltd. (1966). *Pergonal Investigator's Manual.*
SHEARMAN, R. P. (1965). In *Recent Advances in Ovarian and Synthetic Steroids,* p. 26. Ed. Shearman, R. P. Sydney: Globe Commercial Ltd.
SHEARMAN, R. P. (1966). *Australasian Ann. Med.* **15**, 266.
TAYMOR, M. L. (1967). In *Recent Research on Gonadotrophic Hormones,* p. 265. Eds. Bell, E. T. and Loraine, J. A. Edinburgh: Livingstone.
TAYMOR, M. L., STURGIS, S. H., GOLDSTEIN, D. P. & LIEBERMAN, B. (1967). *Fertility Sterility,* **18**, 181.
TOWNSEND, S. L., BROWN, J. B., JOHNSTONE, J. W., ADEY, F. D., EVANS, J. H. & TAFT, H. P. (1966). *J. Obstet. Gynaecol. Brit. Commonwealth,* **73**, 529.
VANDE WIELE, R. L. & TURKSOY, R. N. (1965). *J. Clin. Endocrinol. Metab.* **25**, 369.

CHAPTER IX

Oral Contraception

INTRODUCTION

TOWARDS the end of the nineteenth century a number of investigators including Beard (1897) and Zschokke (1898) recognised that in various animal species ovulation did not occur in an ovary which contained a well-developed corpus luteum, and during the first three decades of the twentieth century further evidence was accumulated indicating that extracts of the corpus luteum were capable of inhibiting ovulation (see Pearl and Surface, 1914 : Haberlandt, 1921 ; Smith, 1929 ; Parkes, 1929). In 1934 there was a major discovery in this field with the isolation by four independent groups of workers of the corpus luteum hormone, progesterone, from sow's ovaries (Butenandt *et al.*, 1934 ; Slotta *et al.*, 1934 ; Allen and Wintersteiner, 1934 ; Hartmann and Wettstein, 1934). Following its isolation the physiological actions of progesterone were intensively studied, and it rapidly became apparent that the hormone was capable of inhibiting ovulation in a variety of animal species including the rabbit and the rat (Makepeace *et al.*, 1937 ; Astwood and Fevold, 1939).

The next important advance in this field was the synthesis by Djerassi *et al.* (1954) of a series of steroids which in their chemical structure resembled both progesterone and the male sex hormone, testosterone (see also Djerassi, 1966 for a historical review). The biological effects of a number of these compounds were elucidated by Pincus and his co-workers (Pincus and Chang, 1953 ; Pincus and Merrill, 1961 ; Pincus *et al.*, 1956) and by Kincl and Dorfman (1963 *a b*). They were shown to produce progestational effects in rabbits and to possess a marked degree of anti-ovulatory activity in various animal species ; the properties of some of these steroids have recently been reviewed by Pincus (1965).

The logical development from the studies in animals was to test the anti-ovulatory activity of these compounds in human subjects. Limited clinical trials were initiated by Pincus and his associates in New England, U.S.A., during 1956, and soon after more extensive trials were commenced in Puerto Rico and Haiti (see Pincus, 1965 for review). The effectiveness of orally administered progestational compounds as contraceptive agents was rapidly established, and over the past decade this form of fertility control has grown widely in popularity throughout the world. At the time of writing it is difficult to estimate with accuracy the total number of women receiving progestogen–oestrogen mixtures as oral contraceptives, but it is not unlikely that the figure exceeds ten million.

The major portion of this chapter deals with what has been termed the " classical" pill, i.e. a progestogen–oestrogen mixture, administered from day 5 of the cycle for a period of 20 or 21 days. The subject matter will be concerned with the types of oral contraceptive available, their effectiveness, side-effects associated with their administration, their mode of action with special reference to the manner in which they affect the endocrine system, and contra-indications to their use in clinical practice. Short sections are also included on the administration of oral contraceptives on a sequential basis and on recent developments in this general field. For further information on some of the subjects considered herein the reader is referred to papers and monographs by Jackson (1963), Goldzieher (1964), Kleinman (1964), Drill (1965, 1966), Mears (1965 a), Pincus (1965), Swyer (1966) and Loraine and Bell (1966). An authoritative summary of the present position will also be found in the W.H.O. Technical Report published in 1966.

TYPES OF ORAL CONTRACEPTIVE

As mentioned previously the typical oral contraceptive consists of a mixture of a progestogen and an oestrogen. The composition of some of the oral contraceptives in current use is shown in Table 15, together with trade names and manufacturers ; the great variety of compounds available should be noted. The oestrogen is added to the contraceptive pill for two main reasons—to control the length of the cycle, and to diminish the incidence of " breakthrough bleeding " (see also p. 268). As will be seen in Table 15 the oestrogens which have been most widely used as constituents of oral contraceptives are ethinyl oestradiol and the 3-methyl ether of this steroid.

Oral contraceptives can be divided into two main categories depending on their chemical nature. These are (a) compounds similar in structure to testosterone and 19-nortestosterone and, (b) compounds related to 17α-hydroxyprogesterone. Typical examples of the structural formulae of compounds in both groups are shown in Figure 111. It will be noted that derivatives of 19-nortestosterone lack the angular methyl group at position 19 between rings A and B of the steroid molecule. These substances possess inherent oestrogenicity and are probably metabolised to oestrogens in the body (Engel et al., 1958 ; Breuer et al., 1960 ; Brown and Blair, 1960). The category of compounds resembling 17α-hydroxyprogesterone are produced by esterification of the 17α-hydroxy group with or without the introduction of other substituents such as a halogen or methyl group at position 6 in the molecule. Such substances tend to be less effective as anti-ovulatory agents and, in addition, they lack inherent oestrogenicity.

261

TABLE 15

TYPES OF ORAL CONTRACEPTIVE CURRENTLY AVAILABLE

(After Mears, 1965 a)

Progestogen		Oestrogen		Trade name	Manufacturer
Compound	dosage (mg.)	Compound	dosage (mg.)		
Norethynodrel (17α-ethinyl-5(10)-estrenolone)	10·0	Mestranol	0·15	Enovid (U.S.A.)	G. D. Searle & Co.
	5·0		0·075	{ Conovid (U.K.) / Enovid (U.S.A.)	
	2·5		0·1	{ Conovid E (U.K.) / Enovid E (U.S.A.) / Previson	Roussel Labs.
Norethindrone / Norethisterone (17α-ethinyl-19-nortestosterone)	10·0	Mestranol	0·06	Ortho-Novum (U.S.A.)	Ortho Pharmaceuticals
	5·0		0·075	Ortho-Novum (Canada)	
	2·0		0·1	{ Ortho-Novum (U.S.A., Canada) / Ortho-Novum (U.K.) / Norinyl	Syntex
Norethindrone acetate / Norethisterone acetate (17α-ethinyl-19-nortestosterone acetate)	4·0	Ethinyl oestradiol	0·05	Anovlar	Schering A.G.
	3·0		0·05	Gynovlar	
	2·5		0·05	Norlestrin	Parke-Davis & Co.

Medroxy progesterone acetate (6α-methyl-17α-hydroxy-progesterone acetate)	10·0 5·0 5·0	Ethinyl oestradiol	0·05 0·05 0·075	Provest Ciclofarlutal Zyklo-Farlutal	Upjohn Farmitalia
Megestrol acetate (17α-acetoxy-6-dehydro-6-methyl progesterone)	5 4·0	Mestranol Ethinyl oestradiol	0·1 0·05	Delpregnin Planovin Volidan Anova	Novo Industri A/S British Drug Houses Teva
Ethinodiol diacetate (17α-ethinylestrene-3β, 17β-diol diacetate)	1·0	Mestranol	0·1	Ovulen	G. D. Searle & Co.
Lynoestrenol (17α-ethinyl-17β-hydroxyestrene)	5·0	Mestranol	0·15	Lyndiol Lindiol (Latin America) Noracyclin	Organon Labs. CIBA
	2·5		0·075	Lyndiol 2·5 Lyndiol Mite (Sweden) Noracyclin	Organon Labs. CIBA (Brazil)

It has already been mentioned that oral contraceptives are generally administered from day 5 of the cycle for 20 or 21 days. Such a regime has two aims, firstly to inhibit ovulation and secondly to establish regular, cyclical menstrual periods.

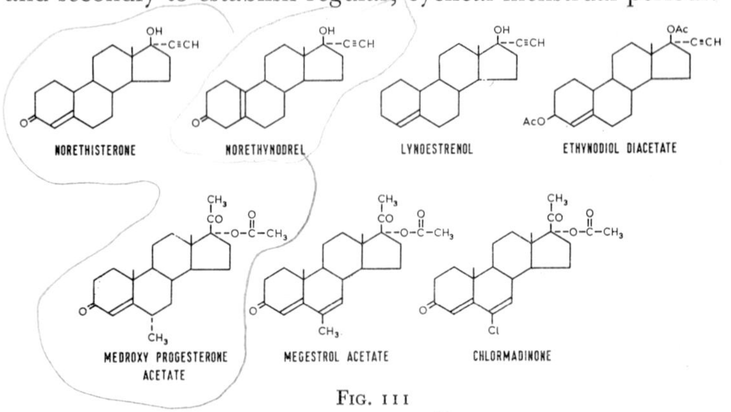

FIG. 111

Structural formulae of various progestogens.

EFFECTIVENESS

There is general agreement that if progestogen–oestrogen mixtures are taken by the patient in the manner described above the form of contraception is virtually 100 per cent effective (see Table 16). If pregnancy occurs this is generally due not to lack of efficacy of the tablets but to the fact that the woman has failed to take the full number. This point is well illustrated in Table 17 which shows experience with combinations of norethynodrel and mestranol and demonstrates the great increase in the pregnancy rate with the number of tablets missed.

SIDE EFFECTS OF ORAL CONTRACEPTIVES

1. Nausea

This symptom occurs fairly frequently at the beginning of therapy with oral contraceptives ; however, its prevalence decreases with continuing medication. If the symptom persists it can frequently be alleviated by changing the product. The incidence of nausea resulting from the administration of a variety of oral contraceptives has been summarised by Venning (1963) and by Drill (1966).

264

TABLE 16

CLINICAL EFFECTIVENESS OF VARIOUS ORAL CONTRACEPTIVES

(After Drill, 1966)

Contraceptive with dose	Women-years* of use	Pregnancy		Pregnancies per 100 women-years* (including missed tablets)
		Number of tablet failures	Number of patient failures (missed tablets)	
Enovid 10 mg.... ...	1,947	1	46	2·4
Enovid 5 mg.	7,821	1	21	0·3
Enovid 2·5 mg. ...	1,115	1	8	0·8
Ortho-Novum 2·5 mg.	1,490	0	0	0
Anovlar 4 mg.... ...	746	0	0	0
Lyndiol 5 mg.	861	0	7	0·8
Ovulen 1 mg.	869	0	3	0·3

* In this and subsequent tables a woman-year is defined as one woman studied over a period of one year.

TABLE 17

PREGNANCY RATE ACCORDING TO NUMBER OF PILLS NOT TAKEN IN PATIENTS IN SAN JUAN

(From Garcia and Pincus, 1965)

Number of pills missed	Dose of progestogen mg./day	Number of women-years*	Number of pregnancies	Pregnancy rate per 100 women-years
0	2·5	411	1*	0·2
	5·0	1,685	4	0·2
	10·0	686	4	0·6
1 to 5	2·5	77	0	0·0
	5·0	154	4	2·6
	10·0	95	3	3·2
6 to 19	2·5	6	4	66·7
	5·0	19	8	42·1
	10·0	31	10	32·3

* Patient took 1·25 mg./day

265

2. Breast Tenderness

Some women complain of breast fullness and tenderness while receiving therapy with oral contraceptives. Conversely, others who normally experience these symptoms towards the end of their menstrual cycle lose them as a result of such medication. Mears (1965 *a*) takes the view that breast tenderness is caused by the progestational component of the tablet. In the experience of Pincus (1965) the incidence of breast tenderness and fullness can vary from 0 to 27 per cent depending on the product used.

3. Increased Appetite and Weight Gain

Increased appetite is by no means invariable. If present it occurs during the first two or three cycles of treatment and gradually disappears with continuing medication. Weight gain may be pronounced in a proportion of women and may sometimes be associated with ankle oedema and abdominal distension. In some subjects the increase in weight is so marked that it is necessary to stop the treatment ; in others, it subsides spontaneously or can be ameliorated by changing to a different product. According to Pincus (1965) who has summarised the experience of various investigations, the percentage of women gaining three pounds or more during therapy varies from 4 to 50.

4. Effects on Libido

Libido is essentially subjective in nature, and it is a matter of considerable difficulty to determine with accuracy how this symptom is affected by oral contraceptives. The effects have been variable, an increase, a decrease and no change in sex drive during treatment having been reported.

5. Alterations in Menstrual Pattern

(*a*) CHANGES IN MENSTRUAL FLOW.—These have been reviewed by Pincus and Garcia (1965) and by Mears (1965 *a*) ; the experience of Pincus and Garcia (1965) is summarised in Table 18. It will be noted that in the majority of women menstrual flow during medication was either the same as, or lighter than, that found prior to treatment ; in only a small proportion of the subjects studied did menstrual bleeding become heavier as a result of therapy.

TABLE 18

CHANGES IN MENSTRUAL FLOW IN WOMEN RECEIVING ENOVID

(From Pincus and Garcia, 1965)

Study conducted in	Treatment	No. of subjects	Percentage change ($\pm$ S.D.) in amount of menstrual flow			
			Heavier	Same	Lighter	Variable
San Juan ...	Enovid 1 to 3 years	398	5±1·1	66±2·4	27±2·2	2±0·7
	Enovid 4 to 7 years	125	2±1·3	69±4·1	29±4·1	0
	Treatment withdrawn	52	4±2·7	69±6·5	21±5·7	6±3·3
Humacao ...	Enovid 1 to 3 years	539	3±0·7	41±2·1	52±2·2	4±0·8
	Enovid 4 to 7 years	112	2±1·3	59±4·7	39±4·6	0
	Treatment withdrawn	35	9±4·9	63±8·3	26±7·5	3±2·9
Haiti ...	Enovid 1 to 3 years	105	4±1·9	31±4·5	60±4·8	5±2·1

TABLE 19

PERCENTAGE INCIDENCE OF BREAKTHROUGH BLEEDING IN SUBJECTS RECEIVING ORAL CONTRACEPTIVES

(From Venning, 1963)

Compound	Source of data	Treatment cycle				
		1st	2nd	3rd	4th–6th	Other
Conovid E ...	Dr. Wiseman ...	37	35	34	25	19
Conovid E ...	Private patients ...	17	10	6	4	3
Conovid... ...	Dr. Bond... ...	24	19	15	14	12
Anovlar	FPA Handbook ...	8	5	4	—	—
SC 11,800 (2 mg.)	Dr. Wiseman ...	9	3	0	0	0
Conovid E ...	Dr. Satterthwaite	18	18	10	12	5
SC 11,800 (1 mg.)	Dr. Satterthwaite	9	0	0	1	—

(*b*) "BREAKTHROUGH BLEEDING."—This is defined as bleeding occurring before the 20 tablets have been taken. It is a major problem during the early months of medication but tends to become less marked the longer the treatment is continued. This point is well illustrated in Table 19 which is taken from a paper by Venning (1963) and in Figure 112 which shows the experience of Hutcherson *et al.* (1966) with the compound Ortho-Novum.

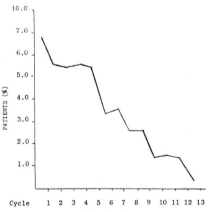

FIG. 112

Incidence of breakthrough bleeding in subjects receiving Ortho-Novum.

(From Hutcherson *et al.*, 1966.)

(c) AMENORRHOEA OR MISSED MENSTRUATION.—Drill (1966) has pointed out that withdrawal bleeding fails to occur in up to 9·7 per cent of all cycles. The incidence varies with the contraceptive administered but is generally below 4 per cent except in the case of Lyndiol. Lack of withdrawal bleeding was especially frequent in the early days of oral contraception when a progestogen alone was administered, and it is now established that the addition of an oestrogen to the tablet has greatly decreased the incidence of this complication. In Figure 113 is shown the hormone excretion pattern in a subject who failed to show a withdrawal bleeding following treatment with norethisterone acetate. It will be noted that in spite of the absence of such bleeding, the cycle occurring during the last 30 days of the investigation was ovulatory in character as judged by assays of oestrogens, pregnanediol and pregnanetriol.

POSSIBLE HARMFUL EFFECTS OF ORAL CONTRACEPTIVES

1. Effects on Subsequent Fertility

At the time of writing there is no evidence to suggest that fertility is decreased in women in whom treatment with oral contraceptives has continued for long periods of time and who have discontinued medication. In the opinion of Goldzieher and his associates (Rice-Wray et al., 1963 a ; Goldzieher, 1964) fertility may actually be increased after cessation of therapy. Goldzieher (1964) has reported that in women discontinuing the use of the oral contraceptive Ortho-Novum the pregnancy rate in the first post-treatment cycle was 62 per cent ; this compares with a figure of 34 per cent in women who stopped using mechanical forms of contraception. These statistics are undoubtedly impressive ; however, it must be remembered that many women discontinue the use of oral contraceptives because of their desire to conceive and, accordingly, the expectation would be that the pregnancy rate in such a group would be relatively high.

On the basis of hormone assay studies Loraine and his associates did not note any deleterious effects of oral contraceptives on ovarian function (Loraine et al., 1963, 1965 ; Bell *et al.*, 1967). These investigators found that, following cessation of treatment, the cycles rapidly reverted to an ovulatory pattern (see also p. 293).

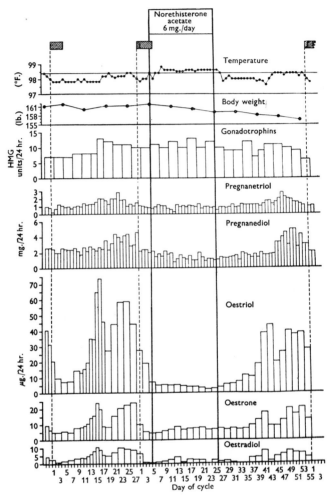

Fig. 113

Hormone excretion pattern in a subject receiving norethisterone acetate.

///// = menstrual bleeding.

(From Brown *et al.*, 1962.)

2. Effects on the Menopause

Fears have been expressed that, because oral contraceptives inhibit ovarian activity and ovulation, they might also postpone the time at which the menopause occurs. This would have the most unfortunate effect that women who had been treated with oral contraceptives for many years and who discontinued medication, might be rendered fertile at an age at which the capacity to conceive was not generally present. Fortunately such fears have proved to be groundless since it is now accepted that the age at which the menopause occurs is dependent on genetic rather than on endocrinological factors. The major feature in the menopausal ovary is atresia of the follicles, and this is known to occur irrespective of whether the ovary is normally active or has been rendered functionally inactive by the administration of oral contraceptives. This view is substantiated by the work of Pincus and Garcia (1965), who on the basis of ovarian biopsies, failed to demonstrate any differences between the numbers of atretic follicles in the ovaries of patients receiving Enovid on the one hand and in those of control subjects on the other. Another point tending to dissociate the occurrence of the menopause from the administration of anti-ovulatory compounds is the well known clinical observation that in women who have borne large numbers of children and in whom ovarian function and ovulation have

TABLE 20

EFFECTS OF ENOVID ON LACTATING WOMEN IN HUMACAO

(From Pincus, 1965)

Dosage of progestogen mg./day	No. of patients	Per cent lactating		
		Less than previously	Same as previously	More than previously
20	22	77	18	5
10	37	38	57	5
5	84	45	45	10
2·5	30	15	70	15

been inhibited for long periods of their reproductive life, the menopause is not delayed and occurs at the same time as in women of low parity.

3. Effects on Lactation

The effect on Enovid on lactation has been studied by Pincus (1965). The results which he obtained are shown in Table 20 from which it will be noted that lactation was slightly depressed when relatively high dosages of the compound were administered. Pincus's findings have been confirmed by other investigators notably Chinnatamby (1963) and Satterthwaite (1964). According to Ferin et al. (1964) the quality of the milk and the growth rate of the baby are not affected by therapy with oral contraceptives.

4. Effects on the Foetus

Masculinisation of the foetus as a result of treatment with progestogens or progestogen–oestrogen mixtures is so rare that such a complication is of little or no importance (see Mears, 1965 a). A few cases of foetal masculinisation have been reported in the literature when such compounds have been administered to pregnant women. However, it must be emphasised that the dosage given to these patients was very much higher than that routinely used for purposes of contraception (see also Jacobson, 1962). Another point which is worthy of emphasis is that this form of contraception is so effective when used properly that the possibility of the woman becoming pregnant is remote ; accordingly, danger to the foetus must be regarded as negligible.

5. Effects on Carbohydrate Metabolism

A number of investigators including Waine et al. (1963), Gershberg et al. (1964), Besch et al. (1965), Javier et al. (1965) and Spellacy and Carlson (1966) have stated that abnormalities in carbohydrate metabolism may occur in women receiving therapy by oral contraceptives. However, other workers, e.g. Copera et al. (1964), have been unable to demonstrate such changes. The main defect found has been the tendency for the blood sugar curve following glucose administration to be of the pre-diabetic type. Such an abnormality has been especially noticeable in women with a family history of diabetes, and in one pre-diabetic patient described by Gershberg *et al.* (1964) actual diabetes developed under therapy with Enovid. It must, however, be emphasised that in patients with established diabetes, the administration of progestogen–oestrogen mixtures has not so far been shown to affect the severity of the disease as judged by insulin requirements.

Spellacy and Carlson (1966), using the radio-immunological assay method for insulin developed by Goetz *et al.* (1963), have estimated plasma levels of this hormone following glucose administration in patients before and during Enovid administration. They noted that insulin concentrations increased when therapy was initiated. This is obviously an interesting finding, but its exact significance remains to be elucidated.

6. Effects on Liver Function

These have been reviewed by Pincus (1965), Mears (1965 *a*), Swyer (1966), Drill (1966), Robertson (1967) and others. In a careful survey Mears (1965 *a*) discussed the effects of oral contraceptives on conventional liver function tests. These included thymol turbidity and cephalin–cholesterol flocculation tests, methods depending on the estimation of serum albumen, globulin, cholesterol esters and bilirubin, and techniques involving the measurement of glutamic-oxaloacetic and glutamic-pyruvic transaminase activities. She concluded that, in women during reproductive life, any changes produced in such tests were transient in character and were of little significance.

Eisalo *et al.* (1964) and Palva and Mustala (1964), working in Finland, have reported alterations in liver function in postmenopausal women receiving the progestogen–oestrogen mixtures Anovlar and Lyndiol. In their series liver function was assessed by tests depending on the serum concentration of glutamic–pyruvic and glutamic–oxaloacetic transaminase. Bakke (1965) failed to demonstrate such alterations in a large series of postmenopausal women treated with oral contraceptives in the U.S.A. The reason for the differing results in Finnish and American women is not at present clear, but it is possible that dietary factors may be at least partly responsible. In a recent publication Robertson (1967) has shown that in women taking oral contraceptives for short periods of time a decrease occurs in serum levels of cholinesterase and albumen, associated with a rise in values for serum α_1-globulin ; the exact significance of these changes is not at present clear.

Swyer (1966) and others have emphasised that in patients in whom liver function was previously normal, medication by progestogen–oestrogen mixtures does not appear to cause jaundice, hepatic necrosis or progressive liver disease. On the other hand, in women with pre-existing liver disease, e.g. infective hepatitis or cirrhosis, there is some evidence suggesting that this form of medication may further impair hepatic function. At the present time the consensus of opinion is that oral contraceptives should not be administered to patients with a history of hereditary or acquired defects of the liver.

7. Effects on Blood Coagulation

Reviews on this topic have been written by Pincus (1965), Mears (1965 a), Swyer (1966) and Drill (1966) ; information is also available in the W.H.O. Technical Report (1966). Pincus (1965) demonstrated that oral contraceptives tend to cause a decrease in the clotting time together with an increase in the blood levels of various substances associated with clotting, especially fibrinogen and fibrinolysin. He also showed that in anaemic patients receiving oral contraceptives an increase both in haemoglobin concentration and in white blood cell count occurred.

Some of the alterations in the blood clotting mechanism which have been reported in users of oral contraceptives are shown in Table 21. It is not yet established whether any of these changes are connected with the occurrence of thromboembolic disease in the human female. However, the balance of evidence currently available would tend to suggest the lack of any such connection (see Drill, 1966).

8. Relationship to Thromboembolic Disease

This condition occurs infrequently in women during reproductive life, and according to Pincus (1966) and others, there is no evidence to suggest that its incidence increases in users of oral contraceptives. In Table 22 which is taken from a paper by Venning (1963) the incidence of thromboembolic disorders in British patients receiving progestogen–oestrogen

TABLE 21

EFFECT OF ORAL CONTRACEPTIVES ON BLOOD CLOTTING FACTORS

(After Swyer, 1966)

Clotting Factor	Effect	Reference
Factor I (fibrinogen)	Increase	Turksoy et al. (1961), Phillips et al. (1961), Pincus (1965)
	No change	Sobrero et al. (1963)
Factor II (prothrombin time)	Reduction	Pincus (1965)
	No change	Sobrero et al. (1963)
Factor V	No change	Pincus (1965)
	Some increase in VII complex	Pincus (1965)
Factor VII	Increase, significant from third month	Thomson and Poller (1965)
Factor VIII (antihaemophilic)	Some increase	Egeberg and Owren (1963)
	No change	Pincus (1965), Thomson and Poller (1965)
Factor X (thromboplastin generating)	No change	Pincus (1965)
Clotting time	No change	Sobrero et al. (1963)
	Reduction	Pincus (1965)
Bleeding time	No change	Pincus (1965)
Fibrinolysin	Increase	Turksoy et al. (1961), Phillips et al. (1961), Pincus (1965)
Antifibrinolysin	Increase	Turksoy et al. (1961), Phillips et al. (1961)
Cephalin time	No change	Thomson and Poller (1965)
	Reduced	Egeberg and Owren (1963)
Proconvertin	Slight increase	Egeberg and Owren (1963)
Plasmin	No change	Sobrero et al. (1963)
Plasmin inhibitor	No change	Sobrero et al. (1963)
Plasminogen	Increase	Pilgeram et al. (1964)
	No change	Brakman and Astrup (1964)
Antithrombin	No change	Brakman and Astrup (1964)

mixtures between the years 1959 and 1962 is shown. It will be noted that the number of reported cases was actually smaller than might have been expected on statistical grounds. A similar conclusion has been reached by Drill (1966).

TABLE 22

THROMBOEMBOLIC DISORDERS REPORTED IN ASSOCIATION WITH NORETHYNODREL AND MESTRANOL (UNITED KINGDOM 1959–1962)

(From Venning, 1963)

Population at risk (Expressed as total cycles of experience)	Women-years of experience (15 cycles per annum)	Expected number of cases*	Reported number of cases
698,281	46,552	102	27

* Based on incidence in women aged 15 to 44 (Morbidity Statistics from General Pratice (1958–1962) H.M.S.O. London).

Recently a Medical Research Council Subcommittee (1967) has investigated possible relationships between the administration of oral contraceptives and the occurrence of thromboembolic disease. The Committee drew conclusions different to those of Venning (1963) and Drill (1966) and stated that " there can be no reasonable doubt that some types of thromboembolic disorder are associated with the use of oral contraceptives ". On the basis of the evidence available the Committee reported that the risk of death which could be attributed to the use of oral contraceptives was approximately three per 100,000 users per year. If the subjects had used forms of contraception other than oral, the failure rate (pregnancy rate) would have been approximately 10 per cent, and of the women becoming pregnant some 12 per 100,000 would have died as a result of thromboembolic complications associated with the pregnancy. The main point of interest in these figures is that the risk of thromboembolic disease is much greater in pregnant women than in subjects receiving oral contraceptives. The Committee also commented on the types of thromboembolic disease to which oral contraceptive users were most prone. The conclusion was that the main correlation existed in the case of venous thrombosis and pulmonary embolism, there being no clear-cut evidence in relation to cerebro-vascular accidents and coronary thrombosis. The recent study of Jennett and Cross (1967) failed to demonstrate a correlation between cerebral thromboembolic disease and the administration of oral contraceptives.

Swyer (1966) has remarked on the fact that in 1964 in the U.S.A. approximately four million women of child-bearing age were receiving treatment with oral contraceptives. In spite of this fact the death rate from cerebral thrombosis in that country was no greater in 1964 than in 1960, a year in which this form of treatment was available on a very limited scale. Swyer (1966) has also made the important comment that the number of deaths attributed to the use of oral contraceptives in the U.S.A. is a very small fraction of the fatalities which would have resulted from the pregnancies which were prevented by this form of treatment.

9. Relationship to Carcinogenesis

(a) CERVICAL CARINOMA.—The consensus of opinion is that hormonal mechanisms play an insignificant role in cancer of the cervix, and that this disease is more closely associated with such factors as poor economic status and inadequate hygiene. According to the W.H.O. Technical Report (1966) there is no evidence indicating an increased incidence of cervical carcinoma in women receiving oral contraceptives. Indeed, the experience of Satterthwaite and Gamble (1962), Mears (1965 a) and others with serial cervical smears indicates that in oral contraceptive users there is in fact a decrease in the number of cells which might be regarded as being suspicious of cervical carcinoma.

(b) ENDOMETRIAL CARCINOMA.—As discussed in Chapter VI it is now generally agreed that the occurrence of this form of neoplasm bears some relationship to the oestrogenic status of the individual. Theoretically, therefore, it might be anticipated that the administration of oral contraceptives over long periods of time might lead to an increased incidence of the disease. Such a hypothesis has not been sustained by clinical experience, and there is now general agreement among investigators in this field that oral contraceptives do not cause endometrial carcinoma. There is even a possibility that the progestogenic component of the tablet may be of value in the treatment of patients with this condition (see Swyer, 1966 for references), and obviously this interesting suggestion requires further study. It appears unlikely that the oestrogenic component of the oral contraceptive would cause endometrial carcinoma in view of the reports of Bishop (1960) and of Wilson (1962) who demonstrated beyond all reasonable doubt that the administration of oestrogens to women over lengthy periods of time did not result in an increased incidence of cancer.

TABLE 23

CASES OF CANCER DURING THE USE OF ORAL CONTRACEPTIVES

(From Drill, 1966)

Compound	Number of women treated	Total cycles studied	Number of cases of cancer observed during treatment		Reference
			Genital	Mammary	
Enovid	830	8,133	0	0	Pincus et al. (1959)
Enovid	550	6,743	2	0	Cook et al. (1961)
Enovid		20,442	1	0	Pincus (1961)
Enovid Ortho-Novum	1,004	33,132*	†	0	Tyler (1961)
Ortho-Novum	210	6,232	0	0	Goldzieher et al. (1962)
Ortho-Novum	364	6,062	0	0	Rice-Wray et al. (1962)
Enovid Ortho-Novum	2,040	22,948‡	0	0	Rice-Wray et al. (1963 b)
Ortho-Novum	829	19,900		0	Tyler et al. (1964)

   * Calculated on basis of 31 months average duration of treatment.
   † No cases reported based on physical and pelvic examination or endometrial biopsy.
   ‡ Enovid or Ortho-Novum employed.

(c) MAMMARY CARCINOMA.—The endocrinology of this disease has been reviewed on a number of occasions in recent years (see Strong, 1958 ; Loraine, 1959 ; Bulbrook, 1965 ; Loraine and Bell, 1966). Although abnormalities in endogenous hormone excretion and in steroid metabolism occur in a proportion of patients with breast cancer the relationship of these changes to the aetiology of the condition remains obscure. Oestrogen administration has been implicated in the causation of mammary carcinoma in certain susceptible strains of mice ; however, there is no evidence to suggest that a similar situation obtains in human subjects.

Clinical experience accumulated so far indicates that the incidence of mammary cancer in women receiving oral contraceptives is low, being no higher than in the general population (see Satterthwaite and Gamble, 1962 ; Mears, 1965 a ; Adams and Spicer, 1965). In the opinion of Pincus (1965) the incidence of the disease may actually be reduced in subjects taking this form of medication. Drill (1966) has summarised the occurrence of genital and mammary carcinoma reported in eight large scale studies on oral contraceptives ; the very low incidence obtained is shown in Table 23.

EFFECTS ON VAGINAL CYTOLOGY

The effects of oral contraceptives on the cytological picture of the vagina have been summarised by Pincus (1965) on the basis of observations made in patients in Puerto Rico and Haiti. He has reported that the incidence of abnormal Papanicoloau smears is lower in oral contraceptive users than in women employing other forms of contraception, e.g. the intra-uterine device. Such an observation must be regarded as reassuring.

A careful study of the effects of oral contraceptives on vaginal cytology is that of Moyer et al. (1964). These investigators administered norethynodrel plus added oestrogen and norethindrone to their patients and compared the results obtained with those in control subjects. They noted that in the women receiving the progestogen–oestrogen mixture differential counts of squamous cells and the karyopyknotic and eosinophilic indices were similar to those in untreated subjects. However, in patients given norethindrone the vaginal smears were less well differentiated than in the other two groups, showing a decrease in superficial cells and a slight increase in intermediate cells. Some of the results obtained by Moyer *et al.* (1964) are illustrated in Figure 114.

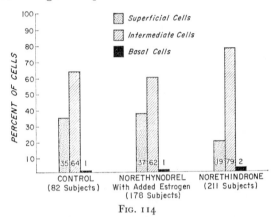

Fig. 114

Mean counts of squamous cells in vaginal smears of control and treated subjects.

(From Moyer *et al.*, 1964.)

EFFECTS ON THE ENDOMETRIUM

Studies of the effect of oral contraceptives on endometrial histology have been reported by Jackson (1963), Maqueo *et al.* (1963), Rice-Wray *et al.* (1963 *b*) and Mears (1965 *a b*). According to Jackson (1963) and Mears (1965 *a*) the endometrial pattern produced is characteristic of the product. On the other hand, Maqueo *et al.* (1963) and Rice-Wray *et al.* (1963 *b*) do not share this view, stating that the endometrial response varies to an insignificant extent from one compound to another.

Mears (1965 *b*) has provided a detailed description of the effect of anti-ovulatory compounds on the endometrium. One of the major alterations is that the endometrium tends to be thinner than normal, and in women who have been receiving therapy for long periods of time it may be difficult to procure tissue at biopsy. The main histological changes during the first few days of treatment are of an early secretory type although glandular development is less well marked than in the normal secretory phase. Basal vacuoles and stromal oedema appear relatively early during the course of treatment ; later there is glandular regression in association with an abundant fibrillary stroma. Towards the end of the 20-day treatment period stromal oedema and a predecidual effect are the predominant features.

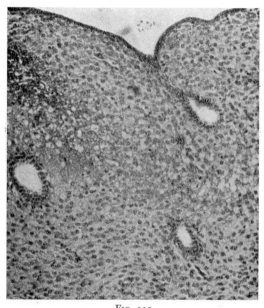

FIG. 115

Endometrial biopsy obtained at approximately midcycle in a subject receiving Ovulen.

(From Mears, 1965 a.)

Typical examples of the effect of oral contraceptives on endometrial patterns are shown in Figures 115 and 116. The subject shown in Figure 115 was under treatment with Ovulen. It will be noted that the glands were small and sparse with flattened cells containing small dark nuclei ; subnuclear vacuolation was not prominent while the stroma was moderately dense and showed the presence of fine oedema. In the woman receiving Conovid (Figure 116) the glands were reasonably well developed and subnuclear vacuolation was present ; the stroma was loose and somewhat oedematous in its middle layers with pseudodecidual changes near the surface.

Long term effects of oral contraceptives on endometrial patterns have been studied by Pincus and Garcia (1965) and by Mears (1965 a). The results obtained by Pincus and Garcia (1965) are shown in Table 24. The main changes noted were (i) a reduction in the proportion of patterns which were

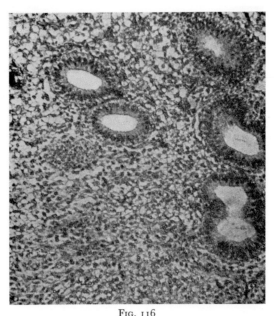

Fig. 116

Endometrial biopsy obtained at approximately midcycle in a subject receiving Conovid.

(From Mears, 1965 a.)

either definitely secretory or proliferative in type, (ii) increase in the proportion of hypoplastic glands, (iii) a tendency to stromal oedema and (iv) a reduced incidence of endometritis and endometrial dysplasia.

Mears (1965 a) has emphasised that, following discontinuation of therapy by oral contraceptives, the histological pattern of the endometrium reverts rapidly to normal. In Figure 117 is shown a biopsy obtained from a patient three weeks after

TABLE 24

ENDOMETRIAL BIOPSY DATA IN WOMEN RECEIVING ENOVID IN SAN JUAN, PUERTO RICO

(From Pincus and Garcia, 1965)

Type of subject	Number of subjects	Proportion of different types of endometrium (%)						
		Proliferative	Secretory	Menstrual	"Hormonal effect"	Dysplastic	Endometritis	Miscellaneous
Prior to treatment	231	44	25	6	10	5	9	2
Post treatment ...	64	33	28	5	22	2	6	5
Enovid 1 year ...	113	13	7	7	70	2	1	0
2 years ...	145	4	8	7	79	1	2	0
3 years ...	131	10	6	9	73	2	1	0
4 years ...	96	10	5	9	72	1	1	0
5 to 8 years	94	9	13	3	69	0	4	2

cessation of therapy with norethisterone. It will be noted that the pattern obtained was secretory in type and was normal in all respects.

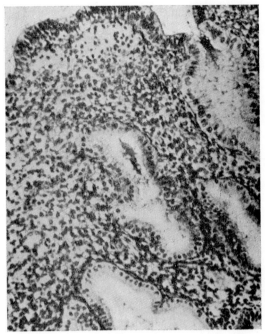

Fig. 117

Endometrial biopsy obtained during the luteal phase in the first post-treatment cycle following therapy with norethisterone.

(From Mears, 1965 *a*.)

EFFECTS ON ENDOCRINE FUNCTION

This section deals with the effect of oral contraceptives on thyroid, adrenocortical, pituitary and ovarian activity. The manner in which they effect ovarian morphology is also discussed.

1. Thyroid Function

It is now well established that an increase in levels of blood protein bound iodine (PBI) and of thyroid binding globulin occurs as a result of therapy with oral contraceptives (see

Wheeler *et al.*, 1960 ; Pincus, 1961 ; Hollander *et al.*, 1963 ; Florsheim and Faircloth, 1964). These changes which are also found during pregnancy and following oestrogen administration, are thought to be due to the oestrogenic component of the tablet, and Roman and Bockner (1963) have found that PBI levels in women receiving oral contraceptives are in the same range as those encountered in normally pregnant women. Following cessation of therapy by oral contraceptives PBI levels return rapidly to normal.

The uptake of tri-iodothyronine by resin is elevated in oral contraceptive users in the absence of clinical signs of hyperthyroidism (Goolden *et al.*, 1967). According to Pincus (1965) there is no marked alteration in the uptake of ^{131}I by the thyroid gland in patients receiving Enovid for long periods of time. Pituitary thyrotrophic function as estimated by serum TSH assays has not yet been studied in patients receiving oral contraceptives, and this remains an important field for future investigation. At the time of writing there is no evidence to support the view that oral contraceptives are capable of causing either clinical hyper- or hypothyroidism (see Swyer, 1966; W.H.O. Technical Report, 1966).

2. Adrenocortical Function

The oestrogenic component of the oral contraceptive causes a rise in plasma levels of transcortin (corticosteroid-binding globulin). This increase is associated with a rise in the total plasma concentration of cortisol, although free cortisol levels remain unchanged (Layne *et al.*, 1962 ; Wallach *et al.*, 1963 ; Metcalf and Beaven, 1963). Pincus (1965) was unable to demonstrate any consistent changes in cortisol production rates between oral contraceptive users and control subjects ; the mean figures in the two groups were 538 ± 238 and 543 ± 135 µg. per 24 hours (S.D.), respectively.

Table 25, which is taken from a publication of Pincus (1965) shows results of urinary steroid assays, together with ACTH stimulation tests, in four patients receiving treatment with Enovid. It will be noted that endogenous levels of 17-OHCS, total 17-oxosteroids, pregnanediol and pregnanetriol prior to ACTH administration were lower in Enovid users than in control subjects. The responsiveness to ACTH in terms of

TABLE 25

MEAN URINARY STEROID EXCRETION (mg. per 24 hr. ±S.D.) AND RESPONSE TO 80 i.u. ACTH (i.m.) OVER TWO CONSECUTIVE DAYS IN FOUR CONTROL SUBJECTS AND IN FOUR WOMEN TREATED WITH ENOVID

(From Pincus, 1965)

Day of study	17-hydroxycorticosteroids		Total 17-oxosteroids		Pregnanetriol		Pregnanediol	
	Enovid treated	Control	Enovid treated	Control	Enovid treated	Control	Enovid treated	Control
Control	3·54±0·35	7·08±0·48	4·90±0·71	7·21±1·16	0·64±0·07	1·74±0·25	0·73±0·06	1·42±0·27
Day 1 ACTH	19·01±3·23	21·33±2·30	12·12±3·09	16·52±4·03	2·48±1·40	5·34±0·82	0·94±0·01	1·90±0·18
Day 2 ACTH	22·94±3·05	22·82±4·26	17·09±0·93	22·74±7·84	4·96±1·52	9·95±2·64	1·44±0·39	3·40±1·02

17-OHCS and 17-oxosteroids was virtually identical in the two groups, but in the case of pregnanediol and pregnanetriol the adrenal response was somewhat less in the patients receiving the contraceptive. Leach and Margulis (1965) have demonstrated that in women taking oral contraceptives, ACTH stimulation tests gave normal results but that the response to Metapyrone was somewhat reduced. Layne *et al.* (1962) found that norethynodrel as well as progesterone and oestrogens themselves were capable of causing a rise in aldosterone secretion rate, while Meyer *et al.* (1961) showed that Enovid caused an increase in the binding of aldosterone to plasma proteins, the binding being greater than that during normal pregnancy.

Recently Starup *et al.* (1966) have studied the effect of megestrol acetate and mestranol on endogenous steroid levels in fourteen normally menstruating women who were treated for periods of time ranging from 3 to 74 weeks. During therapy they observed a decrease in urinary excretion values for both 17-oxogenic steroids and total 17-oxosteroids ; following cessation of treatment a rapid increase in pretreatment levels was noted for both groups of compounds. Østergaard *et al.* (1966) administered megestrol acetate and mestranol from day 20 of the cycle for 20 days to ten normally menstruating women aged from 19 to 32 years. At the end of the treatment period they found a decrease in the output of 17-oxogenic steroids and total 17-oxosteroids ; excretion values for dehydroepiandrosterone, androsterone and aetiocholanolone were also depressed.

3. Ovarian Morphology

Mears (1965 *a*) and Pincus (1965) have summarised the effects of oral contraceptives on the macroscopic and microscopic appearance of the ovaries. A review on this subject is also contained in the W.H.O. Technical Report (1966).

It is now agreed that the macroscopic appearance of the ovary alters rapidly as a result of medication. Morphological changes may occur even during the first cycle of treatment, the ovary shrinking in size and becoming similar to that found at the menopause and postmenopause. In the few women in whom it has so far been possible to conduct the appropriate investigations, the macroscopic appearance of the ovary has returned rapidly to normal following cessation of medication.

Results obtained when ovarian biopsies were performed in subjects receiving Enovid have been reported by Pincus (1965). It was found that, although the ovaries generally failed to show the presence of functional corpora lutea, alterations in the number of primordial or atretic follicles were not observed. At the time of writing there is no evidence to suggest that oral contraceptives cause damage to the oöcytes or that definite pathological changes occur in the ovary as a result of treatment with these compounds.

4. Pituitary and Ovarian Function

This section is concerned with both short and long term effects of oral contraceptives. Only studies in which serial assays of hormones and their metabolites have been performed are quoted, illustrative examples being provided of the types of excretion pattern obtained.

(a) SHORT TERM EFFECTS.—These have been studied by various workers including Brown et al. (1962), Buchholz et al. (1964), Fuchs et al. (1964), Shearman (1963, 1964, 1965), Stevens and Vorys (1965, 1967) and Stevens et al. (1965). One of the more detailed investigations is that of Brown et al.(1962) who performed appropriate estimations in five women; they found that the progestational compounds, norethisterone and norethisterone acetate, could inhibit ovulation as judged by urinary oestrogen, pregnanediol and pregnanetriol assays without affecting HPG output measured by the mouse uterus test. Typical results obtained in this study are shown in Figures 118 and 119.

The patient in Figure 118 was nulliparous, had a previous history of regular 28 day menstrual cycles and had suffered from dysmenorrhoea for many years. The study was conducted over a period of time equivalent to three cycles, during the second of which norethisterone was administered orally from days 5 to 29 at a dose level of 20 mg. per day. The first and third cycles were of a normal ovulatory character as judged by urinary steroid excretion. In the cycle during which treatment was given the pattern of steroid output was of the anovulatory type, this being indicated by the absence of a luteal phase rise in pregnanediol and pregnanetriol excretion and by the absence of midcycle and luteal phase peaks of oestrogen output. It is noteworthy that HPG excretion was maintained throughout the treatment period, the highest readings occurring earlier rather than later in the cycle.

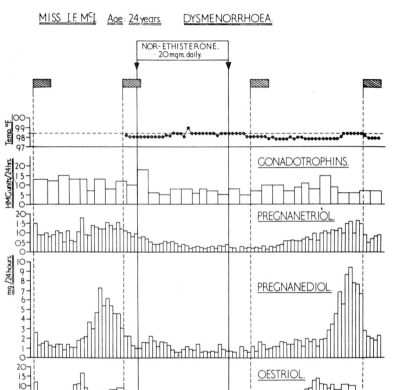

FIG. 118

Hormone excretion pattern in a subject with dysmenorrhoea treated with norethisterone.

//// = menstrual bleeding.

(From Brown *et al.*, 1962.)

The results obtained in a subject treated with norethisterone acetate are shown in Figure 119. This woman, who had a previous history of regular 28 day menstrual cycles with severe premenstrual and menstrual dysmenorrhoea, was studied throughout four cycles, during the second and third of which the compound was administered orally from day 5 to 25 at dose levels of 6 and 12 mg. per day respectively. The two cycles without treatment were of a normal ovulatory character. During the first treatment cycle there was a single oestriol and

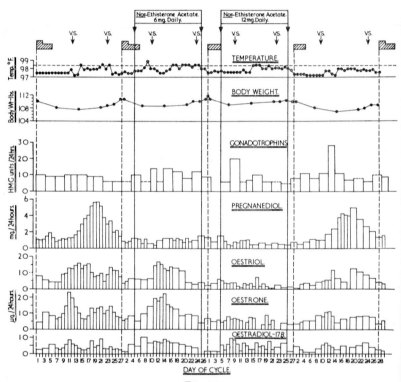

FIG. 119

Hormone excretion pattern in a subject with dysmenorrhoea treated with norethisterone acetate.

//// = menstrual bleeding ; V.S. = vaginal smear ; - - - indicates an HPG reading in which the result is less than the figure quoted.

(From Brown *et al.*, 1962.)

oestrone peak at approximately midcycle but no subsequent rise in oestrogens or pregnanediol ; these results were compatible with the view that luteal but not follicular function had been suppressed. On doubling the dose of norethisterone acetate during the second treatment cycle the output of oestriol, oestrone and pregnanediol remained uniformly low indicating suppression of both follicular and luteal activities. In spite of inhibition of ovulation during both treatment cycles HPG excretion showed little alteration, and the basal temperature record remained biphasic (see also p. 131).

Comment

It has already been emphasised that the bio-assay method for HPG used by Brown *et al.* (1962) and illustrated in Figures 118 and 119 was the mouse uterus test. As indicated in Chapter III this measures " total gonadotrophic activity " and is not specific for either FSH or LH. Since the study of Brown *et al.* (1962) short term effects of oral contraceptives on the differential excretion of FSH and LH have been reported by various investigators including Taymor (1964) and Stevens *et al.* (1965). Taymor (1964), who used the hypophysectomised rat prostate test to measure LH, demonstrated that when norethisterone acetate was administered to normally menstruating women, the midcycle peak of LH output was abolished. A similar result was obtained by Stevens *et al.* (1965) who used the OAAD method to estimate LH and who administered a progestogen–oestrogen mixture containing ethynodiol diacetate (SC. 11,800) and mestranol. Subsequently Vorys *et al.* (1965) reported the effects of a large number of compounds including oestrogens, progestogens and progestogen–oestrogen mixtures on the separate excretion of urinary FSH and LH, and on the basis of their findings drew a number of far-reaching conclusions regarding the differential effects of these substances or urinary gonadotrophin output. Unfortunately, in the study of Vorys *et al.* (1965) each compound was generally tested in one subject only, and because of this fact the conclusions drawn must be accepted with reserve.

(*b*) LONG TERM EFFECTS.—These have been investigated by Loraine *et al.* (1963, 1965), Shearman (1963, 1965), Flowers *et al.* (1966), Ryan *et al.* (1966) and Bell *et al.* (1967). Typical

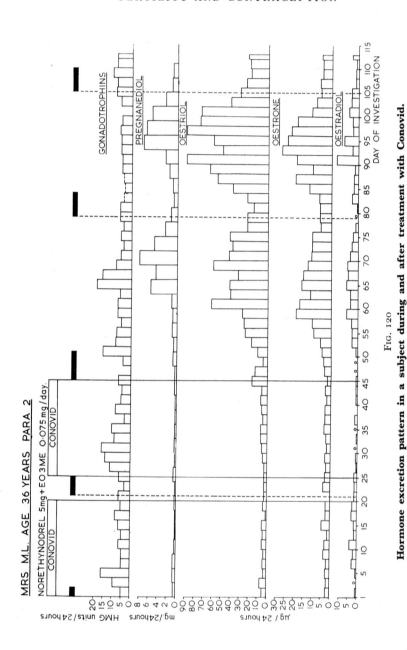

Fig. 120

Hormone excretion pattern in a subject during and after treatment with Conovid.
■ = menstrual bleeding ; - - - indicates an HPG reading in which the result is less than the figure quoted.
(From Loraine *et al.*, 1963.)

examples of the studies conducted by Loraine *et al.* (1963, 1965) in which assays of " total gonadotrophic activity ", oestrogens and pregnanediol were performed are shown in Figures 120 and 121.

Prior to the investigation the subject in Figure 120 had received treatment with Conovid for 57 cycles (44 calendar months). She was studied throughout the last two cycles on treatment and in two succeeding cycles following withdrawal of medication. In the treatment cycles excretion values for oestrogens and pregnanediol were low, indicating suppression of ovarian activity and ovulation. Throughout this period HPG activity was detected in all samples assayed, the readings being within the normal range for a woman during reproductive life. After withdrawal of medication there were two ovulatory cycles, the first from day 46 to 79, and the second from day 80 to 105 of the investigation. In both, peaks of oestrogen excretion at midcycle and in the luteal phase were well defined, with higher values in the second cycle during which oestriol readings in the ovulatory and luteal phases were above the range generally encountered in normally menstruating women. Most of the pregnanediol values were within normal limits, but the figures between days 94 and 96 were at the upper end of the normal range. HPG excretion values were similar to those observed during the periods of Conovid therapy.

In Figure 121 are shown the results in a woman who prior to the period of investigation, had been treated with Lyndiol for 20 calendar months. Assays were performed during the last two courses of treatment and in the first two cycles following cessation of therapy. It will be noted that the two treatment cycles were anovular as judged by the pattern of urinary steroid excretion ; nevertheless, HPG activity was present in the majority of samples tested, most of the readings being within the normal range for a woman during reproductive life. The two cycles immediately following medication were of a normal ovulatory character, showing midcycle and luteal phase peaks of oestrogen excretion together with a luteal phase rise in pregnanediol output, the latter being more marked in the second than in the first post-treatment cycle.

The studies illustrated in Figures 120 and 121 indicated that following long term therapy with oral contraceptives the cycles

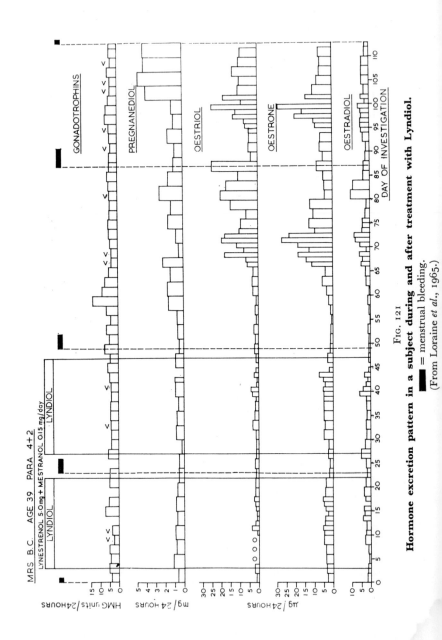

FIG. 121

Hormone excretion pattern in a subject during and after treatment with Lyndiol.

■ = menstrual bleeding.

(From Loraine *et al.*, 1965.)

rapidly reverted to an ovulatory pattern. They also demonstrated that such therapy produced little or no effect on " total gonadotrophic activity " as measured by the mouse uterus test. More recent studies by the Edinburgh group (see Bell *et al.*,

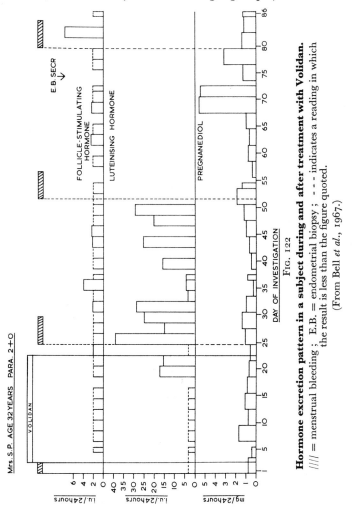

Hormone excretion pattern in a subject during and after treatment with Volidan.

//// = menstrual bleeding ; E.B. = endometrial biopsy ; - - - indicates a reading in which the result is less than the figure quoted.

(From Bell *et al.*, 1967.)

FIG. 122

1967) have concentrated on the long term effects of oral contraceptives on the differential excretion of FSH and LH, the former hormone being measured by the mouse ovarian augmentation test and the latter by the OAAD method.

Results obtained in two such investigations are illustrated in Figures 122 and 123.

The woman shown in Figure 122 was aged 32 years and previously had been treated with Volidan for 30 cycles. The last cycle on treatment was anovular in character as judged by urinary pregnanediol output. During this time FSH levels

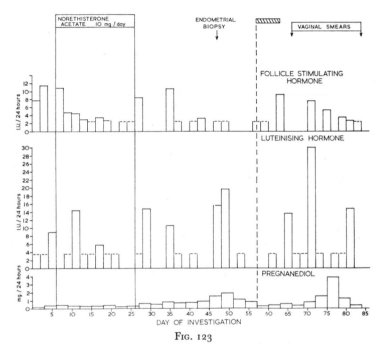

Mrs E.S.: AGE 41 YEARS: PARA 5 + 1

FIG. 123

Hormone excretion pattern in a subject during and after treatment with norethisterone acetate.

/// = menstrual bleeding ; - - - indicates a reading in which the result is less than the figure quoted.

(From Bell *et al.*, 1967.)

were undetectable and LH could be measured in the last two samples only. The first post-treatment cycle from days 25 to 51 of the study was also anovular on the basis of pregnanediol output. FSH activity at this time was either very low or unmeasurable ; on the other hand, LH activity was detectable throughout, readings being relatively high at the beginning and the end of the cycle, and low at midcycle. In the second post-treatment cycle which lasted for 28 days a marked increase in pregnanediol output on days 68 to 72 of the study indicated that ovulation had taken place. The occurrence of ovulation was further supported by the finding of a secretory endometrium when a biopsy was performed on the 74th day. During this cycle FSH levels were again either low or undetectable, while LH assays could not be conducted because of the toxicity of the urinary extracts to the experimental animals.

The results shown in Figure 123 were obtained in a 41 year old subject who had been treated with norethisterone acetate for 89 cycles (61 calendar months) prior to the commencement of the study. The first 26 days of the investigation included the last treatment period. During this time ovulation did not occur, pregnanediol levels remaining low and constant. FSH and LH activities were present in a proportion of the urine samples assayed. For the remaining 58 days of the investigation no medication was given, and two ovulatory menstrual cycles occurred on the basis of pregnanediol output; these lasted 31 and 27 days respectively. In both cycles FSH and LH could be detected in a proportion of the samples tested. In general, levels of these hormones were similar to those encountered in the last treatment cycle; the marked day-to-day fluctuations in LH excretion are noteworthy. The occurrence of ovulation in the first post-treatment cycle was further confirmed by the finding of a secretory endometrium when a biopsy was performed on the 48th day. The series of vaginal smears taken during the second post-treatment cycle gave results compatible with the presence of ovulation.

The data of Bell et al. (1967) indicate that the long term administration of oral contraceptives does not produce a consistent effect on FSH and LH excretion. Thus in Figure 122 the progestogen–oestrogen mixture Volidan abolished FSH activity from the urine, while in Figure 123 in which a progestogen alone was administered, FSH activity could be detected in the majority of samples assayed during the last treatment cycle. LH levels in the last treatment cycle of the subject receiving Volidan were low, while activity was detectable more frequently in the patient receiving the " pure " progestogen, northisterone acetate.

The long term effects of the progestogen–oestrogen mixture, Ovulen, on pituitary gonadotrophic function have been investigated by Flowers *et al.* (1966), and Figure 124 shows a composite pattern of the results reported by these workers in four patients. It will be noted that during treatment, levels of both hormones remained consistently low. Flowers *et al.* (1966) have also studied gonadotrophin output in cycles following cessation of medication. A consistent pattern of FSH and LH excretion was not observed, readings varying considerably from one subject to another.

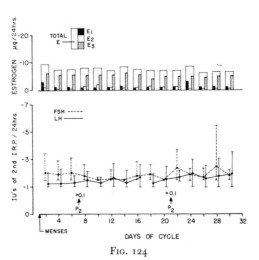

FIG. 124

Mean excretion of FSH, LH, oestrogens and pregnanediol (P) in four subjects receiving an oestrogen–progestogen mixture for periods of 12 to 27 months.

Vertical lines represent S.E.

(From Flowers *et al.*, 1966.)

(*c*) ATYPICAL HORMONE EXCRETION PATTERNS DURING LONG TERM THERAPY WITH ORAL CONTRACEPTIVES.—In this sub-section two patients are described. The first was a woman studied by Loraine *et al.* (1965) who showed the phenomenon of " breakthrough ovulation " i.e. ovulation occurring during treatment with anti-ovulatory compounds. The second was a subject investigated by Shearman (1963) in whom an abnormal pattern of oestrogen excretion during therapy was noted.

The woman in Figure 125 was aged 38 years and had had four children. Prior to the period of investigation she had been treated with norethisterone acetate for 67 cycles extending over a period of 44 calendar months. Steroid and gonadotrophin assays were performed during the last treatment cycle and in two cycles immediately following withdrawal of medication. The main point of note is the occurrence during the second half of the treatment cycle of a rise in pregnanediol output, indicating the presence of " breakthrough ovulation ". In the two cycles immediately following cessation of medication the luteal phase increases in pregnanediol output were more pronounced than in the treatment cycle. HPG activity, estimated by the mouse uterus test, was present in all samples assayed, the readings being within the normal range.

" Breakthrough ovulation " during therapy with oral contraceptives is a recognised although infrequent occurrence (see Mears 1965 a). The fact that the woman shown in Figure 125 did not become pregnant in spite of repeated sexual intercourse during the cycle in which "breakthrough ovulation" occurred confirms the belief that, in addition to affecting pituitary and ovarian function, oral contraceptives may produce effects at other sites e.g. at the level of the cervix or the uterus (see also p. 308).

In Figure 126 is shown Shearman's patient in whom an atypical pattern of oestrogen output was observed during the fifth month of treatment by Anovlar. It will be noted that oestrogen readings were high and showed considerable fluctuations, levels being maximal from days 9 to 15 of the investigation. The high oestrogen levels were associated with low and relatively constant pregnanediol values indicating that a functional corpus luteum had not been formed. After cessation of therapy bleeding occurred, and this was followed by a normal ovulatory cycle on the basis of urinary steroid output.

CONTRA-INDICATIONS TO THERAPY BY ORAL CONTRACEPTIVES

These have been discussed by Mears (1965 a), Swyer (1966) and others, and have been reviewed in the W.H.O. Technical Report (1966). The consensus of opinion is that

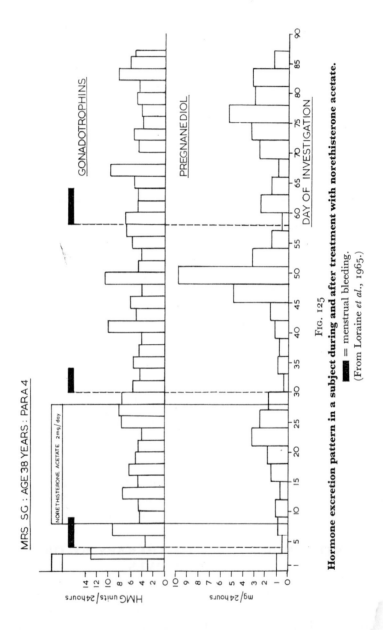

FIG. 125

Hormone excretion pattern in a subject during and after treatment with norethisterone acetate.

■ = menstrual bleeding.

(From Loraine *et al.*, 1965.)

there are few if any absolute contra-indications to the administration of oral contraceptives. It is recommended that such
compounds should not be given to women with acquired and
hereditary hepatic disease as typified by the syndromes of
Dubin-Johnson and Rotor. In addition, most clinicians would
be reluctant to prescribe this form of medication in subjects
suffering from mammary and genital carcinoma and in
women with a previous history of thromboembolic disease.

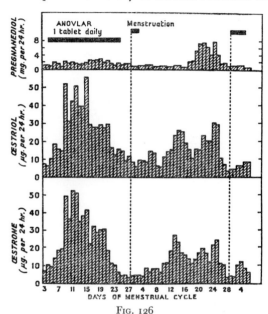

FIG. 126

Steroid excretion pattern in a subject receiving Anovlar.
(From Shearman, 1963.)

SEQUENTIAL THERAPY BY ORAL CONTRACEPTIVES

The sequential form of oral contraception involves the
administration of an oestrogen alone for the first part of the
treatment period (e.g. for 15 days), this being followed by combined therapy by an oestrogen and a progestogen generally for
five days. Such a regime would appear to have certain theo-
retical advantages over the administration of the "classical"
pill as it would more closely mimic the endocrine background

TABLE 26

TYPES OF SEQUENTIAL ORAL CONTRACEPTIVE CURRENTLY AVAILABLE

(After Mears, 1965 a)

Compounds	Composition of pill and dosage	Duration of treatment (days)	Trade name	Manufacturer
Megestrol acetate and ethinyl oestradiol	Ethinyl oestradiol 0·1 mg. Ethinyl oestradiol 0·1 mg. plus megestrol acetate 5·0 mg. Inert tablets	16 5 7	Ovisec (New Zealand)	British Drug Houses
Norethynodrel and mestranol	Mestranol 0·1 mg. Mestranol 0·1 mg. plus norethynodrel 5·0 mg.	15 5	Feminor	London Rubber Industries
Chlormadinone acetate and mestranol	Mestranol 0·08 mg. Mestranol 0·08 mg. plus chlormadinone acetate 2·0 mg.	15 5	Serventox (Mexico)	Syntex
	Mestranol 0·08 mg. Mestranol 0·08 mg. plus chlormadinone 2·0 mg.	15 5	Sequens	Eli Lilly
Dimethisterone and ethinyl oestradiol	Ethinyl oestradiol 0·1 mg. Ethinyl oestradiol 0·1 mg. plus dimethisterone 25 mg.	16 5	Ovin Oracon	Chas. Macdonald Mead Johnson

of the normal menstrual cycle. Various types of sequential regime have been proposed and these, together with some of the compounds in current use, are listed in Table 26. Investigators who have reported experience with the sequential form of oral contraceptive therapy include Greenblatt (1961), Aydar and Greenblatt (1961), Goldzieher (1964), Rice-Wray (1964), Liggins (1964), Board and Borland (1964), Mears (1965 *a b*) and Greenblatt *et al.* (1966).

The main aims of the present section are firstly to attempt to evaluate the effectiveness of the sequential form of treatment, secondly to discuss side effects associated with the use of the regime, and finally to describe the effects of sequential therapy on endometrial histology and endocrine function. At the time of writing possible harmful effects of the sequential regime have been investigated in much less detail than is the case for progestogen–oestrogen mixtures, and accordingly a section comparable to that on pages 269 to 279 is not included.

1. Effectiveness

There is still some divergence of opinion amongst clinicians regarding the relative merits of the sequential and " classical " forms of oral contraception. Maas (1966) believes that the former method " compares favourably " with the classical technique. Goldzieher (1964), using a sequential regime involving mestranol and chlormadinone, quoted a failure rate of 1·28 per 100 women years in a series of 25,000 cycles. Rice-Wray (1964), employing the same regime during 13,000 cycles, found no pregnancies in women who took the tablets regularly. On the other hand, Mears (1965 *a*) who studied a number of types of sequential therapy, reported a relatively high pregnancy rate of 5 per 100 women years, these being associated with failure to take the tablets.

It is now recognised that " breakthrough ovulation " occurs in a significant proportion of women receiving sequential therapy. The incidences quoted by Goldzieher (1964) and by Liggins (1964) were 2·2 and 9 per cent respectively ; the corresponding figure reported by Mears (1965 *a*) was 8 per cent. An example of the endocrine changes present when breakthrough ovulation occurs is shown in Figures 125 and 129 (see pp. 303 and 307).

2. Side Effects

Present evidence suggests that the incidence of side effects is lower with the sequential than with the " classical " regime of oral contraception (see Mears, 1965 *b* ; Maas, 1966). The most frequent symptom is again nausea which, according to Goldzieher *et al.* (1964), has an overall incidence of 2·5 per cent. Rare side effects include headache, premenstrual tension, breast tenderness and abdominal distension.

Mears (1965 *a*) has noted a higher incidence of amenorrhoea with the 15/5 than with 10/11 sequential regime. She also states that withdrawal bleedings tend to be heavier with sequential than with " classical " oral contraception. Maas (1966) and others have stressed that the overall incidence of " breakthrough bleeding " is much lower with sequential therapy than with progestogen–oestrogen mixtures.

3. Effect on the Endometrium

One of the earlier studies of the effects of sequentially administered oral contraceptives on the endometrium is that of Maqueo *et al.* (1964) who gave mestranol and chlormadinone on a 20/5 basis. They noted that when biopsies were taken during the period of mestranol administration, the pattern was proliferative in type and that within two days of commencing chlormadinone, secretory changes were observed. Towards the end of the treatment period the secretory changes in the endometrium were found to be less marked than at a comparable time during the normal ovulatory menstrual cycle, biopsies taken after day 26 being similar in their histological appearance to those of the 18th and 19th days of a normal cycle.

The effect of sequential therapy on the endometrium has also been investigated by Board and Borland (1966) who used a 14/6 regime involving mestranol and 3-deoxy-6α-methyl-17α-acetoxyprogesterone (DMAP). These workers demonstrated that the endometrial pattern produced resembled the menstrual cycle more closely than that found when the classical form of oral contraception was administered. A similar conclusion was drawn by Mears (1965 *b*) who used a 10/11 regime consisting of mestranol and chlormadinone.

Endometrial histology produced by a 15/5 sequential regime of mestranol and chlormadinone has been intensively studied by Mears (1965 *b*) and the patterns shown in Figures 127 and 128 are illustrative of her findings. The endometrium in Figure 127 was obtained on day 10 of the cycle after 5 days of mestranol therapy. The presence of a large number of glands will be noted ; mitoses are frequent and there is some stromal oedema. With the addition of the progestogen some secretory changes appear in the glands but a fully developed secretory pattern is not observed. This latter point is well illustrated in Figure 128 in which the endometrium was obtained on the 26th day of the cycle.

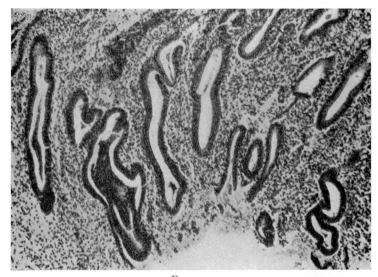

FIG. 127

Endometrial biopsy obtained on day 10 of the cycle in a subject receiving sequential therapy with mestranol and chlormadionone.

(From Mears, 1965 *b*.)

4. Effects on Endocrine Function

At the time of writing the literature contains little or no information on the manner in which the sequential form of contraception affects thyroid and adrenocortical function. Stevens (1967) has reported some preliminary data on the effect a sequential combination consisting of mestranol and Lormin on pituitary gonadotrophic activity. He found low levels of urinary FSH in the second half of the cycle, at which time excretion values for LH tended to rise.

In Figure 129 are shown urinary steroid excretion patterns in a subject studied by the Edinburgh group and receiving an 11/10 sequential regime consisting of mestranol and chlormadinone. The pretreatment cycle was of a typical ovulatory character ; it is of special interest that during treatment ovulation, as judged by pregnanediol assays, certainly occurred. Sexual intercourse took place during the treatment cycle but in spite of this the woman did not become pregnant, again suggesting that the contraceptive regime was producing its effect at sites other than the ovary and the pituitary.

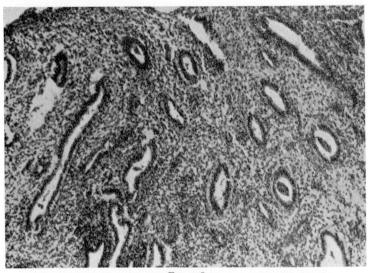

Fig. 128

Endometrial biopsy obtained on day 26 of the cycle in a subject receiving sequential therapy with mestranol and chlormadinone.

(From Mears, 1965 b.)

SITE OF ACTION OF ORAL CONTRACEPTIVES

The most detailed publications on the subject are probably those of Lunenfeld et al. (1963), Diczfalusy (1965), Mears (1965 a c) and Drill (1966). Diczfalusy (1965) has emphasised that oral contraceptives might produce their effects in a variety of ways. For example, they could render abnormal the character of the cervical mucus so that the latter became relatively " hostile " to penetration by spermatozoa. Again they might produce changes in tubal motility or cause alterations in the endometrium which could result in the failure of a fertilised ovum to implant. A direct effect on the ovary, rendering this organ insensitive to stimulation by endogenously

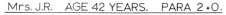

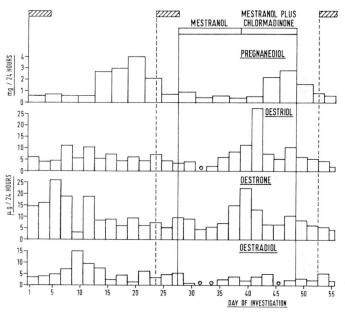

Fig. 129

Steroid excretion pattern in a subject receiving mestranol and chlormadinone.

//// = menstrual bleeding.

produced gonadotrophins is another possibility as is a direct inhibitory effect on the secretion of gonadotrophins by the anterior pituitary. Yet another site of action might be at a relatively high level influencing the secretion of gonadotrophin-releasing factors from the hypothalamus, and it is even possible that the compounds act on the central nervous system itself. Previous sections of this chapter have dealt with the action of oral contraceptives on the differential excretion of FSH and LH, and the ensuing discussion will be mainly concerned with effects of these compounds on cervical mucus and on the response of the ovaries to stimulation with exogenously administered gonadotrophins.

One of the most detailed studies of the action of oral contraceptives on cervical mucus is that of Zañartu (1964). This investigator administered a variety of progestogen–oestrogen mixtures to a series of 70 young women of proven high fertility, and performed Sims-Hubner tests for sperm penetration from 2 to 12 hours after coitus. He observed that as a result of such treatment the cervical mucus rapidly became progestational in character (see p. 116) and because of its increased viscosity became more hostile to sperm penetration. Ferin (1964) conducted post-coital tests in 13 women receiving the progestogen–oestrogen mixture, Lyndiol. He also noted the absence of ovulatory mucus, and demonstrated that as a result of therapy hostility to spermatozoa was greatly increased.

There is at present controversy in the literature regarding the manner by which oral contraceptives affect the response of the ovaries to stimulation by exogenously administered gonadotrophins. Lunenfeld and his collaborators (Lunenfeld, 1964 ; Lunenfeld et al., 1963) based their evidence on urinary steroid assays. They found that in patients in whom ovulation had been induced by therapy with Pergonal and HCG, the administration of a progestogen–oestrogen mixture, containing 6α-methyl-17α-acetoxy-progesterone and ethinyl oestradiol, inhibited this phenomenon. Their conclusion was that the main site of action of the oral contraceptive was a direct one on the ovaries. On the other hand, Johannisson et al. (1965), who studied a number of progestogen–oestrogen mixtures, failed to abolish the ovarian response to exogenously administered gonadotrophins and concluded that the main site of action was at the pituitary rather than the ovarian level.

Comment

At the time of writing the balance of evidence would favour the view that the major site of action of oral contraceptives is at the pituitary level and that the main effect produced is an inhibition of LH secretion. However, it is likely that, in addition, such compounds may act directly on the ovaries and on the cervical mucus. The data currently available favour the view that factors such as the composition of the tablet and the duration of therapy are likely to be of importance as far as the site and mode of action of oral contraceptives are concerned.

RECENT DEVELOPMENTS IN ORAL CONTRACEPTION

1. Low Dosage Oral Progestogens

Such compounds have been administered by Rudel *et al.* (1965) and by Martinez-Manautou *et al.* (1966). The latter group of authors administered chlormadinone acetate at a dose level of 0·5 mg. per day either from day 5 to 24 of the cycle or continuously ; some 1,600 cycles in 415 women were studied. They noted that ovulation, judged by urinary pregnanediol excretion, endometrial biopsies and the findings on culdoscopy, took place in a relatively high proportion of their subjects (approximately 60 per cent). In spite of the occurrence of ovulation this form of contraception was found to be highly effective, there being only one failure among the patients who took all the tablets.

Reliable information regarding the mode of action of low dosage progestogens is not at present available. Mears (1965 *a*) has suggested a direct effect on the cervical mucus or an action of the endometrium making it impossible for the fertilised ovum to implant. Her interesting suggestions require further study.

2. Injectable Contraceptives

These have been investigated by Felton *et al.* (1965) who administered the progestogen–oestrogen mixture, Deladroxate (16α-dihydroxy-progesterone acetophenide), together with oestradiol oenanthate intramuscularly once per month. No pregnancies occurred in a series of 590 cycles in 127 women. The major disadvantage of this form of medication is its tendency to produce cycles of variable length. The treatment has been recommended by Felton *et al.* (1965) for women in whom regular pill-taking is difficult or impossible, and it is possible that this form of contraception may be especially useful in patients with psychiatric disorders.

3. " Once-a-Month Pill "

Suggestions have been made that it might be feasible to develop a tablet which could be taken once per month instead of regularly throughout the cycle. A preliminary report of such a form of contraception has recently been published by Greenblatt (1967).

4. Encapsulated Steroids

Another possibility that has been suggested is the use of encapsulated steroids similar to those which have been used by Segal of New York City in animals (see Kleinman, 1967). In his animal experiments Segal found that the active material from such a capsule was absorbed very slowly, and that the contraceptive effect was of long duration. If this type of contraception could be made available for human use it might prove popular in women who desire protection from child-bearing for long periods of their reproductive life.

5. Post-Coital and Post-Ovulatory Pills

Pills of this type could be taken after intercourse or following ovulation ; they would presumably inhibit implantation of the fertilised ovum and might have a wide sphere of applicability. At the time of writing research in this field remains at a very preliminary stage.

SUMMARY AND CONCLUSIONS

A great variety of oral contraceptives are now available for clinical use. The majority of these are progestogen–oestrogen mixtures which are generally given from the fifth day of the cycle for 20 days. This constitutes the " classical " form of oral contraception.

If the tablets are taken in the manner prescribed the " classical " form of oral contraception is virtually 100 per cent effective.

The main side effects associated with the administration of oral contraceptives are nausea, weight gain and alterations in the menstrual pattern, with special reference to " breakthrough bleeding ".

Possible harmful effects of oral contraceptives are reviewed including relationships to subsequent fertility, postponement of the menopause, biochemical abnormalities and the occurrence of thromboembolic and neoplastic disease. It is concluded that there is little or no evidence suggesting that the administration of these compounds produces any lasting deleterious effects.

No major changes in thyroid or adrenocortical function result from therapy with oral contraceptives.

When administered on a short-term basis progestogen–oestrogen mixtures produce anovulatory cycles as judged by urinary steroid excretion and obliterate the midcycle peak of LH output. Their effects on urinary FSH levels are variable.

Following withdrawal of oral contraception after long-term medication, cycles rapidly revert to an ovulatory pattern. In a small proportion of women receiving long-term treatment " breakthrough ovulation " occurs. Long-term effects of oral contraceptives on urinary FSH and LH output are variable.

The sequential form of oral contraception is probably somewhat less effective than the " classical" regime, but is associated with a lower incidence of side effects.

The consensus of opinion at present is that the main site of action of oral contraceptives is at the pituitary level, causing an inhibition of LH secretion. It is, however, probable that the compounds have alternative sites of action, especially at the ovarian level and on the cervical mucus.

Important future developments in the field of oral contraception will be the introduction of encapsulated steroids for long-term use and the manufacture of the post-coital pill.

REFERENCES

ADAMS, M. J. T. & SPICER, C. C. (1965). *Lancet*, **ii,** 732.
ALLEN, W. M. & WINTERSTEINER, O. (1934). *Science*, **80,** 190.
ASTWOOD, E. B. & FEVOLD, H. L. (1939). *Am. J. Physiol.* **127,** 192.
AYDAR, C. K. & GREENBLATT, R. B. (1961). *J. Med. Assoc. Alabama*, **31,** 53.
BAKKE, J. L. (1965). *Brit. Med. J.* **i,** 631.
BEARD, J. (1897). Cited by Asdell, S. A. (1928). *Physiol. Rev.* **8,** 325.
BELL, E. T., HERBST, A. L., KRISHNAMURTI, M., LORAINE, J. A., MEARS, E., JACKSON, M. C. N. & GARCIA, C-R. (1967). *Acta Endocrinol.* **54,** 96.
BESCH, P. K., VORYS, N., ULLERY, J. C., STEVENS, V. C. & BARRY, R. D. (1965). *Metabolism*, **14,** 387.
BISHOP, P. M. F. (1960). *Clin. Obstet. Gynecol.* **3,** 1109.
BOARD, J. A. & BORLAND, D. S. (1964). *Obstet. Gynecol.* **24,** 655.
BOARD, J. A. & BORLAND, D. S. (1966). *Fertility Sterility*, **17,** 234.
BRAKMAN, P. & ASTRUP, T. (1964). *Lancet*, **ii,** 10.
BREUER, H., DARDENNE, U. & NOCKE, W. (1960). *Acta Endocrinol*, **33,** 10.
BROWN, J. B. & BLAIR, H. A. F. (1960). *Proc. Roy. Soc. Med.* **53,** 433.

BROWN, J. B., FOTHERBY, K. & LORAINE, J. A. (1962). *J. Endocrinol.* **25,** 331.
BUCHHOLZ, R., NOCKE, L. & NOCKE, W. (1964). *Intern. J. Fertility*, **9,** 231.
BULBROOK, R. D. (1965). *Vitamins Hormones*, **23,** 329.
BUTENANDT, A., WESTPHAL, U. & HOHLWEG, W. (1934). *Hoppe-Seylers. Z. Physiol. Chem.* **227,** 84.
CHINNATAMBY, S. (1963). Quoted by Mears, E. (1965). *Handbook on Oral Contraception.* London : Churchill.
COOK, H. H., GAMBLE, C. J. & SATTERTHWAITE, A. P. (1961). *Am. J. Obstet. Gynecol.* **82,** 437.
DICZFALUSY, E. (1965). *Brit. Med. J.* **2,** 1394.
DJERASSI, C. (1966). *Science*, **151,** 1055.
DJERASSI, C., MIRAMONTES, L., ROSENKRANZ, G. & SONDHEIMER, F. (1954). *J. Am. Chem. Soc.* **76,** 4092.
DRILL, V. A. (1965). *Metabolism*, **14,** 295.
DRILL, V. A. (1966). *Oral Contraceptives.* New York : McGraw-Hill.
EGEBERG, O. & OWREN, P. A. (1963). *Brit. Med. J.* **1,** 220.
EISALO, A., JÄRVINEN, P. A. & LUUKKAINEN, T. (1964). *Brit. Med. J.* **2,** 426.
ENGEL, L. L., ALEXANDER, J. & WHEELER, M. (1958). *J. Biol. Chem.* **231,** 159.
FELTON, H. T., HOELSCHER, E. W. & SWARTZ, D. P. (1965). *Fertility Sterility*, **16,** 665.
FERIN, J. (1964). *Intern. J. Fertil.* **9,** 29.
FERIN, J., CHARLES, J., ROMMELART, G. & BEUSELINCK, A. (1964). *Intern. J. Fertil.* **9,** 41.
FLORSHEIM, W. H. & FAIRCLOTH, M. A. (1964). *Proc. Soc. Exp. Biol. Med.* **117,** 56.
FLOWERS, C. E., VORYS, N., STEVENS, V. C., MILLER, A. T. & JENSEN, L. (1966). *Am. J. Obstet. Gynecol.* **96,** 784.
FUCHS, A-R., FUCHS, F. & JOHNSEN, S. G. (1964). *Intern. J. Fertil.* **9,** 139.
GARCIA, C-R. & PINCUS, G. (1965). *Intern. J. Fertil.* **9,** 95.
GERSHBERG, H., JAVIER, Z. C. & HULSE, M. (1964). *Diabetes*, **13,** 378.
GOETZ, F. C., GREENBERG, B. Z., ELLS, J. & MEINERT, C. (1963). *J. Clin. Endocrinol. Metab.* **23,** 1237.
GOLDZIEHER, J. W. (1964). *Med. Clin. N. Am.* **48,** 529.
GOLDZIEHER, J. W., MOSES, L. E. & ELLIS, L. T. (1962). *J. Am. Med. Assoc.* **180,** 359.
GOLDZIEHER, J. W., BECERRA, C., GUAL, C., LIVINGSTON, N. B. Jr., MAQUEO, M., MOSES, L. E. & TIETZE, C. (1964). *Am. J. Obstet. Gynecol.* **90,** 404.
GOOLDEN, A. W. G., GARTSIDE, J. M. & SANDERSON, C. (1967). *Lancet*, **i,** 12.
GREENBLATT, R. B. (1961). *Med. Clin. N. Am.* **45,** 973.
GREENBLATT, R. B. (1967). *Fertility Sterility*, **18,** 207.
GREENBLATT, R. B., ZARATE, A. & JUNGCK, E. C. (1966). In *Ovulation*, p. 216. Ed. Greenblatt, R. B. Philadelphia : Lippincott.
HABERLANDT, L. (1921). *München Med. Wochschr.* **68,** 1577.
HARTMANN, M. & WETTSTEIN, A. (1934). *Helv. Chim. Acta.* **17,** 1365.
HOLLANDER, C. S., GARCIA, A. M., STURGIS, S. H. & SELENKOW, H. A. (1963). *New Engl. J. Med.* **269,** 501.
HUTCHERSON, W. P., SCHWARTZ, H. A. & WEATHERS, W. Jr. (1966). *Fertility Sterility*, **17,** 59.
JACKSON, M. C. N. (1963). *J. Reprod. Fertil.* **6,** 153.
JACOBSON, B. D. (1962). *Am. J. Obstet. Gynecol.* **84,** 962.
JAVIER, Z. C., HULSE, M. & GERSHBERG, H. (1965). *Diabetes*, **14,** 458.
JENNETT, W. B. & CROSS, J. N. (1967). *Lancet*, **i,** 1019.
JOHANNISSON, E., TILLINGER, K-G. & DICZFALUSY, E. (1965). *Fertility Sterility*, **16,** 292.
KINCL, F. A. & DORFMAN, R. I. (1963 a). *Acta Endocrinol. Suppl.* **73,** 3.
KINCL, F. A. & DORFMAN, R. I. (1963 b). *Acta Endocrinol. Suppl.* **73,** 17.
KLEINMAN, R. L. (1964). *Medical Handbook on Contraception.* London : International Planned Parenthood Federation.
KLEINMAN, R. L. (1967). *I.P.P.F. Med. Bull.* **1,** No. 2.
KOPERA, H., DUKES, M. N. G. & IJZERMAN, G. L. (1964). *Intern. J. Fertility*, **9,** 69.
LAYNE, D. S., MEYER, C. J., VAISHWANAR, P. S. & PINCUS, G. (1962). *J. Clin. Endocrinol. Metab.* **22,** 107.

312

LEACH, R. B. & MARGULIS, R. R. (1965). *Am. J. Obstet. Gynecol.* **92**, 762.
LIGGINS, G. C. (1964). Quoted by Mears, E. (1965). *Handbook on Oral Contraception.* London : Churchill.
LORAINE, J. A. (1959). In *Cancer*, vol. 6, p. 160. London : Butterworth.
LORAINE, J. A. & BELL, E. T. (1966). *Hormone Assays and their Clinical Application.* Second Ed. Edinburgh : Livingstone.
LORAINE, J. A., BELL, E. T., HARKNESS, R. A., MEARS, E. & JACKSON, M. C. N. (1963). *Lancet*, **ii**, 902.
LORAINE, J. A., BELL, E. T., HARKNESS, R. A., MEARS, E. & JACKSON, M. C. N. (1965). *Acta Endocrinol.* **50**, 15.
LUNENFELD, B. (1964). *Intern. J. Fertil.* **9**, 167.
LUNENFELD, B., SULIMOVICI, S. & RABAU, E. (1963). *J. Clin. Endocrinol. Metab.* **23**, 391.
MAAS, J. M. (1966). In *Ovulation*, p. 206. Ed. Greenblatt, R. B. Philadelphia : Lippincott.
MAKEPEACE, A. W., WEINSTEIN, G. L. & FRIEDMAN, M. H. (1937). *Am. J. Physiol.* **119**, 512.
MAQUEO, M., PEREZ-VEGA, E., GOLDZIEHER, J. W., MARTINEZ-MANAUTOU, J. & RUDEL, H. (1963). *Am. J. Obstet. Gynecol.* **85**, 427.
MAQUEO, M., BECERRA, C., MUNGUIA, H. & GOLDZIEHER, J. W. (1964). *Am. J. Obstet. Gynecol.* **90**, 395.
MARTINEZ-MANAUTOU, J., CORTEZ, V., GINER, J., AZNAR, R., CASASOLA, J. & RUDEL, H. W. (1966). *Fertility Sterility*, **17**, 49.
MEARS, E. (1965 *a*). *Handbook on Oral Contraception.* London : Churchill.
MEARS, E. (1965 *b*). In *Biological Council Symposium on Agents Affecting Fertility*, p. 211. Eds. Austin, C. R. and Perry, J. S. London : Churchill.
MEARS, E. (1965 *c*). *Eugenics Rev.* **56**, 195.
MEDICAL RESEARCH COUNCIL (1967). *Brit. Med. J.* **2**, 355.
METCALF, M. G. & BEAVEN, D. W. (1963). *Lancet*, **ii**, 1095.
MEYER, C. J., LAYNE, D. S., TAIT, J. F. & PINCUS, G. (1961). *J. Clin. Invest.* **40**, 163.
MOYER, D. L., TYLER, E. T., OLSON, H. J. & ZELDIS, J. (1964). *Fertility Sterility*, **15**, 164.
ØSTERGAARD, E., ARENDS, J., HAMBURGER, C. & JOHNSEN, S. G. (1966). *Acta Endocrinol.* **53**, 13.
PARKES, A. S. (1929). *The Internal Secretions of the Ovary.* London : Longmans Green.
PALVA, I. P. & MUSTALA, O. O. (1964). *Brit. Med. J.* **2**, 688.
PEARL, R. & SURFACE, F. M. (1914). *J. Biol. Chem.* **19**, 263.
PHILLIPS, L. L., TURKSOY, R. N. & SOUTHAM, A. L. (1961). *Am. J. Obstet. Gynecol.* **82**, 1216.
PILGERAM, L. O., AMUNDSON, B. A. & LOFGREN, P. E. (1964). *Thromb. Diath. Haemorrhag.* **11**, 94.
PINCUS, G. (1961). In *Modern Trends in Endocrinology*, Second Series, p. 231. Eds. Gardiner-Hill, H. London : Butterworth.
PINCUS, G. (1965). *The Control of Fertility.* New York : Academic Press.
PINCUS, G. (1966). In *Ovulation*, p. 200. Ed. Greenblatt, R. B. Philadelphia : Lippincott.
PINCUS, G. & CHANG, M. C. (1953). *Acta Physiol. Latinoam.* **3**, 177.
PINCUS, G. & GARCIA, C-R. (1965). In *Recent Advances in Ovarian and Synthetic Steroids*, p. 104. Ed. Shearman, R. P. Sydney : Globe Commercial.
PINCUS, G. & MERRILL, A. P. (1961). In *Control of Ovulation*, p. 37. Ed. Villee, C. W. New York : Pergamon Press.
PINCUS, G., CHANG, M. C., ZARROW, M. X., HAFEZ, E. S. E. & MERRILL, A. P. (1956). *Endocrinology*, **59**, 695.
PINCUS, G., GARCIA, C-R., ROCK, J., PANIAGUA, M., PENDLETON, A., LARAQUE, F., NICOLAS, R., BORNO, R. & PEAN, V. (1959). *Science*, **130**, 81.
RICE-WRAY, E. (1964). Quoted by Mears, E. (1965). *Handbook on Oral Contraception.* London : Churchill.
RICE-WRAY, E., ARANDA-ROSELL, A., MAQUEO, M. & GOLDZIEHER, J. W. (1963 *a*). *Am. J. Obstet. Gynecol.* **87**, 429.

RICE-WRAY, E., GOLDZIEHER, J. W. & ARANDA-ROSELL, A. (1963 *b*). *Fertility Sterility*, **14,** 402.

RICE-WRAY, E., SCHULZ-CONTRERAS, M., GUERRERO, I. & ARANDA-ROSELL, A. (1962). *J. Am. Med. Assoc.* **180,** 355.

ROBERTSON, G. S. (1967). *Lancet*, **i,** 232.

ROMAN, W. & BOCKNER, V. (1963). Quoted by Mears, E. (1965). *Handbook on Oral Contraception.* London : Churchill.

RUDEL, H. W., MARTINEZ-MANAUTOU, J. & MAQUEO-TOPETE, M. (1965). *Fertility Sterility*, **16,** 158.

RYAN, G. M., Jr., GOSS, D. A. & REID, D. E. (1966). *Am. J. Obstet. Gynecol.* **94,** 515.

SATTERTHWAITE, A. P. (1964). Quoted by Mears, E. (1965). *Handbook on Oral Contraception.* London : Churchill.

SATTERTHWAITE, A. P. & GAMBLE, C. J. (1962). *J. Am. Med. Women's Assoc.* **17,** 797.

SHEARMAN, R. P. (1963). *Lancet*, **i,** 197.

SHEARMAN, R. P. (1964). *Lancet*, **ii,** 557.

SHEARMAN, R. P. (1965). In *Recent Advances in Ovarian and Synthetic Steroids*, p. 26. Ed. Shearman, R. P. Sydney : Globe Commercial.

SLOTTA, K. H., ROSCHIG, H. & FELS, E. (1934). *Ber. Dtsch. Chem. Ges.* **67** (b), 1270.

SMITH, G. V. (1929). *Ann. Rept. Free Hospital Women*, **54,** 39.

SOBRERO, A. J., FENICHEL, R. L. & SINGHER, H. O. (1963). *J. Am. Med. Assoc.* **185,** 136.

SPELLACY, W. N. & CARLSON, K. L. (1966). *Am. J. Obstet. Gynecol.* **95,** 474.

STARUP, J., SELE, V. & BUUS, O. (1966). *Acta Endocrinol.* **53,** 1.

STEVENS, V. C. (1967). In *Recent Research on Gonadotrophic Hormones*, p. 246. Eds. Bell, E. T. and Loraine, J. A. Edinburgh : Livingstone.

STEVENS, V. C. & VORYS, N. (1965). In *Recent Advances in Ovarian and Synthetic Steroids*, p. 49. Ed. Shearman, R. P. Sydney : Globe Commercial.

STEVENS, V. C. & VORYS, N. (1967). *Obstet. Gynec. Surv.* **22,** 781.

STEVENS, V. C., VORYS, N., BESCH, P. K. & BARRY, R. D. (1965). *Metabolism*, **14,** 327.

STRONG, J. A. (1958). In *Endocrine Aspects of Breast Cancer*, p. 141. Eds. Currie, A. R. and Illingworth, C. F. W. Edinburgh : Livingstone.

SWYER, G. I. M. (1966). In *Current Medicine and Drugs.* London : Butterworth.

TAYMOR, M. L. (1964). *J. Clin. Endocrinol. Metab.* **24,** 803.

THOMSON, J. M. & POLLER, L. (1965). *Brit. Med. J.* **2,** 270.

TURKSOY, R. N., PHILLIPS, L. L. & SOUTHAM, A. L. (1961). *Am. J. Obstet. Gynecol.* **81,** 1211.

TYLER, E. T. (1961). *J. Am. Med. Assoc.* **175,** 225.

TYLER, E. T., OLSON, H. J., GOTLIB, M., LEVIN, M. & BEHME, D. (1964). *Clin. Med.* **71,** 997.

VENNING, G. R. (1963). In *Proc. Symposium Oral Contraception*, p. 43. G. D. Searle and Co.

VORYS, N., ULLERY, J. C. & STEVENS, V. C. (1965). *Am. J. Obstet. Gynecol.* **93,** 641.

WAINE, H., FRIEDEN, E. H., CAPLAN, H. I. & COLE, T. (1963). *Arthritis Rheumat.* **6,** 796.

WALLACH, E. E., GARCIA, C-R., KISTNER, R. W. & PINCUS, G. (1963). *Am. J. Obstet. Gynecol.* **87,** 991.

WHEELER, H. O., MELTZER, J. & BRADLEY, S. E. (1960). *J. Clin. Invest.* **39,** 1131.

WILSON, R. A. (1962). *J. Am. Med. Assoc.* **182,** 327.

World Health Organisation Technical Report Series No. 326 (1966).

ZAÑARTU, J. (1964). *Intern. J. Fertil.* **9,** 225.

ZSCHOKKE, E. (1898). *Landwirtsch. Jahrb. Schweiz.* **4,** 252.

CHAPTER X

Contraception by the Intra-Uterine Device

INTRODUCTION

HISTORICAL aspects of intra-uterine contraception have been reviewed by many authors including Southam (1965), Tietze (1965), Guttmacher (1965), Jackson (1965) and Borell (1966). There can be no doubt that this form of contraception was practised many centuries ago, possibly even before the dawn of the Christian era. It is of interest to recall that one of the earliest applications of the technique was to prevent excessive fertility in camels, and it is well documented that Arabian and Turkish camel drivers were in the habit of inserting a round stone into the uterus of their animals prior to long journeys through the desert. During the 19th century intra-uterine devices (IUD's) were used on a limited scale, in the early part of the century for the treatment of uterine displacement and for menstrual abnormalities, and subsequently for contraceptive purposes (see Hartwig, 1874 ; Rothacker, 1883). The 1920's and early 1930's saw a revival of interest in contraception by means of the IUD. Pust (1923) developed a ring-shaped pessary made of loops of silk-worm gut and incorporating a tailed cervical extension connected to a glass button which covered the external os. Experience with Pust's device was reported by various clinicians including Ohnesorge (1927), Strassman (1928) and Küstner (1931). However, the technique of contraception did not win favour because of the relatively high incidence of pelvic inflammatory disease in women in whom the device had been inserted.

In 1929 the German gynaecologist Gräfenberg (1929 *a b*) introduced a new type of device which could be placed completely in the uterus. This was in the form of a ring made originally of silk-worm gut and later of coiled silver or gold wire. In 1934 Ota in Japan described a modification of the Gräfenberg ring ; this was a coil with a small, hollow capsule suspended from three radial springs. Following their introduction into clinical practice neither the Gräfenberg nor the Ota ring found general acceptance because it was supposed that their insertion was associated with a relatively high incidence of pelvic inflammatory disease. Due to their rejection by the majority of clinicians there was a decrease in interest in intra-uterine contraception, and from the early 1930's until the late 1950's few papers on this subject appeared in the literature.

The modern era of intra-uterine contraception can be said to have begun in 1959 with the publications of Oppenheimer in Israel and Ishihama in Japan. Oppenheimer (1959), using a modification of the original Gräfenberg ring, reported results in a series of 329 women who were equipped with a total of 866 rings. In his experience the method proved both safe and reliable, and in particular, pelvic inflammatory disease was not encountered ; the failure rate (pregnancy rate) was low, amounting to 2·5 per 100 women years (see p. 265). The experience of Ishihama (1959), using the IUD introduced by Ota (1934), was similar in all respects to that of Oppenheimer. The work of Oppenheimer and Ishihama caused a great resurgence of interest in the IUD as a method of contraception, with the result that the literature on this subject in the past eight years has become very extensive.

This chapter deals exclusively with the newer devices which have been introduced in the 1960's. Most of these are made of the plastic material, polyethylene, and unlike the Gräfenberg silver ring which had to be removed periodically, they can remain in the uterus almost indefinitely. After a description of the devices themselves consideration is given to their efficacy, to complications associated with their use and finally to their possible mechanisms of action. For further details on some of the topics discussed herein articles by Tietze (1965), Kleinman (1966) and others along with the W. H. O. Technical Report (1966) should be consulted.

TYPES OF INTRA-UTERINE DEVICE

The following devices which are illustrated in Figure 130 will be considered :

1. The Margulies spiral.
2. The Lippes loop.
3. The Birnberg bow.
4. The Hall-Stone ring.
5. The Zipper nylon ring.

1. The Margulies Spiral

This was introduced into clinical practice in 1960, and came into relatively wide use during 1961. It is made of

317

polyethylene plastic and is equipped with a tail. Experience with the Margulies spiral has been described by its originator (Margulies, 1962, 1964) and by others.

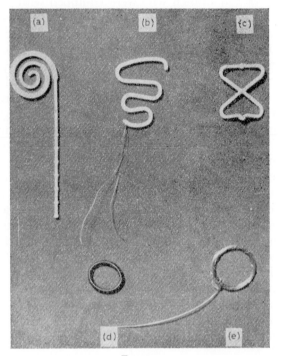

FIG. 130

Various types of IUD (a) Margulies spiral (b) Lippes loop (c) Birnberg bow (d) Hall-Stone ring (e) Zipper nylon ring : all three-quarters actual size.

(From Guttmacher, 1965.)

2. The Lippes Loop

This is also a plastic device which is made in at least four sizes ; like the spiral, it is equipped with a tail. It became available in the early part of 1961 and has been more extensively used than any other device (see Table 27). At the time of writing the model of choice in this category is the Lippes loop D (see also Lippes, 1962, 1965).

TABLE 27

NUMBER OF INSERTIONS AND DURATION OF USE OF VARIOUS INTRA-UTERINE DEVICES

(After Tietze, 1966)

Type of device	Number of insertions	Months of use
Lippes loop A	1,073	19,935
Lippes loop B	350	4,456
Lippes loop C	2,882	29,334
Lippes loop D	7,399	105,186
Margulies spiral-small	480	6,966
Margulies spiral-large	2,535	36,146
Birnberg bow-small	1,732	21,111
Birnberg bow-large	2,557	33,211
Hall-Stone steel ring	1,851	31,447
Other devices	1,544	19,639
Total	22,403	307,441

3. The Birnberg Bow

Like the spiral and the loop the bow is made of polyethylene plastic. It consists of two triangles joined at the top. Nine sizes of the bow have been described (see Birnberg and Burnhill, 1964 ; Burnhill and Birnberg, 1965). Those in current use are No. 5 (large) and No. 3 (small).

4. The Hall-Stone Ring

This consists of a coiled ring made of steel wire. It is available only in a single size, which is approximately that of a sixpence. Experience with the Hall-Stone ring has been described by its originators (H. H. Hall and Stone, 1962) and by H. H. Hall et al. (1964).

5. The Zipper Nylon Ring

This closely resembles the old Gräfenberg ring, but is made from nylon fishing line instead of silk-worm gut. Zipper et al. (1965) have discussed its value in clinical practice.

6. General Considerations Regarding Intra-Uterine Devices

As mentioned previously the spiral and the loop are equipped with an appendage or tail which passes through the cervical canal into the vagina. This facilitates easy removal and enables the patient to determine whether or not the device remains in place. The steel ring and most models of the bow do not possess tails and must be removed from the uterus by a hook similar to that used for the original Gräfenberg ring. From early 1966 onwards the bow has been equipped with a tail, but as yet, extensive clinical experience with this form of IUD has not been reported.

Since the spiral, loop and bow are made from polyethylene plastic to which a barium salt has been added, they are radio-opaque ; accordingly, their presence can be detected on X-ray examination. All three devices can be stretched into a linear form and threaded into a tephlon tube. The latter is passed through the cervical canal, just beyond the internal os ; then the plunger is inserted and the device is forced into the uterine cavity. When *in situ* in the uterus the device reshapes itself into its original form.

The time of insertion of the IUD is of considerable importance, and it is now generally agreed that in women with regular menstrual cycles the optimal time is at or just before the end of a period. This ensures that the device is not inserted in a subject who is already pregnant. Following delivery, the optimal time for insertion is approximately six weeks after parturition ; after an abortion, a similar time should be allowed to elapse . In the case of a Caesarean section a delay of eight weeks is generally recommended (see also Kleinman, 1966 ; W. H. O. Technical Report, 1966).

EFFECTIVENESS OF INTRA-UTERINE DEVICES

This has been studied by numerous investigators, including H. H. Hall and Stone (1962), Fuchs *et al.* (1964), H. H. Hall *et al.* (1964), Margulies (1964), Lay (1965), Lippes (1965), Willson *et al.* (1965 a), Lehfeldt *et al.* (1965), Lee and Wei (1965), Malkani *et al.* (1965), Shin (1965), R. E. Hall (1965, 1966), Satterthwaite *et al.* (1965), Nash (1965), Brooks and

Horne (1966), H. H. Hall (1966), Blott and Radcliffe (1966), Johnson *et al.* (1966), Israel and Davis (1966) and Haller *et al.* (1966). The most comprehensive reviews currently available in the literature are those of Guttmacher (1965), Tietze (1965, 1966), Tietze and Lewit (1965) and Borell (1966).

Tietze (1966) has reviewed the experience of a large number of investigators who have inserted various types of IUD. His composite data are presented in Table 27 from which it will be noted that the device most widely used in clinical practice to date has been the Lippes Loop D.

TABLE 28

PREGNANCY RATE AND NUMBER OF EXPULSIONS PER 100 FIRST INSERTIONS DURING THE FIRST YEAR OF USE

(After Tietze, 1966)

Type of device	Pregnancy rate	Number of first expulsions
Lippes loop A	4·9	19·7
Lippes loop B	3·8	15·2
Lippes loop C	2·5	14·0
Lippes loop D	2·8	10·4
Margulies spiral-small	3·4	30·1
Margulies spiral-large	1·6	19·3
Birnberg bow-small	11·3	3·6
Birnberg bow-large	5·3	1·8
Hall-stone steel ring	6·9	13·9

In Table 28, which is also taken from Tietze's paper, are shown the pregnancy and expulsion rates for various IUD's. The pregnancy rate for loop D during the first year of use was 2·8 per cent; the corresponding figures for the large spiral and the large bow were 1·6 and 5·3 per cent respectively. The table also shows that, in general, smaller sizes of IUD are associated with higher failure rates. Approximately one-third of the pregnancies occur with the device *in situ*; pregnancy rates tend to be lower after the first year of use, and Tietze (1966) has reported that, with the Lippes loop D, the figures for the first, second and third years are respectively 2·8, 1·4 and 1·1 per cent. Cumulative pregnancy rates obtained by R. E. Hall (1966) for four types of IUD are shown in Figure 131. The relatively high rate in the case of the Birnberg bow (No. 3, small) is noteworthy.

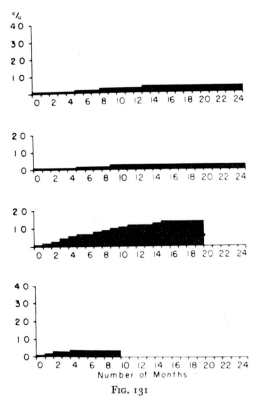

FIG. 131

Cumulative pregnancy rate following first insertion of, from top to bottom, Margulies spiral-large, Lippes loop D, Birnberg bow-small and Birnberg bow-large.

(From R. E. Hall, 1966.)

Expulsion is one of the major problems associated with the use of the IUD. According to the Co-operative Statistical Programme organised in the U.S.A. for the evaluation of such devices this term includes " complete expulsion into or from the vagina and partial expulsions requiring removal of the IUD from the cervix, whether noticed or unnoticed by the wearer ".

The percentage of women in whom expulsion occurs once (first expulsion) varies from 1·8 to 30·1 per cent depending on the type of device inserted (see Table 28). The incidence of first expulsion becomes less the longer the device remains *in situ*, and, for the Lippes loop D, Tietze (1966) quotes a figure of 10·4 per cent for the first year, and figures of 1·6 and 0·7 per cent for the second and third years respectively. Some 50 per cent of expulsions occur within the first three months following insertion, the majority taking place during menstruation. Reinsertion after expulsion is usually associated with a higher risk of subsequent expulsion than is a first insertion. Expulsions which are not noticed by the patient are likely to be followed by a pregnancy, and this represents one of the major hazards of intra-uterine contraception. In Figure 132 is shown the relationship of the age and parity of the subject to the expulsion rate for the Lippes loop D. The major points to emerge are the high incidence of expulsions in young women and in subjects of low parity.

COMPLICATIONS ASSOCIATED WITH THE USE OF INTRA-UTERINE DEVICES

These have been commented on by numerous investigators, including H. H. Hall and Stone (1962), Fuchs *et al.* (1964), H. H. Hall *et al.* (1964), Margulies (1964), Lay (1965), Lippes (1965), Willson *et al.* (1965 a), Lehfeldt *et al.* (1965), Lee and Wei (1965), Malkani *et al.* (1965), Shin (1965), R. E. Hall (1965, 1966), Satterthwaite *et al.* (1965), Brooks and Horne (1966), Blott and Radcliffe (1966), Johnson *et al.* (1966), Haller *et al.* (1966) and Mischell *et al.* (1966). Review articles dealing with complications include those of Guttmacher (1965), Borell (1966), Tietze (1965, 1966), Tietze and Lewit (1965) and Kleinman (1966) as well as the W.H.O. Technical Report (1966). The most frequent side effects are undoubtedly bleeding and pain ; pelvic inflammatory disease occurs occasionally, while the most serious complication following the insertion of an IUD is perforation of the uterus. Major complications and side effects noted at various times after the first insertion of a number of types of device in the 2,330 patients studied by R. E. Hall (1966) are shown in Table 29.

1. Bleeding

Following the insertion of an IUD some bleeding generally takes place ; this must be regarded as a normal reaction of little or no significance. Intermenstrual bleeding at varying times during the cycle can occur relatively soon after the device has been placed in the uterine cavity. Such bleeding normally lasts for a few months only and seldom necessitates removal of the IUD. The first few periods following the insertion of the device may be associated with excessive blood loss. Generally, the degree of loss diminishes with time. Occasionally, however, it becomes increasingly severe and if this happens there is little or no alternative to removal of the IUD.

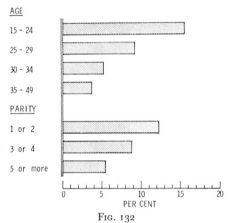

FIG. 132

Expulsion rate of Lippes loop D during the first year of use according to age and parity.

(From Tietze, 1966.)

2. Pain

Soon after the device has been inserted cramp-like pain or low backache may be noted. These symptoms are sometimes associated with bleeding or vaginal discharge, and they generally abate spontaneously or as a result of therapy with suitable analgesics. Acute pain immediately following insertion is relatively rare except in nulliparous women in whom the pain may be associated with syncope. The occurrence of pain and bleeding some months after insertion of the IUD and following an asymptomatic period should be carefully noted as such complaints may herald the impending expulsion of the device.

3. Vaginal Discharge

This occurs rather frequently and probably represents the initial reaction of the endometrium to the lodgement of the IUD. The discharge is transient in character and usually subsides after the first or second menstrual period.

4. Perforation of the Uterus

This is a rare but serious complication. It was noted in 43 (0·2 per cent) out of the 22,403 cases reported by Tietze (1966). Thirty-four occurred with the bow, six with the loop, two with the steel ring and one with the spiral. The relatively high incidence of uterine perforation with the bow is noteworthy, the risk of this complication being maximal if the device is inserted within six weeks of delivery. In a small number of patients the terminal bead of the tail of the Margulies spiral

TABLE 29

CUMULATIVE INCIDENCE (%) OF FIRST COMPLAINTS FOLLOWING FIRST INSERTION OF VARIOUS DEVICES

(After R. E. Hall, 1966)

Device	Margulies spiral-large			Lippes loop D			Birnberg bow		
							small		large
Time after insertion (months)	9	12	24	9	12	24	9	12	9
Complaint									
Severe bleeding...	38·7	43·1	45·4	8·8	10·1	12·0	7·8	8·8	6·7
Mild bleeding ...	17·4	20·2	28·4	7·0	8·3	13·2	3·6	5·6	3·2
Severe pain ...	14·0	15·7	17·1	5·4	5·7	6·7	3·2	3·7	1·0
Mild pain ...	11·2	12·9	16·6	3·8	5·4	0·3	1·3	2·7	3·5
Excess number of beads	14·5	16·2	17·7	0	0	0	0	0	0
Inability to feel tail	4·8	4·8	6·3	3·5	3·8	3·8	0	0	0
Male discomfort	6·5	6·5	8·7	0	0	0	0	0	0
Miscellaneous ...	8·0	12·4	24·9	5·5	5·8	7·7	9·8	5·3	5·0
Infections ...	5·4	6·5	10·9	0·8	1·4	1·4	1·6	2·4	1·0
Serious complications	0	1·1	2·6	1·7	1·7	1·7	0·6	1·4	1·0

may be found embedded in the vaginal mucosa ; however, such an occurrence is rarely associated with a uterine perforation. Tietze (1966) has emphasised that the majority of perforations are asymptomatic, being noted on routine examination or following delivery.

5. Pelvic Inflammatory Disease

This well recognised complication has been described by many investigators. In Tietze's (1966) series it occurred in 606 out of 22,403 women (2·7 per cent), but in only one-sixth of these cases was the disease classified as severe. The extensive experience of R. E. Hall (1966) involving 2,330 patients is summarised in Table 30. In some women the complication represents an exacerbation of a pre-existing condition ; in a few there is a previous history of gonococcal infection and in others a septic abortion may have occurred. The majority of women who show pelvic inflammatory disease with a device *in situ* respond satisfactorily to treatment with antibiotics. In those who do not it is frequently necessary to remove the IUD.

It is not yet established with certainty whether the insertion of an IUD into a completely healthy uterus can of itself cause pelvic inflammatory disease. This point requires further investigation before a definite conclusion can be reached.

6. Genital Carcinoma

There is at present no evidence to suggest that patients in whom an IUD has been inserted have any greater risk of developing endometrial carcinoma than the general population. Furthermore, serial studies of cervical and vaginal cytology in women wearing IUD's have failed to demonstrate an increase in the frequency of the abnormal cell types indicative of cervical carcinoma. A final conclusion regarding the true incidence of genital carcinoma in women with devices *in situ* must await more clinical experience, but, at the time of writing, there would appear to be no necessity for apprehension on this account.

7. Male Discomfort during Intercourse

This occasionally occurs in association with devices bearing a tail. It is seldom severe and actual injury to the penis is extremely rare.

TABLE 30

INCIDENCE OF PELVIC INFECTION (%) IN 2,330 PATIENTS FITTED WITH VARIOUS DEVICES

(After R. E. Hall, 1966)

	Margulies spiral-large	Lippes loop A	Lippes loop D	Birnberg bow small	Birnberg bow large	Hall-Stone steel ring	Zipper nylon ring	Total
Total incidence of pelvic infection ...	0·81	0·13	0·47	0·69	0·21	0·26	0·04	2·62
Patients admitted to hospital	0·13	0·04	0·08	0·13	0·13	0·04	0	0·56
Patients treated with antibiotic	0·56	0·13	0·39	0·43	0·13	0·21	0·04	1·89
IUD removed	0·43	0·04	0·08	0·26	0·04	0·08	0	0·94
Previous pelvic inflammation ...	0·17	0·04	0	0	0·08	0·04	0	0·34

8. Side Effects Leading to Removal

The major symptom necessitating removal on medical grounds is bleeding ; next come cramp-like uterine pains and low backache. In the Co-operative Statistical Programme in the U.S.A. the removal rate because of bleeding and/or pain during the first year of use was 11 per cent for the loop, 16 per cent for the spiral and 7 per cent for the bow. The rates were slightly lower for the small loop and spiral than for the larger sizes ; however, they were higher for the small bow. The rate for the steel ring was 7 per cent in the first year.

OTHER EFFECTS OF INTRA-UTERINE DEVICES

1. On Vaginal Cytology

The effect of IUD's on vaginal cytology has been studied by various investigators including Margulies (1964), Lippes (1965), Ishihama and Kagabu (1965) and Vorys et al. (1965). In a series of 4,800 women reviewed by Tietze (1966) only 105 (2·2 per cent) showed abnormal vaginal smears. Most of these smears were of the Class III Papanicolaou type (see p. 126), and the majority returned spontaneously to normal within a year. No correlation appears to exist between the presence of an IUD and the development of carcinoma of the cervix or vagina. According to Vorys et al. (1965) cytological evidence indicates that ovulatory cycles occur in the majority of women in whom IUD's have been inserted.

2. On Endometrial Histology

Detailed studies on this subject have been made by H. H. Hall et al. (1964), Willson et al. (1965 b), Lehfeldt et al. (1965), Vorys et al. (1965), Moyer and Mishell (1965), Sujan-Tejuja et al. (1965) and Israel and Davis (1966). In the report of Willson et al. (1965 b) the Margulies spiral was used, and the most consistent change noted was increased superficial vascularity associated with stromal oedema ; cellular changes suggestive of the development of neoplasia were absent. In Figure 133 is shown an endometrial biopsy taken from a patient on the 25th day of the cycle with an IUD in situ ; the most notable feature is the change in vascularity.

Moyer and Mishell (1965) investigated the effect of the Lippes loop on tissue reactions of the endometrium and myometrium in 29 patients. In a proportion of their subjects they noted slight infiltration of the subepithelial layers with leucocytes ; in others, there were diffuse chronic inflammatory lesions involving the endometrium and myometrium. The changes described were generally not associated with any symptoms, and their exact significance remains obscure. Sujan-Tejuja *et al.* (1965) found both proliferative and

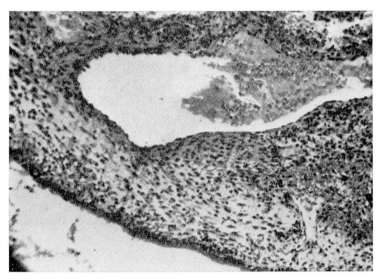

FIG. 133
Endometrial biopsy showing large thin walled vascular sinuses
(From Willson *et al.*, 1965 *b.*)

secretory types of endometrium in patients with IUD's *in situ* and concluded that ovulation occurred normally in such women. An endometrial biopsy taken on day 23 of the menstrual cycle, 18 months after the insertion of an IUD is shown in Figure 134 ; the presence of a secretory pattern and of stromal oedema should be noted. Histochemical studies on the endometrium of patients fitted with an IUD, have been performed by Vorys *et al.* (1965) ; no significant abnormalities were detected.

3. On the Fallopian Tubes

The effect of intra-uterine insertion of the Margulies Spiral on the activity of the Fallopian tube has been studied by Siegler and Hellman (1964) in four subjects. Tubal activity was not altered, and no mechanical obstruction of the tube was noted in any of the volunteers.

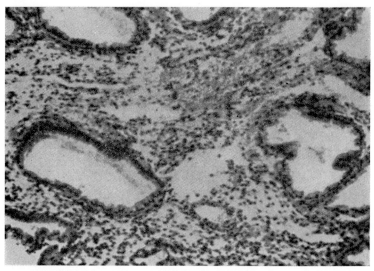

FIG. 134

Endometrial biopsy showing a secretory pattern and stromal oedema.

(From Sujan-Tejuja *et al.*, 1965.)

4. On Hormone Excretion

At the time of writing very little information is available on this subject. Vorys *et al.* (1965) claimed that FSH levels during the cycle tended to be high in women in whom a Margulies spiral had been inserted. They also reported that the peak of LH output, which generally occurs at midcycle, was of longer duration in patients with an IUD *in situ* than in their control series. In a recent study conducted by the Edinburgh group in a subject in whom a Lippes loop D had been inserted for three months before the institution of hormone assays two ovulatory cycles were noted on the basis of oestrogen and pregnanediol output.

330

5. On Spermatozoa

The major study in this field is probably that of Morgenstern *et al.* (1966). The most important conclusion to emerge from this paper was that insertion of an IUD did not prevent the transport of spermatozoa to the site of fertilisation of the ovum in the Fallopian tubes.

INTRA-UTERINE DEVICES IN RELATION TO PREGNANCY

1. Outcome of Pregnancy in Patients with an IUD

It is generally agreed that pregnancies occurring with a device *in situ* terminate more frequently in abortion than those in which the device has previously been expelled. Kleinman (1966) quotes an incidence of abortion of 41 per cent in pregnancies with a device *in situ* as compared with 33 per cent in patients in whom the device has been expelled. The incidence of ectopic pregnancy is also higher in patients wearing an IUD than in a control group, and in a series of 1,028 unintended pregnancies with a device *in situ* 26 (2·5 per cent) were ectopic in type (see Tietze, 1966). It is obvious that in terms of total numbers, the incidence of ectopic pregnancy reported by Tietze (1966) is relatively low ; this is, of course, due to the fact that the device is acting as a reasonably efficient method of contraception. Malformations of the foetus have not so far been attributed to the wearing of an IUD.

2. Effect on Fertility

Clinical experience indicates that, following removal of an IUD, fertility is not impaired. Kleinman (1966) found that 75 per cent of women conceived within six months of removing the device ; after one year the figure had reached 90 per cent. Such pregnancy rates are entirely normal.

3. Effect on Lactation

This has been investigated by Gomez-Rogers *et al.* (1965) who demonstrated that lactation was not impaired when an IUD was inserted immediately or soon after delivery.

CONTRA-INDICATIONS TO THE USE OF INTRA-UTERINE DEVICES

These have been summarised by Kleinman (1966) and by the W.H.O. Technical Report (1966). The most important contra-indications are pelvic infection and pregnancy.

1. Pelvic Infection

In the presence of active infection, e.g. salpingitis, endometritis and cervicitis, the insertion of an IUD should be postponed until the infection has been appropriately treated. On the other hand, the finding of *Trichomonas vaginalis* or *Candida albicans* in the absence of clinical signs is not an absolute contra-indication to the insertion of a device. If at all possible, such infections should be treated before insertion, but if this is not practicable, therapy should be commenced immediately after the IUD has been put in place.

2. Pregnancy

Obviously an IUD should not be inserted into the gravid uterus, and strict precautions must be taken by the clinician to ensure that the patient is not pregnant at the time at which this form of contraception is requested. Reliable evidence is still lacking on the effects produced on the conceptus by the insertion of a device.

3. Nulliparity

Nulliparity is no longer regarded as a contra-indication to this form of contraception. It is, however, generally necessary under such circumstances to dilate the cervix and to use models of smaller size. Because of the need to use smaller devices the risks of expulsion and consequent pregnancy are higher in nulliparous than in multiparous women.

4. Miscellaneous

In patients with *abnormal uterine bleeding* the cause of this symptom should be sought before an IUD is inserted. In women with *fibromyomata of the uterus* intra-uterine contraception is probably not indicated, while in subjects with *genital carcinoma* treatment should be directed to the primary condition before this form of birth control is considered.

MECHANISM OF ACTION OF INTRA-UTERINE DEVICES

Although various modes of action have been postulated by different investigators, the precise mechanism whereby the IUD produces its contraceptive effect in human subjects remains obscure. Among the mechanisms suggested are alterations in tubal and uterine mobility, lack of fertilisation of the ovum, failure of implantation of the fertilised ovum and acceleration of the transport of ova through the Fallopian tubes. A recent and attractive theory of " tubal-uterine asynchrony " has been put forward by Bonney *et al.* (1966) to explain the mode of action of IUD's. According to their hypothesis the device causes an alteration in the pattern of endometrial maturation so that when the ovum reaches the uterus, implantation cannot occur. This interesting suggestion requires further investigation before any firm conclusion can be drawn regarding its validity.

The mode of action of IUD's in animals is somewhat better understood than in humans and has been summarised by Guttmacher (1965) and in the W.H.O. Technical Report (1966). In monkeys the work of Mastroianni and Hongsomand (1965) with the Margulies Spiral has indicated that the major action of the IUD is to accelerate the transport of ova through the Fallopian tube so that passage is effected in one day or less rather than in three or four days. In ruminants, e.g. sheep and cattle, devices appear to affect the ovary directly, causing deficient ovulation and inadequate luteal function ; in addition, they may inhibit transport of spermatozoa. In rats, mice, rabbits, and ferrets the main effect of the IUD appears to be to prevent implantation of the fertilised ovum.

SUMMARY AND CONCLUSIONS

Historical aspects of contraception by the intra-uterine device (IUD) have been briefly reviewed, and it is emphasised that there have been many major advances in this field.

The five main types of IUD available for use are the Margulies spiral, the Lippes loop, the Birnberg bow, the Hall-Stone ring and the Zipper nylon ring. The device most widely employed in clinical practice is the Lippes loop D.

The effectiveness of the various types of IUD is discussed, and it is emphasised that one of the major limitations of this form of contraception is expulsion during the first year of use.

The most frequent side effects associated with the presence of an IUD are bleeding and pain. Pelvic inflammatory disease is a relatively rare complication and perforation of the uterus is even rarer.

In women in whom conception occurs with an IUD *in situ* the incidence both of abortion and of ectopic pregnancy is relatively high.

The IUD does not produce consistent effects on vaginal cytology. Changes in endometrial histology occur, but the exact significance of these is not at present clear.

Information is lacking on the mechanism by which the IUD produces its contraceptive effect in the human female.

REFERENCES

BIRNBERG, C. H. & BURNHILL, M. S. (1964). *Am. J. Obstet. Gynecol.* **89,** 137.
BLOTT, G. R. & RADCLIFFE, R. W. (1966). *Fertility Sterility*, **17,** 332.
BONNEY, W. A. Jr., GLASSER, S. R., CLEWE, T. H., NOYES, R. W. & COOPER, C. L. (1966). *Am. J. Obstet. Gynecol.* **96,** 101.
BORELL, U. (1966). *Acta Obstet. Gynecol. Scand.* **45,** Suppl. 1, 5.
BROOKS, P. G. & HORNE, H. W. Jr. (1966). *Fertility Sterility*, **17,** 267.
BURNHILL, M. S. & BIRNBERG, C. H. (1965). In *Excerpta Med. Intern. Cong. Series*, No. 86, p. 127. Amsterdam : Excerpta Medica Foundation.
FUCHS, K., GRÜNSTEIN, S. & PERETZ, A. (1964). *Fertility Sterility*, **15,** 338.
GÓMEZ-ROGERS, C., GUILOFF, E. & ZAÑARTU, J. (1965). *Excerpta Med. Intern. Cong. Series*, No. 86, p. 142. Amsterdam : Excerpta Medica Foundation.
GRÄFENBERG, E. (1929 a). In *Geburtenretelung : Vorträge und Verhandlungen des Ärztekursus*, p. 50. Ed. Bendix, K. Berlin : Selbstverlag.
GRÄFENBERG, E. (1929 b). In *Proc. Third Congr. League for Sexual Reform*, p. 116.
GUTTMACHER, A. F. (1965). *J. Reprod. Fertility*, **10,** 115.
HALL, H. H. (1966). *Am. J. Obstet. Gynecol.* **95,** 879.
HALL, H. H. & STONE, M. L. (1962). *Am. J. Obstet. Gynecol.* **83,** 683.
HALL, H. H., STONE, M. L., SEDLIS, A. & CHABON, I. (1964). *Fertility Sterility*, **15,** 618.
HALL, R. E. (1965). In *Excerpta Med. Intern. Cong. Series*, No. 86, p. 66. Amsterdam: Excerpta Medica Foundation.
HALL, R. E. (1966). *Am. J. Obstet. Gynecol.* **94,** 65.
HALLER, Y. I., JONES, G. F., MARGOLIS, A. J. & WELLINGTON, C. J. (1966). *J. Am. Med. Women's Assoc.* **21,** 398.
HARTWIG, M. (1874). *Berlin Klin. Wochschr.* **11,** 351.
ISHIHAMA, A. (1959). *Yokohama Med. J.* **10,** 89.
ISHIHAMA, A. & KAGABU, T. (1965). *Am. J. Obstet. Gynecol.* **91,** 576.
ISRAEL, R. & DAVIS, H. J. (1966). *J. Am. Med. Assoc.* **195,** 764.
JACKSON, M. C. N. (1965). *Practitioner*, **194,** 485.
JOHNSON, F. L., DOERFFER, F. R. & TYSON, J. E. A. (1966). *Can. Med. Assoc. J.* **95,** 14.
KLEINMAN, R. L. (1966). *Intra-uterine Contraception*, 1966. London : International Planned Parenthood Federation.

334

CONTRACEPTION—INTRA-UTERINE DEVICE

KÜSTNER, (1931). *Arch. Gynaekol.* **144,** 375.
LAY, C. L. (1965). *Am. J. Obstet. Gynecol.* **93,** 330.
LEE, C. H. & WEI, P. Y. (1965). In *Excerpta Med. Intern. Cong. Series*, No. 86, p. 23. Amsterdam : Excerpta Medica Foundation.
LEHFELDT, H., KULKA, E. W. & LIEBMANN, H. G. (1965). *Obstet. Gynecol.* **26,** 679.
LIPPES, J. (1962). In *Excerpta Med. Intern. Cong. Series*, No. 54, p. 69. Amsterdam : Excerpta Medica Foundation.
LIPPES, J. (1965). *Am. J. Obstet. Gynecol.* **93,** 1024.
MALKANI, P. K., VIRICK, R. K. & SUJAN-TEJUJA, S. (1965). In *Excerpta Med. Intern. Cong. Series*, No. 86, p. 34. Amsterdam : Excerpta Medica Foundation.
MARGULIES, L. C. (1962). In *Excerpta Med. Intern. Cong. Series*, No. 64, p. 61. Amsterdam : Excerpta Medica Foundation.
MARGULIES, L. C. (1964). *Obstet. Gynecol.* **24,** 515.
MASTROIANNI, L. Jr. & HONGSONAND, C. (1965). *Excerpta Med. Intern. Cong. Series*, No. 86, p. 194. Amsterdam : Excerpta Medica Foundation.
MISHELL, D. R. Jr., BELL, J. H., GOOD, R. G., & MOYER, D. L. (1966). *Am. J. Obstet. Gynecol*, **96,** 119.
MORGENSTERN, L. L., ORGEBIN-CRIST, M-C., CLEWE, T. H., BONNEY, W. A., Jr. & NOYES, R. W. (1966). *Am. J. Obstet. Gynecol.* **96,** 114.
MOYER, D. L. & MISHELL, D. R., Jr. (1965). *Excerpta Med. Intern. Cong. Series*, No. 86, p. 159. Amsterdam : Excerpta Medica Foundation.
NASH, W. (1965). *N.Y. State J. Med.* **65,** 1872.
OHNESORGE, V. (1927). *Münch. Med. Wochschr.* **74,** 419.
OPPENHEIMER, W. (1959). *Am. J. Obstet. Gynecol.* **78,** 446.
OTA, T. (1934). *Japan J. Obstet. Gynecol.* **17,** 210.
PUST, K. (1923). *Dtsch. Med. Wochschr.* **49,** 952.
ROTHACKER, W. A. (1883). *Cincinnati Lancet and Clinic New Series*, **10,** 287.
SATTERTHWAITE, A. P., ARANDES, E. & NEGRON, M. E. (1965). In *Excerpta Med. Intern. Cong. Series*, No. 86, p. 76. Amsterdam : Excerpta Medica Foundation.
SHIN, H. S. (1965). In *Excerpta Med. Intern. Cong. Series*, No. 86, p. 45. Amsterdam : Excerpta Medica Foundation.
SIEGLER, A. M. & HELLMAN, L. M. (1964). *Obstet. Gynecol.* **23,** 173.
SOUTHAM, A. L. (1965). In *Excerpta Med. Intern. Cong. Series*, No. 86, p. 3. Amsterdam : Excerpta Medica Foundation.
STRASSMAN, P. (1928). *Deut. Z. Ges. Gerichtl. Med.* **12,** 278.
SUJAN-TEJUJA, S., VIRICK, R. K. & MALKANI, P. K. (1965). *Excerpta Med. Intern. Cong. Series*, No. 86, p. 172. Amsterdam : Excerpta Medica Foundation.
TIETZE, C. (1965). *J. Chronic Diseases*, **18,** 1147.
TIETZE, C. (1966). *Am. J. Obstet. Gynecol.* **96,** 1043.
TIETZE, C. & LEWIT, S. (1965). In *Excerpta Med. Intern. Cong. Series*, No. 86, p. 98. Amsterdam : Excerpta Medica Foundation.
VORYS, N., DE NEEF, J. C., BOUTSELIS, J. G., DETTMANN, F. G., SCOTT, W. P., STEVENS, V. C. & BESCH, P. K. (1965). *Excerpta Med. Intern. Cong. Series*, No. 86, p. 147. Amsterdam : Excerpta Medica Foundation.
WILLSON, J. R., LEDGER, W. J. & ANDROS, G. J. (1965 b). *Am. J. Obstet. Gynecol.* **93,** 802.
WILLSON, J. R., LEDGER, W. J., BOLLINGER, C. C. & ANDROS, G. J. (1965 a). *Am. J. Obstet. Gynecol.* **92,** 62.
World Health Organisation *Technical Report Series*, (1966) No. 332. Geneva : World Health Organisation.
ZIPPER, J., GARCIA, M. L. & PASTENE, L. L. (1965). In *Excerpta Med. Intern. Cong. Series*, No. 86, p. 88. Amsterdam : Excerpta Medica Foundation.

335

CHAPTER XI

Overpopulation and Contraception

INTRODUCTION

THE subjects of fertility and contraception are inextricably interwoven with the greatest problem facing the universe in the 20th century, namely the crisis of overpopulation. In the opinion of many, including the present authors, this problem has now reached such catastrophic proportions that it outranks all other threats to the survival of mankind, even that involving nuclear warfare. This final chapter is included in order to emphasise that some of the topics dealt with in previous sections of this book are not only of strictly medical but also of global significance. To those who are deeply concerned about the world population crisis, one of the most frustrating features of the situation is the fact that, with the introduction of new and really efficient methods of birth control, notably by oral contraception and by the intra-uterine device, together with the liberalisation of abortion laws in many countries, the problem would appear, in the long term, to be capable of solution. Such a solution is at present being prevented by factors which are essentially non-medical in type and include inadequate standards of education, the teaching of various religious faiths and the mistaken belief which is by no means confined to the underdeveloped countries of the world, that the production of a large number of children is desirable from the point of view of society.

The first topic to be considered herein is the growth of man's numbers from the dawn of history until the present time ; subsequently, the population problem as it affects the United Kingdom* is briefly reviewed. The final section deals with contraception in the 1960's and includes a comparison of the efficiency of the various methods of birth control currently in use. The literature on overpopulation is now voluminous, and readers with a special interest in this topic are referred to recent papers and monographs by Baird (1965), Draper (1965), Venning (1966), Fox (1966 *a b*), Stycos (1966), Hall (1966), Ritchie-Calder (1966) Ehlrich (1967) and Currie (1967). A comprehensive account of the subject is also given in the publications of the Population Reference Bureau, those from 1962 onwards being especially informative.

THE CRISIS OF WORLD POPULATION

There can be no question that large areas of the world are now affected by an exceedingly grave problem of over-population. Such pressures are especially severe in India and in other far eastern countries, but the situation is now assuming menacing proportions in Latin America and in certain parts of Africa. In Europe and in North America a definite crisis in man's numbers has not yet been reached. However, there is good evidence to support the view that the steady increase in population in these latter areas over the last few decades is gradually impairing what has been so aptly termed by J. K. Galbraith " the quality of life ". Furthermore, it can be predicted with assurance that, unless appropriate remedial action is rapidly taken, an overpopulation problem of considerable magnitude is likely to exist in areas of Europe and North America by the end of the present century.

* The United Kingdom is taken to include England, Scotland, Wales and Northern Ireland.

It is generally agreed that the population explosion has not occurred because of an increase in human fertility. The major cause of the present situation has been the rapid advances in medical science resulting in a decrease in the death rate. Among the more spectacular of these have been the virtual eradication of malaria and other diseases from large areas of the world together with marked decreases in the neonatal and infantile mortality rates. Between 1953 and 1959 deaths from malaria in India fell from 800,000 to 10,000 per year, and the life span of great numbers of people was correspondingly increased (see Hall, 1966). In Ceylon in 1946 the expectation of life at birth was 43 years; by the end of 1947 it had risen to 52 and in 1956 stood at 61. An excellent example of the effect of the modern chemotherapy for malaria on population growth has been given by Burnet (1961) who studied the results obtained in the island community of Mauritius. Between 1946 and 1948 there was an intensive and highly successful campaign to eliminate malaria from Mauritius using modern chemotherapy along with D.D.T. Over a ten year period this programme resulted in a reduction of the infantile mortality rate from 150 to 50 per thousand. During this time the death rate fell from 28 to 10 per thousand, the birth rate remained approximately constant and the population rose by 40 per cent.

A diagram of the world population from the early Stone Age to the year A.D. 2,000 is shown in Figure 135 while a more detailed representation of population trends between 1800 and 2000 A.D. is presented in Figure 136. It will be noted that it has taken the whole of man's existence to reach the present figure of 3,300,000,000. However, at the anticipated rate of increase the population will have more than doubled in another 35 years by which time it will approximate 7,000,000,000. A population of 1,000,000,000 was not reached until the 1830's, and a further 100 years passed before the second thousand million was added. The contrast in the present century is obvious, a third thousand million being added in the 30 years between 1930 and 1960 and a fourth being expected in the 15 years between 1960 and 1975.

According to Hauser (1965) population growth for the 600,000 years constituting the old Stone Age was very low, approximating two per cent per 1,000 years. This contrasts

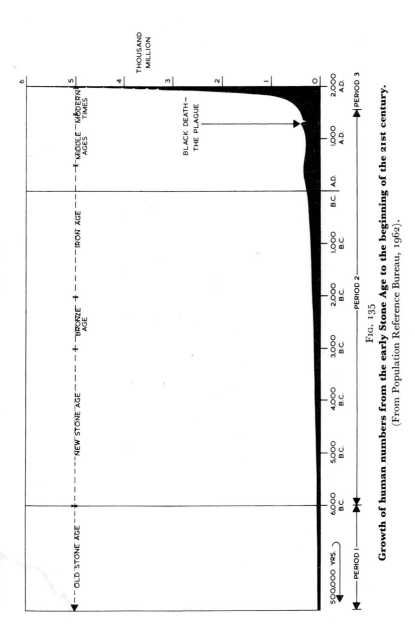

FIG. 135

Growth of human numbers from the early Stone Age to the beginning of the 21st century.

(From Population Reference Bureau, 1962).

markedly with the situation in the 1960's, when the increase is some thousandfold greater, being in the neighbourhood of two per cent per annum. Hauser (1965) has stated that during the second half of the twentieth century there will be a much greater rise in world population than took place in all the millennia of human existence up to the present time.

In recent years there have been many pronouncements both from organisations and from individuals in responsible positions emphasising the dangers of the population explosion. Three typical examples of such statements will be given. According to the Department of Economic and Social Affairs

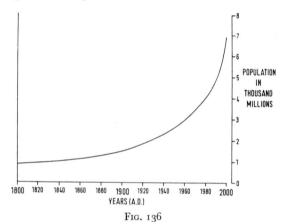

FIG. 136

Growth of human numbers between A.D. 1800 and 2000.

(After Fox, 1966 *b*).

at the United Nations " The growth of world population in the next 25 years has an importance which transcends economic and social considerations. It is at the very heart of the problem of our existence ". The United States Academy of Sciences (1963) has bluntly stated " Either the birth rate of the world must come down or the death rate must go back up ". Lord Caradon (1965), permanent British representative at the United Nations Organisation, has succinctly emphasised the gravity of the situation in the following memorable words, " If tackling the problem is left too late, all our political and economic achievements will be swept away like sand castles before the advancing tide ".

In Figures 137 and 138 are shown contrasts in the age constitution of the population in a developing agricultural country, Pakistan and in a highly industrialised community, the United Kingdom. It is noteworthy that the proportion of the population below the age of 10 is much higher in Pakistan than in the U.K., and because of this fact, is it clear that those of working age in Pakistan must support many more children than the comparable segment of the community in the U.K. Reduction in the birth rate in Pakistan and in other countries with a similar problem would have obvious beneficial effects. By this means the number of dependent children would be diminished and, as a consequence, proportionately more of

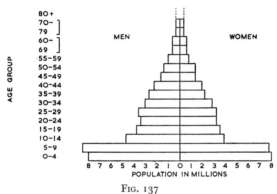

FIG. 137

Age constitution of the population in Pakistan.

(From Florence, 1964).

the nation's gross national product would be available for investment in industry and in agriculture.

In relation to the population explosion in the under-developed countries President Lyndon Johnston (1965) has stated " Let us face forthrightly the multiplying problems of our multiplying populations and seek the answer to this most profound challenge to the future of the world. Let us act on the fact that $5 invested in population control in developing countries is worth $100 invested in economic growth ". Also worthy of mention in this connection is the comment of President Ayub Khan of Pakistan " It may be better for our future economy if the greater part of our development was spent on popularising and encouraging family planning ".

Birth and death rates vary considerably in different areas of the world, and this fact obviously has a marked influence on population trends. Table 31 presents statistics on birth and death rates in various countries together with data on population growth. The relatively small increase in population anticipated in European countries as compared with that in Africa, Asia and South America is noteworthy.

The distribution of population in different parts of the world between the years A.D. 1,000 and 2,000 is shown in Figure 139. In A.D. 1,000 it was estimated that Asia accounted

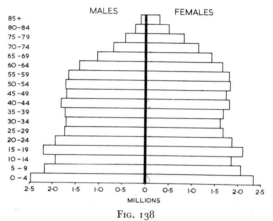

Fig. 138

Age constitution of the population in the United Kingdom.

Ordinate = age group.

for some 60 per cent of the world's population, the corresponding figures for Europe including Russia, Africa and the Americas being respectively 17, 18 and 5 per cent. By 1960 the percentage of the world's population resident in Asia and Africa had fallen slightly to 57 and 8 per cent respectively ; on the other hand, that of Europe and the USSR and of the Americas had increased to 21 and 14 per cent. By the year 2,000 demographers predict that Asia may comprise 62 per cent of the total, Europe and the USSR 15 per cent, the Americas 15 per cent and Africa 8 per cent.

WORLD POPULATION AND FOOD SUPPLIES

It is now generally agreed that world food production is failing to keep pace with population growth, and this fact has been emphasised in a number of recent publications (see Cook, 1964 ; Paddock and Paddock, 1964 ; Cépède et al., 1964 ; Harrar, 1965 ; Revelle, 1966 ; Food and Agricultural Organisation (FAO) Report, 1966). Harrar (1965) is amongst those who have stressed the state of imbalance which exists between the underdeveloped and developed countries of the world in relation to food production. He has pointed out that the less developed countries which accommodate some 70 per cent of the population produce only 47 per cent of the world's grain, while the developed nations with only 30 per cent of the population grow approximately 53 per cent of the grain. Harrar (1965) has emphasised that, in spite of all the major advances in science and technology which have characterised the 20th century, a greater number of people throughout the world live in hunger and deprivation in the 1960's than in the early 1900's.

The report of the FAO for 1966 is frankly pessimistic regarding the relationship between world food supplies and population. The memorandum states that in the years 1964/65 and 1965/66 world food production remained virtually static, despite the fact that in the latter year there were some 70,000,000 more mouths to feed. The perilous nature of this situation needs no emphasis, and it can only be assumed that the near famine conditions prevailing in Bihar in India during the spring and summer of 1967 are likely to be repeated in other parts of the world. Thomas Malthus, in his now classical " Essay on the Principle of Population " written in 1798 (see also Cook, 1966 ; Morris, 1966), postulated the existence of " positive checks " on population growth in the form of famine, disease and war. The importance of the first of these checks is certainly being illustrated by the experience of the underdeveloped world in the 1960's.

POPULATION TRENDS IN THE UNITED KINGDOM

Until recently there was little appreciation of the fact that a problem of overpopulation exists in the U.K., and it is only within the last few years that a number of articles on this

TABLE 31

DATA ON WORLD POPULATION (MID-1965)

(After Population Reference Bureau, 1966)

Continent	Country	Population millions	Annual rate of increase %	Number of years to double population	Per 1,000 population	
					Birth rate	Death rate
Africa	Guinea	3·5	3·0	24	53–57	33–35
	Madagascar	6·4	3·0	24	42–50	17–21
	Senegal	3·5	2·3	31	40–47	23–29
	U.A.R.	29·6	2·5	28	41–44	17–19
Asia	Ceylon	11·2	2·5	28	35–41	8·7
	India	482·5	2·3	31	40–43	21–23
	Indonesia	104·6	2·3	31	43–48	19–23
	Israel	2·6	3·5	20	25·7	6·3
	Japan	97·8	0·9	78	17·7	6·9
	Malaysia	9·4	3·2	22	39–44	8·9
	Singapore	1·9	3·2	22	33·2	5·8
	South Korea	28·4	2·8	25	40–45	12–16
	Thailand	30·6	3·0	24	42–48	19–21

America	Argentina	22·4	1·6	44	21·7	8·1
	Bolivia	3·7	1·4	50	41-45	20-25
	Brazil	81·1	3·1	23	43-47	11-16
	Canada	19·6	2·0	35	23·5	7·6
	Costa Rica	1·4	4·5	16	47-50	8·8
	Mexico	40·9	3·2	22	45·4	10·3
	Paraguay	2·0	2·4	29	45-50	12-16
	United States	194·6	1·6	44	21·1	9·4
Europe	Austria	7·3	0·6	117	18·6	12·3
	Czechoslovakia	14·1	0·7	100	17·1	9·6
	France	48·8	1·3	54	18·1	10·7
	Hungary	10·1	0·4	175	13·1	10·0
	Ireland	2·8	−0·1		22·5	11·4
	Italy	52·6	0·6	117	20·0	9·6
	Spain	31·6	0·8	88	22·2	8·7
	Sweden	7·7	0·5	140	16·0	10·0
	United Kingdom	54·4	0·7	100	18·8	11·3
Oceania	Australia	11·4	2·1	33	20·6	9·0
	New Zealand	2·7	2·2	32	24·1	8·8
USSR		234·0	1·7	41	19·6	6·9

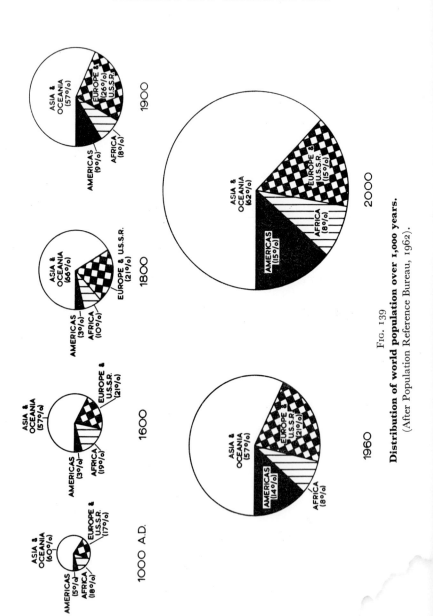

FIG. 139

Distribution of world population over 1,000 years.

(After Population Reference Bureau, 1962).

subject have been written (see Fox, 1966 *b* ; Hutchinson, 1966 ; Renton, 1967 *a b c*). According to the Monthly Digest of Statistics (1967) the population of the U.K. in June 1966 was 54,895,600, and it is estimated that, if present demographic trends continue, the figure by the year 2,000 will have reached approximately 75,000,000. Figure 140 which is based upon data taken from the Monthly Digest of Statistics (1966) shows population trends for the U.K. from 1965 up to 2000.

There can be no question that many of the problems with which successive governments in the U.K. are unsuccessfully

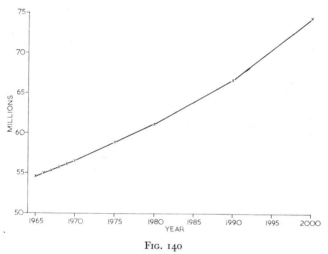

FIG. 140
Estimated total population of the United Kingdom.

attempting to grapple, arise directly from the increasing population of these islands. These include the shortage of houses and land, the pressures on the educational and health services and the increasing congestion on the roads ; in addition, there is the problem of the ever-extending urban sprawl which results in erosion of the green belt areas of cities and destruction of the countryside. Renton (1967 *a b c*), in a series of letters to the Prime Minister, Mr Harold Wilson, has expressed grave concern regarding the amount of farmland in the U.K. which will eventually be urbanised. He states that within the next 10 years an area the size of Leicestershire will be " converted to tarmacadam, concrete or bricks and mortar ". Renton (1967 c) also considers that, if present demographic trends continue, the next 30 years will see the construction of 20 more cities the size of Birmingham, the present population of which is 1,106,040. Although other authorities take a somewhat less pessimistic view than Renton regarding the degree of urbanisation of the U.K. by the year 2000 (see Hall, 1966), the potential dangers of such a situation to a country which must of necessity import a relatively high proportion of its foodstuffs, are self evident.

In his presidential address to the British Association for the Advancement of Science in 1966 Hutchinson has reviewed the overpopulation problem as it affects the U.K. Approaching the subject from the point of view of an agriculturist, Hutchinson has suggested that an optimal population for these islands would be in the region of 40,000,000. However, he is of the opinion that such a figure might take two centuries to attain. Maxwell (1967), in a letter to all Members of Parliament written on behalf of the Edinburgh branch of the World Population Crisis Campaign, an affiliate of the International Planned Parenthood Federation (I.P.P.F.), has also stressed the perils of current population growth in the U.K., and has requested the Government to establish a Royal Commission to investigate the whole subject in detail. In this connection it is somewhat ironic to recollect that the last Royal Commission on Population, the deliberations of which were published in 1949, predicted a fall in the population of the United Kingdom by the end of the twentieth century, expressed concern on this account and recommended an increase in children's allowances as one means of reversing this trend !

In a recent article Currie (1967) has criticised present legislation in many countries by means of which family allowances are paid by governments and income tax relief is given on behalf of children. Watts (1966) has suggested that curtailment of such allowances might aid in the solution of the population problem of the U.K. There can be no question that legislation of this type was originally introduced for humanitarian motives. At the same time, it must be emphasised that in the world of the 1960's which is characterised by excessive population growth and in which reliable methods of contraception are readily available, such relief is probably less appropriate than in previous decades of this century.

Within the past two years there have been three important developments in the U.K. which may ultimately have a significant bearing on the population problem of that country. The first is the recent passage through Parliament of the National Health Service (Family Planning) Bill for England and Wales which makes it possible for Local Health Authorities to give advice on contraception and to supply contraceptive applicances. The second is the establishment in various cities, notably London, Cambridge and Birmingham, of so-called Brook Advisory Centres one of the functions of which is to provide contraceptive advice for the unmarried and in this way to tackle the ever-increasing problems of illegal abortion and illegitimate births (see *Family Planning*, 1966). In England and Wales the figures for illegitimate births in 1966 stood at 66,312, and it has been estimated that there may be as many as 100,000 criminal abortions each year in the U.K. (*Brit. Med. J.* 1966). The third important development is the attempt that is currently in progress to liberalise the existing law governing abortion (see *Brit. Med. J.* 1966). In the U.K. abortion for social reasons was pioneered by Baird in his now classical studies conducted in the Aberdeen area of Scotland and recently summarised by him (see Baird, 1965). That a liberal abortion law is a potent factor in reducing the birth rate of a country and thus attenuating population growth is illustrated by the experience of Japan from the late 1940's onwards and more recently by the results reported from various eastern European countries, notably Hungary, Czechoslovakia and Yugoslavia (see Tietze 1963, 1965 for references).

At the time of writing some 800,000 women in the U.K. are believed to be receiving medication by oral contraceptives, and it is tempting to postulate that this fact is in some way connected with the slight fall in the British birth rate which has recently been reported (see *Economist* 1967). It must, however, be emphasised that the reasons for minor fluctuations in birth rates are notoriously difficult to interpret, and obviously further information on this subject is required before any definite conclusions can be drawn.

CONTRACEPTION IN THE 1960's

In few other fields of medical endeavour has progress in recent years been so rapid as in that involving techniques of birth control. Up to the mid 1950's the outlook in this area was very unpromising, many of the methods available having the major disadvantages of poor acceptability and relatively low efficiency. However, within the last 10 years, the situation has been completely revolutionised, firstly by the introduction of the oral contraceptive pill and secondly by improved methods of intra-uterine contraception. At the time of writing the impetus to research in the field of contraception is so great that it can be predicted with confidence that in the forseeable future even more satisfactory methods of birth control are likely to become generally available. (See also p. 309)

TABLE 32

AVAILABLE METHODS OF CONTRACEPTION

1. Mechanical methods
   (a) Diaphragm (cap)
   (b) Condom (sheath)
   (c) Intra-uterine device
2. Chemical spermicides
3. Oral contraception in females
4. Oral contraception in males
5. Non-appliance methods
   (a) Coitus interruptus
   (b) Coitus reservatus
   (c) Rhythm method (Safe period)
6. Sterilisation
   (a) Males
   (b) Females

In Table 32 are shown some of the methods of contraception in current use. Techniques depending on the intra-uterine device, on oral contraception in females and on the rhythm method have been described in previous sections of this book and will not be considered herein. Many of the other methods listed, e.g. those depending on diaphragms, condoms, chemical spermicides, coitus interruptus and coitus reservatus, are of a traditional nature and have been in widespread use for very many years. A detailed description of such procedures, together with their advantages and limitations, is available to the reader in the monograph edited by Kleinman (1964) on behalf of the I.P.P.F. Sterilisation in males is generally performed by the operation of vasectomy, an account of which is also given by Kleinman (1964). Obviously this is a highly effective method of birth control but, in many cases, the operation is irreversible. Up till now experience with vasectomy has been mainly confined to Southern India (see Chitre, 1964 ; Venning, 1966) and the technique has had no opportunity of influencing the global problem of overpopulation..

Sterilisation in females by tubal section and tubal ligation has been employed by Baird (1965) in Scotland as a method of family planning, and has also been used for this purpose in other countries including Switzerland, Japan and Puerto Rico (see Stycos, 1954 ; Ekblad, 1961 ; Tietze, 1965). For details of the operative procedures involved together with the social and psychiatric implications of female sterilisation, articles by Ekblad (1961), Jeffcoate (1962) and Baird (1965) should be consulted.

There remain for consideration two other methods of contraception which, although of considerable potential significance, are currently at a very early stage of development. These are oral contraception in males by compounds capable of inhibiting spermatogenesis, and the possibility of an immunological approach to contraception.

In recent years the effect of numerous compounds on spermatogenesis in a variety of animal species and in human subjects has been investigated (see Nelson, 1965 ; Nelson and Patanelli, 1965 ; MacLeod, 1965 ; Jackson, 1966 ; Venning, 1966). Such substances have included natural and synthetic oestrogens, androgens and progestogens together with non-steroidal compounds such as nitrofurans, thiophenes, bis-diamines and dinitropyrroles. Nitrofurans and thiophenes cannot be used clinically because of their relatively high toxicity. Compounds of the bis-(dichloroacetyl) diamine series have been employed in limited clinical trials and have been shown to be capable of inhibiting spermatogenesis in men. (Heller *et al.*, 1961 ; MacLeod, 1965). However, these substances when administered together with alcohol, produce unpleasant side effects similar to those experienced with

Antabuse, and this has limited their widespread use in clinical practice. A number of investigators have reported that immunological factors may be of importance in problems of infertility in woman (see Schwimmer *et al.*, 1967 for references). In view of this suggestion the possibility exists that fertility in women might be controlled by the administration of antibodies to spermatozoa and to other constituents of semen (see Venning, 1966). At the time of writing a satisfactory method of contraception based on an immunological reaction does not exist, and further work in this important area will be awaited with considerable interest.

EFFECTIVENESS OF VARIOUS METHODS OF CONTRACEPTION

Comparisons of the effectiveness of a variety of contraceptive techniques have been made by numerous investigators including Tietze (1959), Venning (1961) and Westoff *et al.* (1961). The results shown in Table 33 are based on data reported by Venning (1961), Kleinman (1964) and Pincus (1965). The following points should be noted :

1. Contraceptive techniques utilising the rhythm method and post coital douching are associated with relatively high failure rates.

2. Procedures involving the diaphragm, the condom and coitus interruptus are more satisfactory than those in the first category but still have considerable limitations in terms of efficiency.

3. Much the most reliable methods are those dependent on oral contraception in females and on the intra-uterine device, the efficacy of the former being virtually 100 per cent.

4. All the contraceptive procedures listed reduce the pregnancy rate as compared with subjects in whom no precautions are taken.

CONCLUDING COMMENT

The major aim of this chapter has been to stress the catastrophic consequences which are likely to ensue as a result of the rapid increase in world population. At the same time, the point has been made that the past few years have witnessed great advances in the field of contraception. It now remains for individual governments and for international organisations to exploit these technological advances to the full. If this is done there still remains the possibility that the quality of life will not be unduly impaired, and that existence will still be tolerable for those destined to inhabit this planet in the twenty-first and subsequent centuries.

TABLE 33

FAILURE RATE OF VARIOUS METHODS OF CONTRACEPTION

(After Venning, 1961 ; Kleinman, 1964 ; Pincus, 1965)

Method	Average pregnancy rate per 100 women-years
None used	115
Douche	31
Rhythm method	24
Coitus interruptus	18
Condom	14
Diaphragm	12
Intra-uterine device	3·4
Oral contraception	1

REFERENCES

BAIRD, Sir D. (1965). *Brit. Med. J.* **2**, 1141.
Brit. Med. J. (1966). **1**, 850.
BURNET, F. M. (1961). *Eugen. Rev.* **45**, 139.
CARADON LORD (1965). Speech to *Economic and Social Council of United Nations*, July 5th.
CÉPÈDE, M., HOUTART, F. & GROND, L. (1964). *Population and Food*, New York : Sheed and Ward.
CHITRE, K. T. (1964). *J. Fam. Welf.* **10**, 25.
COOK, R. C. (1964). *Pop. Bull.* **20**, 205.
COOK, R. C. (1966). *Pop. Bull.* **22**, 1.
CURRIE, L. (1967). *Pop. Bull.* **23**, 25.
DRAPER, E. (1965). *Birth Control in the Modern World*, Harmondsworth : Penguin Books.
Economist (1967). p. 1336, June 24th.
EHRLICH, P. (1967). *New Scientist*, **36**, 652.
EKBLAD, M. (1961). *Acta Psychiat. Scand.* **37**, *Suppl.* 161.
Family Planning (1966). **15**, 47.
FLORENCE, P. S. (1964). *Eugen. Rev.* **56**, 143.
Food and Agriculture Organisation, (1966). *Annual Report.*

Fox, Sir T. (1966 *a*). *Lancet,* **ii,** 175.

Fox, Sir T. (1966 *b*). *Lancet,* **ii,** 1238.

HALL, P. (1966). *Sunday Times,* March 20th.

HARRAR, J. G. (1965). *The Race between Procreation and Food Production,* New York : The Rockefeller Foundation.

HAUSER, P. M. (1965). cited by Currie, L. (1967). *Pop. Bull.* **23,** 25.

HELLER, C. G., MOORE, D. J. & PAULSEN, C. A. (1961). *Toxicol. Appl. Pharmacol.* **3,** 1.

HUTCHISON, J. (1966). *The Listener,* p. 303.

JACKSON, H. (1966). *Antifertility Compounds in the Male and Female.* Springfield : Thomas.

JEFFCOATE, T. N. A. (1962). *Principles of Gynaecology,* Second Ed. London : Butterworths.

JOHNSON, L. B. (1965). quoted by Caradon, Lord (1965) Speech to *Economic and Social Council of United Nations* July 5th.

KLEINMAN, R. L. (1964). *Medical Handbook on Contraception,* London : International Planned Parenthood Federation.

MacLEOD, J. (1965). In *Agents Affecting Fertility,* p. 93 Eds. Austin, C. R. and Perry, J. S., London : Churchill.

MAXWELL, E. (1967). *Personal communication.*

Monthly Digest of Statistics (1966). No. 244, London, H.M.S.O.

Monthly Digest of Statistics (1967). No. 256, London, H.M.S.O.

MORRIS, J. K. (1966). *Pop. Bull.* **22,** 7.

NELSON, W. O. (1965). In *Excerpta Med. Intern. Cong. Series* No. 83, p. 794. Amsterdam : Excerpta Medica Foundation.

NELSON, W. O. & PATANELLI, D. J. (1965). In *Agents Affecting Fertility,* p. 78. Eds. Austin, C. R. and Perry, J. S., London : Churchill.

PADDOCK, P. & PADDOCK, W. (1964). *Hungry Nations,* Boston : Little Brown.

PINCUS, G. (1965). *The Control of Fertility,* New York : Academic Press.

Population Reference Bureau (1962), *Pop. Bull.* **18,** 1.

RENTON, Sir D. (1967 *a*). *The New Horizon,* January, p. 5.

RENTON, Sir D. (1967 *b*). *The New Horizon,* February, p. 7.

RENTON, Sir D. (1967 *c*). *The New Horizon,* April, p. 5.

REVELLE, R. (1966). *Proc. Nat. Acad. Sci.* **56,** 328.

RITCHIE-CALDER, LORD (1966) *The Scotsman,* December 24th.

SCHWIMMER, W. B., USTAY, K. A. & BEHRMAN, S. J. (1967). *Fertility Sterility,* **18,** 167.

STYCOS, J. M. (1954). *Eugen. Quart.* **1,** 3.

STYCOS, J. M. (1966). *Family Planning,* **14,** 87.

TIETZE, C. (1959). *Am. J. Obstet. Gynecol.* **78,** 650.

TIETZE, C. (1963). In *Human Fertility and Population Problems,* p. 222. Ed. Greep, R. O. Cambridge, Massachusetts : Schenkman.

TIETZE, C. (1965). *J. Chron. Dis.* **18,** 1161.

United States National Academy of Sciences (1963). *Report on Growth of World Population.*

VENNING, G. R. (1961). *Brit. Med. J.* **2,** 899.

VENNING, G. R. (1966). In *Ovulation,* p. 178. Ed. Greenblatt, R. B. Philadelphia : Lippincott.

WATTS, M. (1966). *The Observer,* March 13th.

WESTOFF, C. F., POTTER, R. G., SAGI, P. C. & MISHLER, E. G. (1961). *Family Planning in Metropolitan America,* Princeton : Princeton University Press.

ACKNOWLEDGEMENTS OF ILLUSTRATIONS

The authors wish to express their thanks to the authors, editors and publishers listed below for permission to reproduce illustrations.

JOURNALS

Acta Endocrinologica

Fig. 18 Nocke, W. & Breuer, H. (1963). **44,** 47. Fig. 5.

Figs. 27 & 28 Bell, E. T., Mukerji, S. Loraine, J. A. & Lunn, S. F. (1966). **51,** 578. Figs. 3 & 4.

Fig. 30 Svendsen, R. & Sørensen, B. (1964). **47,** 245. Fig. 2.

Fig. 89 Loraine, J. A., Bell, E. T., Harkness, R. A. & Harrison, M. T. (1966). **52,** 527. Fig. 2.

Fig. 100 Crooke, A. C., Butt, W. R. & Bertrand, P. V. (1966). Suppl. 111. Fig. 6.

Fig. 107 Diczfalusy, E., Johannisson, E., Tillinger, K-G. & Bettendorf, G. (1964). Suppl. **90,** 35. Fig. 3.

Fig. 121 & 125 Loraine, J. A., Bell. E, T., Harkness, R. A., Mears, E. & Jackson, M. C. N. (1965). **50,** 15. Figs. 4 & 6.

Figs. 122 & 123 Bell, E. T., Herbst, A. L., Krishnamurti, M., Loraine, J. A., Mears, E., Jackson, M. C. N. & Garcia, C-R. (1967). **54,** 96. Figs. 3 & 4.

American Journal of Obstetrics and Gynecology

Fig. 31 Woolever, C. A. (1963). **84,** 981. Fig. 3.

Fig. 39 Viergiver, E. & Pommerenke, W. T. (1944). **48,** 321. Fig. 3.

Fig. 43 Moghissi, K. S. & Neuhaus, O. W. (1966). **96,** 91. Fig. 4.

Fig. 45 McSweeney, D. J. & Sbarra, A. J. (1964). **88,** 705. Fig. 1.

Figs. 83 & 84 Charles, D., Bell, E. T., Loraine, J. A. & Harkness, R. A. (1965). **91,** 1050. Figs. 1 & 4.

Figs. 95 & 96 Charles, D., Barr, W., Bell, E. T., Brown, J. B., Fotherby, K. & Loraine, J. A. (1963). **86,** 913. Figs. 1 & 3.

Fig. 102 Buxton, C. L. & Herrmann, W. (1961). **81,** 584. Fig. 4.

Fig. 124 Flowers, C. E., Vorys, N., Stevens, V. C., Miller, A. T. & Jensen, L. (1966). **96,** 784. Fig. 4.

Fig. 131 Hall, R. E. (1966). **94,** 65. Fig. 4.

Fig. 132 Tietze, C. (1966). **96,** 1043. Fig. 7.

Fig. 133 Willson, J. R., Ledger, W. J. & Andros, G. J. (1965). **93,** 802. Fig. 1.

Australasian Annals of Medicine

Figs. 88, 105 & 106 Shearman, R. P. (1966). **15,** 266. Figs. 7, 2 & 3.

Biochemical Journal

Table 4 Ismail, A. A. A. & Harkness, R. A. (1966). **99,** 717. Table 4.

British Journal of Nutrition

Fig. 54 Watson, P. E. & Robinson, M. F. (1965). **19,** 237. Fig. 1.

Compte Rendu de la Societe Francaise de Gynecologie

Fig. 108 Lunenfeld, B., Sulimovici, S., Rabau, E. & Eshkol, A. (1962). **32,** 346. Fig. 2.

Endocrinology

Fig. 32 Midgley, A. R. Jr. (1966). **79,** 10. Fig. 4.

The Eugenics Review

Fig. 137 Florence, P. S. (1964). **56,** 143.

Fertility and Sterility

Fig. 44 Herzberg, M., Joël, C. A. & Katchalsky, A. (1964). **15,** 684. Fig. 2.

Fig. 86 Charles, D., Loraine, J. A., Bell, E. T. & Harkness, R. A. (1966). **17,** 351. Fig. 2.

Fig. 92 Roy, S., Greenblatt, R. B., Mahesh, V. B. & Jungck, E. C. (1963). **14,** 575. Fig. 12.

Fig. 112 Hutcherson, W. P., Schwartz, H. A. & Weathers, W. Jr. (1966). **17,** 59. Fig. 2.

Fig. 114 Moyer, D. L., Tyler, E. T., Olson, H. J. & Zeldis, J. (1964). **15,** 164. Fig. 1.

ACKNOWLEDGEMENTS OF ILLUSTRATIONS

International Journal of Fertility
Table 17 Garcia C-R. & Pincus, G. (1963). **9,** 95. Table 1.

Journal of Clinical Endocrinology and Metabolism
Fig. 17 Eechaute, W. & Demeester, C. (1965). **25,** 480. Fig. 4.
Fig. 33 Midgley, A. R. Jr. & Jaffe, R. B. (1966). **26,** 1375. Fig. 5.
Fig. 50 Castallanos, H. & Sturgis, S. H. (1958). **18,** 1369. Fig. 2.
Fig. 103 Johannisson, E., Gemzell, C. A. & Diczfalusy, E. (1961). **21,** 1068. Fig. 2.

The Journal of Endocrinology
Fig. 3 Bullough, W. S. (1942). **3,** 150. Fig. 1.
Fig. 52 Brown, J. B., Klopper, A. & Loraine, J. A. (1958). **17,** 410. Fig. 2.
Figs. 113, 118 & 119 Brown, J. B., Fotherby, K. & Loraine, J. A. (1962). **25,** 331. Figs. 5, 4 & 1.

Journal of Obstetrics and Gynaecology of the British Commonwealth
Figs. 19, 20 & 21 Klopper, A. (1957). **64,** 504. Figs. 2, 1 & 3.
Fig. 51 Tompkins, P. (1945). **52,** 241. Chart 1.
Fig. 56 Loraine, J. A. & Bell, E. T. (1968). *In Press.*
Figs. 73 & 80 Brown, J. B., Kellar, R. J. & Matthew, G. D. (1959). **66,** 177. Figs. 25 & 11.
Figs. 87 & 91 Bell, E. T., Loraine, J. A., Harkness, R. A. & Foss, G. L. (1966). **73,** 766. Figs. 2 & 1.
Figs. 98, 99 & 104. Townsend, S. L., Brown, J. B., Johnstone, J. W., Adey, F. D., Evans, J. H. & Taft, H. P. (1966). **73,** 529. Figs. 6, 7 & 11.
Figs. 109 & 110 Bell, E. T., Loraine, J. A. & Strong, J. A. (1968). *In Press.*

Journal of Reproduction and Fertility
Fig. 130 Guttmacher, A. F. (1965). **10,** 115. Plate 1.

Obstetrical and Gynecological Survey
Figs. 29, 67, 68, 69, 70, 74, 75, 76, 77, 78, Tables 5, 6 & 7. Loraine, J. A. & Bell, E. T. (1967). **22,** 463. Figs. 2, 5, 6, 7, 8, 10, 11, 13, 15, 17, Tables 1, 3 & 6.

357

Population Bulletin
  Fig. 135 (1962). **18,** 1. Fig. 1.

Proceedings of the Royal Society of Medicine
  Fig. 41 Clift, A. F. (1945). **39,** 1. Fig. 2.

Steroids
  Figs. 24 & 26 Apostolakis, M., Becker, H. & Voigt, K. D. (1966). **7,** 146. Figs. 1 & 2.

The Lancet
  Figs. 15 & 16 Brown, J. B. (1955). **i,** 320. Figs. 1 & 3.
  Fig. 55 Zilva, J. F. & Patston, V. J. (1966). **i,** 459. Fig. 3.
  Fig. 63 Bell, E. T. & Loraine, J. A. (1966). **ii,** 519. Fig. 1.
  Figs. 93 & 94 Charles, D. (1962). **ii,** 278. Figs. 3 & 4.
  Fig. 101 Crooke, A. C., Butt, W. R., Carrington, S. P., Morris, R., Palmer, R. F. & Edwards, R. L. (1964). **i,** 184. Fig. 2.
  Fig. 120 Loraine, J. A., Bell, E. T., Harkness, R. A., Mears, E. & Jackson, M. C. N. (1963). **ii,** 902. Fig. 3.
  Fig. 126 Shearman, R. P. (1963). **i,** 197. Fig. 3.
  Table 3 Bell, E. T. & Loraine, J. A. (1965). **i,** 1029. Table 1.

The Practitioner
  Fig. 53 Brown, P. F. E. (1965). **194,** 525. Fig. 9.

Vitamins and Hormones
  Fig. 97 Gemzell, C. A. (1964). **22,** 129. Fig. 2.

BOOKS

  Fig. 12 Blandua, R. J. (1966). In *Ovulation.* Fig. 1. Ed. Greenblatt, R. B. Philadelphia : Lippincott.
  Figs. 34 & 53 Browne, F. J. & McClure Browne, J. C. (1964). *Postgraduate Obstetrics and Gynaecology,* 3rd ed. Figs. 24 & 19. London : Butterworth.
  Fig. 90 Charles, D., Loraine, J. A., Bell, E. T. & Harkness, R. A. *Proceedings of Fifth World Congress on Fertility and Sterility. Stockholm* 1966. Excerpta Med. Intern. Cong. Series No. 133 p. 92 Amsterdam: Excerpta Medica Foundation.

Fig. 40 Cohen, M. R. (1966). In *Ovulation*. Fig. p. 293. Ed. Greenblatt, R. B. Philadelphia : Lippincott.

Fig. 49 De Allende, I. L. C. & Orías, O. (1950). *Cytology of the Human Vagina*, Fig. 25. New York: Harper & Row.

Table 23 Drill, V. A. (1966). *Oral Contraceptives*. New York : McGraw-Hill.

Fig. 7 Eshkol, A. (1967). In *Recent Research on Gonadotrophic Hormones*. Fig. 104. Eds. Bell, E. T. & Loraine, J. A. Edinburgh : Livingstone.

Table 11 Greenblatt, R. B. & Mahesh, V. B. In Yearbook of Endocrinology. Ed. Schwartz, T. B. 1964–5. Table 1.

Fig. 1 Ham, A. W. (1965). *Histology*, 5th ed. Fig. 29–6. Philadelphia : Lippincott.

Fig. 6 Patten, B. M. (1953) *Human Embryology* 2nd Ed. Fig. 11. New York: McGraw-Hill.

Figs. 115, 116 & 117 Mears, E. (1965). *Handbook on Oral Contraceptives*. Plate 1 Fig. IV, Plate 1 Fig. V, Plate 4 Fig. 11. London : Churchill.

Figs. 127 & 128 Mears, E. (1965). In *Agents Affecting Fertility*. Figs. 1 & 3. Eds. Austin, C. R. & Perry, J. S. London : Churchill.

Figs. 2, 4, 5, 36 & 37 Novak, E. R. & Woodruff, J. D. (1962). *Gynecologic and Obstetric Pathology*, 5th ed. Figs. 350, 358, 359, 148 & 147. Philadelphia : Saunders.

Fig. 38 Noyes, R. W. (1966). In *Ovulation*. Fig. 1. Ed. Greenblatt, R. B. Philadelphia : Lippincott.

Tables 20 & 25 Pincus, G. (1965). *Control of Fertility*, Tables 64 & 72. New York : Academic Press.

Tables 18 & 24 Pincus, G. & Garcia, C. L. R. (1965). In *Recent Advances in Ovarian and Synthetic Steroids*, Tables 12 & 5. Ed. Shearman, R. P. High Wycombe : Searle.

Fig. 42 Riley, G. M. (1959). *Gynecologic Endocrinology*, Fig. 67. New York : Harper & Row.

Figs. 8, 9 & 10 Savard, K. (1967). In *Recent Research on Gonadotrophic Hormones*, Figs. 90, 91 & 92. Eds. Bell, E. T. & Loraine, J. A. Edinburgh : Livingstone.

Fig. 25 Stevens, V. C. (1967). In *Recent Research on Gonadotrophic Hormones*, Fig. 121. Eds. Bell, E. T. & Loraine, J. A. Edinburgh : Livingstone.

Fig. 134 Sujan-Tejuja, S., Virick, R. K. & Malkani, P. K. (1965). *Proceedings of the Second International Conference on Intra-Uterine Contraception.* New York, 1964. Amsterdam : Excerpta Medica Foundation.

Tables 19 & 22 Venning, G. R. (1963). In *Symposium on Oral Contraception*, Tables 4 & 2. High Wycombe : Searle.

Index of Authors

Index of Subjects

A

Abdominal discomfort, incidence of following Clomiphene, 223

Adenosine monophosphate cyclic, effect of LH on, 15

Adrenal cortex, secretion by, of oestrogens, 32
of pregnanetriol, 50
of progesterone, 43

Adrenal hyperplasia, incidence of ovulation following Clomiphene, 206

Adrenocortical function, effect of oral contraception on, 285–287

Adrenogential syndrome, treatment of, by Clomiphene, 200

Amenorrhoea, associated with oral contraception, 269
using sequential administration, 304
ovarian, definition of, 168
pituitary, definition of, 168
primary, definition of, 168
treatment of, by Clomiphene, 200
by gonadotrophins, 231
urinary levels, of HPG in, 168
of oestrogens in, 168
of pregnanediol in, 169
secondary, definition of, 168
effect of Clomiphene on urinary levels, of FSH, 213
of HPG, 209–214
of LH, 213
of oestrogens, 209–214
of pregnanediol, 209–214
effect of pituitary gonadotrophins on urinary levels, of HCG, 240
of oestrogens, 234–241
of 17-OHCS, 235
of 17-oxosteroids, 235
of pregnanediol, 234–241
effect of TACE on urinary levels, of HPG in, 209
of oestrogens, 209
of pregnanediol, 209
effect of urinary gonadotrophins on urinary levels, of oestrogens, 247

of pregnanediol, 247
incidence of ovulation following Clomiphene, 206
treatment of, by Clomiphene, 200
by gonadotrophins, 231
urinary levels, of HPG in, 170–176
of oestrogens in, 170–176
of pregnanediol in, 170–176

Anovulatory cycles, definition of, 145
incidence of ovulation following Clomiphene, 206
urinary levels, of HPG in, 146–150
of LH in, 148
of oestrogens in, 146–150
of pregnanediol in, 146–150
of pregnanetriol in, 146–150

Appetite, increase of, associated with oral contraception, 266

Arborisation of cervical mucus, changes in during normal menstrual cycle, 118

Arrhenoblastoma, plasma levels of testosterone in, 189
urinary levels, of DHA in, 189
of 17-oxosteroids in, 188

Atresia, of primary follicles, 3

B

Basal body temperature, during normal menstrual cycle, 127–133
measurement of, cranial, 129
oral, 129
rectal, 129
vaginal, 129
relationship of, to ovulation, 129–133
to "safe" period of cycle, 133
to urinary levels of oestrogens, 130
use of, in contraception, 131

Birnberg bow, *See* Intra-uterine device

Birth rate, in various countries, 344

Blood, inorganic constituents of during normal menstrual cycle, 134

Blood coagulation, effect of oral contraception on, 274

Body temperature, *See* Basal body temperature

373

375

Follicle, effect on rupture,
  of peptidase, 26
  of phosphatase, 26
  of pronase, 26
  of trypsin, 26
  growth of, effect of FSH on, 10
  mature, histology of, 4
  primary, atresia of, 3
    histology of, 3–5
    number of, 2
  rupture of, 2
Follicle-stimulating hormone, assay
    of, by ovarian augmentation,
    in mice, 61
    in rats, 60
  by radio-immunological methods,
    61
  by uterine weight in hypophysec-
    tomized mice, 61
  biochemical effects of, 16
  biological effects of, 10
  blood levels of in normally menstrua-
    ting women, 103
  effect of, on follicular growth, 10
    on ovarian steroid synthesis, 10
    on uterine growth, 10
  effect on urinary levels, of Clomi-
    phene, 213, 215, 225
  of oral contraception, 291–299
  preparation of, from pituitary tissue,
    232
    from urine, 245
  urinary levels of, in normally men-
    struating women, 89–91, 94
Follicular fluid, chemical composition
    of, 24
  release of, at ovulation, 23
  secondary, formation of, 20
Follicular phase, changes during, in
    endometrial histology, 111
  in urinary cytology, 127
  in vaginal cytology, 124
Follicular pressure and ovulation, 23
Food, world population and supplies
    of, 343
Forbes syndrome, *See also* Galac-
    torrhoea
  effect of urinary gonadotrophins on
    urinary levels, of oestrogens,
    247
  of pregnanediol, 247
FSH, *See* Follicle-stimulating hormone

G

Galactorrhoea, effect of Clomiphene
    on urinary levels, of DHA,
    214
  of FSH, 215
  of HPG, 214
  of LH, 215
  of oestrogens, 214–216
  of 17-OHCS, 214
  of 17-oxosteroids, 214
  of pregnanediol, 214
  of pregnanetriol, 214
  urinary levels, of DHA in, 177
  of HPG in, 177
  of oestrogens in, 177
  of 17-OHCS in, 177
  of 17-oxosteroids in, 177
  of pregnanediol in, 177
Gonadotrophin, *See* Human chorionic
    gonadotrophin *and* Human
    pituitary gonadotrophins
Gonadotrophin therapy, by pituitary
    gonadotrophins, comparison
    of effect on hormone excretion
    with Clomiphene, 244
  dosage of administered material,
    233
  effect of, on endometrial histology,
    240
    on hormone excretion in amenor-
      rhoeic women, 234–240
    on urinary levels, of HCG, 240
      of oestrogens, 234–241
      of 17-OHCS, 235
      of 17-oxosteroids, 235
      of pregnanediol, 234–241
    on vaginal cytology, 242
  incidence of multiple pregnancy
    following, 242
  ovulation following, 234
  prediction of response following,
    245
  pregnancy following, 234
  preparation of administered
    material, 232
  side effects following, 244
  by urinary gonadotrophins, com-
    parison of effects on hormone
    excretion with Clomiphene,
    253
  dosage of administered material,
    245

379

Ovulation, observation of, 23
rate of ovum extrusion and, 23
relationship of, to basal body
temperature, 129–133
to body weight, 133
stigma formation and, 22
time of, in relation to urinary levels
of oestrogens, 79–82
17-oxosteroids, effect on urinary
levels, of Clomiphene, 214,
219, 226, 253
of oral contraception, 287
of pituitary gonadotrophins, 235
of urinary gonadotrophins, 249
urinary levels of, in arrhenoblastoma,
188
in endometrial carcinoma, 190–
194
in galactorrhoea, 177
in granulosa cell tumour, 188
in Stein-Leventhal syndrome, 179–
183
11-oxygenated-17-oxosteroids,
effect on urinary levels of
Clomiphene, 219

P

Pain, associated with contraception by
intra-uterine device, 324
Parabasal cells, occurrence of in
vaginal smear, 123
Pelvic inflammatory disease, associated with contraception by
intra-uterine device, 326
Polycystic ovary syndrome, See
Stein-Leventhal syndrome
Population, abortion and control of,
349
age constitution of, in Pakistan, 341
in United Kingdom, 341
crisis of world, 337
distribution by continents, 346
effect of medical science on, 338
food supplies and world, 343
number of years to double in various
countries, 345
of United Kingdom, 347
rate of increase, 347
oral contraception and control of, 349
rate of increase of world, 338
Precornified cells, occurrence of in
vaginal smear, 123

Pregnancy, effect of intra-uterine
device on outcome of, 331
incidence of following therapy, with
Clomiphene, 208
with pituitary gonadotrophins, 234
with urinary gonadotrophins,
246
multiple, following therapy by pituitary gonadotrophins, 242
relation of, to urinary levels, of
oestrogens, 242
of pregnanediol, 242
following therapy by urinary, gonadotrophins, 247
rate, associated with contraception
by intra-uterine device, 321
associated with oral contraception,
264
associated with oral contraception
using sequential administration, 303
Pregnanediol, conjugation of, 45
effect on urinary levels, of Clomiphene, 209–219, 226, 244, 253
of oral contraception, 287–299
of pituitary gonadotrophins, 234–
241
of urinary gonadotrophins, 247–
252, 255
estimation of, in blood, 49
in urine, by colorimetric methods,
46–48
by gas chromatographic
methods, 48
by isotopic methods, 49
metabolite of progesterone, 45
structural formula of, 42
urinary levels of, in amenorrhoea,
primary, 169
secondary, 170–176
in anovulatory cycles, 146–150
in dysfunctional uterine haemorrhage, 183–187
in dysmenorrhoea, 150–156
in galactorrhoea, 177
in granulosa cell tumour, 188
in normally menstruating women,
82–85, 91–98, 141–145
in oligomenorrhoea, 156–167
in pregnancy following gonadotrophin therapy, 240, 242, 251
in Stein-Leventhal syndrome, 179–
183

Stigma, occurrence of, 22

Stratum granulosum, changes in prior to ovulation, 20

Sterilisation for contraception, of females, 351
of males, 351

Steroidogenesis, effect on, of Clomiphene, 227
of LH, 12–16
in bovine corpus luteum, 13
in human corpus luteum, 13
site of action of LH on, 14

Superficial cells, occurrence of in vaginal smear, 123

T

TACE, effect of on urinary levels, of HPG, 209
of oestrogens, 209
of pregnanediol, 209

Tack, of cervical mucus, changes in during normal menstrual cycle, 117

Temperature, *See* Basal body temperature

Testosterone, blood levels of in normally menstruating women, 101
conjugation of, 51
estimation of, in blood, by fluorimetric method, 54
by gas chromatographic method, 54
by isotopic methods, 55, 69
in urine, by colorimetric method, 52
by fluorimetric method, 52
by gas chromatographic methods, 53
plasma levels of in arrhenoblastoma, 189
urinary levels of, in oligomenorrhoea, 163–167
in normally menstruating women, 85–87, 92
secretion of, 51
structural formula of, 51

Testosterone derivatives, use of in oral contraception, 261

Tetrahydrocorticosteroids, effect on urinary levels of Clomiphene, 219

Thecal cell tumour, urinary levels of oestrogens in, 188

Thromboembolic disease, relationship of oral contraception to, 274–277

Thyroid function, effect of oral contraception on, 284

"Total oestrogens", definition of, 30

U

Uterus, bleeding of, associated with contraception by intra-uterine device, 324
carcinoma of, use of vaginal cytology in, 126
effect on growth, of FSH, 11
of LH, 11
perforation of, associated with contraception by intra-uterine device, 325

Urinary cytology, cell types in, 126
during normal menstrual cycle, 126

V

Vaginal cytology, cell types in, 122
cytological indices employed, 123
during normal menstrual cycle, 121–126
effect on, of Clomiphene, 221
of intra-uterine device, 328
of oral contraception, 279
of therapy, by pituitary gonadotrophins, 242
by urinary gonadotrophins, 250, 252
use of,
in cervical carcinoma, 126
in endometrial carcinoma, 194
in uterine carcinoma, 126

Vaginal discharge, associated with contraception by intra-uterine device, 325

Viscosity of cervical mucus, changes in, during normal menstrual cycle, 116

Visual complaints, incidence of following Clomiphene, 223

Vomiting, incidence of following Clomiphene, 223

Printed by Neill and Co. Ltd., Edinburgh